Counseling and Psychotherapy for South Asian Americans

This essential text explores what it means to be a South Asian American living in the US while seeking, navigating and receiving psychological, behavioral or counseling services. It delves into a range of issues including cultural identity, racism, colorism, immigration, gender, sexuality, parenting, and caring for older adults.

Chapter authors provide research literature, clinical and cultural considerations for interviewing and treatment planning, case examples, questions for reflection, suggested readings, and resources. The book also includes insights on the future of South Asian American mental health, social justice, advocacy, and public policy.

Integrating theory, research, and application, this book serves as a clinical guide for therapists, instructors, professors, and supervisors in school/university counseling centers working with South Asian American clients, as well as for counseling students.

Ulash Thakore-Dunlap is a licensed Marriage and Family Therapist, faculty at the Wright Institute MA Counseling Psychology Program, and is a current doctoral student in the Educational Leadership program at San Francisco State University (anticipated to graduate, 2023).

Dr. Devika Srivastava is a licensed Psychologist who has significant research, policy, programming, and clinical experience in mental health and is a former Psychiatry professor who is currently in private practice (Devika Srivastava Ph.D. LLC) in Texas and Florida. She focused on issues of Asian Americans, people of color, children of immigrants, and diasphoric communities.

Dr. Nita Tewari is a consultant, educator and former Staff Psychologist and lecturer at the University of California, Irvine with publications in Asian American Psychology and South Asian American mental health.

Counseling and Psychotherapy for South Asian Americans

Identity, Psychology, and Clinical Implications

**Edited by Ulash Thakore-Dunlap,
Devika Srivastava, and Nita Tewari**

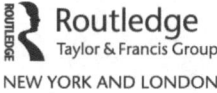
Routledge
Taylor & Francis Group

NEW YORK AND LONDON

Cover image: Getty Images

First published 2023
by Routledge
605 Third Avenue, New York, NY 10158

and by Routledge
4 Park Square, Milton Park, Abingdon, Oxon, OX14 4RN

Routledge is an imprint of the Taylor & Francis Group, an informa business

ISBN: 978-0-367-53350-2 (hbk)
ISBN: 978-0-367-53349-6 (pbk)
ISBN: 978-1-003-08154-8 (ebk)

DOI: 10.4324/9781003081548

Typeset in Times New Roman
by MPS Limited, Dehradun

Contents

Preface

This book has been a culmination of decades of experience as psychologists, therapists, counseling and clinical psychology educators, clinical supervisors, and most importantly, South Asian American women who have the lived experience of what it means to be a South Asian American, navigating mental health and accessing psychological, counseling, and behavioral services.

Although the three of us (Ulash, Devika and Nita) have known each other for over 10 years, several years ago we decided the time was long overdue in filling a gap in publishing a book that addresses clinical and counseling issues needs from a South Asian American cultural perspective for those learning to work with and are providing mental health services for South Asian American communities. Our peers in the field of counseling, mental health, and psychology have encouraged us to publish a book where contributing authors not only understand our culture, but are also experts in unique cultural topics in an evolving field given our expanding and varied South Asian American populations. As editors, we manifested our frustration and excitement towards the creation of the first book of its kind, so here we are.

We primarily created this book due to the limited journal articles and books focusing on the nuances and intersectionalities of South Asian Americans. As mental health providers and educators, there is not one book or resource entirely dedicated to learning about South Asian American Counseling and Psychology. In our research, we could not find a definition of South Asian American Counseling and Psychology, therefore created one for our field of study for educators and clinicians. In our personal and professional experiences, South Asian and South Asian American mental health resources have been limited with regard to training, textbooks, classroom vignettes, graduate and medical course curriculum, and community mental health.

We created this book with three main intentions. First, this book is intended for students and providers, instructors/professors, and supervisors in community mental health, school/university counseling centers, professional graduate schools, medical schools, and for clinicians and supervisors dedicated to expanding their knowledge, education and culturally competent care in working with diasporic South Asian American populations. Second, we created this book to serve as a clinical guide. Third, we created this book with the intention that readers in ethnic studies, allied health care, law, and other disciplines would find the content useful as well when studying, working with and advocating for South Asian Americans.

We organized our book in five parts, comprising 14 chapters. In crafting a book of this scope, we attempt to provide chapter topics that may be most interesting and relevant to your interest and exploration. The book begins with Part I: Foundation and Roots of Asian American Psychology and the History and Evolution of South Asian American Counseling and Psychology to explore the influences and history of South Asian American Counseling and Psychology. Part II: Immigration, Acculturation, and Identity Development explores the ways immigration, racism, the current sociopolitical climate, South Asian American Multiracial, Multi-Heritage, and Diaspora Identities impacts South Asian American individuals and their communities. Part III: Gender, Sexuality, and Cultural Influences in Psychological Adaptation explores ways gender, sexuality, gender socialization, religion and spirituality, dating and marriage impact South Asian Americans and clinical considerations. Part IV: Raising Families, Working with Elders and Providing Counseling Services explores clinicals considerations in supporting and working with South Asian American parents, children and adolescents, older adults and the clinical nuances of South Asian/South Asian American therapists working with South Asian American clients. Part V: Future of South Asian American Mental Health addresses the future of South Asian American behavioral and mental health as it relates to advocacy, social Justice, and public policy.

Each chapter begins with a case overview; this case study is weaved into the chapter where possible to illustrate application of assessment and interventions to concepts and themes discussed by the authors. We believe one of the strengths of this book is the ability to explore South Asian American topics by using clinical cases throughout the chapters to bridge the gap between scholarship and practice. As editors, we hope the abstracts come to life as you learn about ideas and concepts that relate to the everyday lives of South Asian Americans. Towards the end of the chapters, authors provide reflection questions for further thought to encourage broadening your knowledge. Chapters end with resources to build and widen your resource bank when working with South Asian American clients.

Last, but not least, we are grateful to our contributors who agreed to take part in creating such a book. It is not often where South Asian American leading experts, emerging scholars, and practitioners dedicated to mental health come together in a shared space to make a collective difference for clients and our diverse community.

We hope you will share this book with others, and feel inspired to find new ways to support our people. Most importantly, if you see a gap somewhere in our evolving South Asian American Counseling and Psychology, we hope you too, will find a way to collaborate and work to fill the gap where you see it. Our wish for those coming after us is that you continue to move our field onward, upward and forward.

Ulash Thakore-Dunlap MS
Devika Srivastava Ph.D.
Nita Tewari Ph.D.

Foreword

The sociocultural and psychological experience of South Asian immigrant communities cannot be complete without a nuanced and multilevel understanding of this diverse diasporic community. Given that South Asian Americans are the fastest growing community in the United States, approximating 21% (4.6 million) of the total Asian American population it is important to raise awareness of the unique aspects of this community.

This is the first book to present a comprehensive resource that highlights the complicated intersection of migrational histories, generations, ethnicities, races, religions, genders and sexualities. Situated against the backdrop of colonialism, casteism, and colorism, authors highlight the impact of these factors on the identity and mental wellbeing of this group. The attention to the South Asian American lifespan (youth to the elderly) through an intersectional lens and the inherent interlocking systems of oppression not only has implications for the entire field of counseling and psychology, but also challenges the universal experience of this immigrant community. Moving beyond acculturation and mono-racial identity development, the chapters draw on critical race theory, liberation psychology, and a decolonized counseling approach to understand and engage with South Asian Americans. These foci signify an important shift in the clinical literature.

As a South Asian woman who has spent her entire academic journey researching the experience of this immigrant group, I applaud the editors and the authors for their excellent knowledge, critique, and practical exemplification of South Asian identities and experiences. Set against the backdrop of important historical, socio-political, and contemporary narratives for this community, this book is unique in its analysis of the South Asian experience. Going beyond a description of the similarities and differences in cultural values and lifestyles, the authors illustrate the cultural, social, economic, and political issues confronting the mental health of South Asian Americans through exemplar vignettes, case analysis, and reflection questions that readers will find extremely helpful. There is no other comprehensive account that discusses the totality of the South Asian experience in such a personal and humane manner. The book is a must read for educators, practitioners, scholars, and students interested in the South Asian American experience.

Arpana G. Inman, Ph.D.
Rutgers University, New Brunswick, New Jersey

Acknowledgments

So many people have paved the way to create this book and supported me throughout this process. I am thankful to my parents, family, mentors, and friends who have shown me that with unconditional love and support, change is possible. To my husband Oliver who has been incredibly supportive, and from the start believed that anything is possible, including writing this book. I have been inspired by my teen son, Ezra who is Asian Indian and White—we often talk about being multiracial and how proud we are to be South Asian/South Asian American. Our conversations bring me hope that this book will support our current and next generation of South Asian Americans who sometimes feel invisible. I want to personally acknowledge each author who wrote for this book—thank you, your work is so important in elevating South Asian American needs. And to the amazing South Asian American co-editors Devika and Nita—I have been in awe of your creativity, energy, expertise, and commitment in creating the first book of its kind. Devika and Nita, we are stronger together, so thankful and honored to be on this journey with you. ~ Ulash Thakore-Dunlap, MS

The creation of this book is of great meaning and passion to me as it is about my parents, family, friends, community, and me. This work is a dedication to my family, my mother, Dr. Lekha Srivastava, and brother, Shiv Srivastava, and in loving memory of my father, Dr. Brij Srivastava, who passed away while I was working on this. My parents left everyone and everything they knew to start a family in America. Their values of compassion, service, equality, and community is what colored my personal and professional passions. They taught me to be strong, to speak up, to create space for myself and others. This is also what motivated me to work on this book, and to drive for change. I would also like to thank my younger brother, Shiv, who is my best friend and role model and who is changing the world in so many important ways. I am also honored to be working on this book with my wonderful co-editors, Ulash and Nita, with whom I share a vision to improve the lives of the members of our community, who are amazing people. ~ Devika Srivastava, Ph.D.

I would like to first thank my parents for paving the way in the U.S. for providing me with opportunities different than their own and to South Asian American psychologists, Asian American psychologists, and multicultural elders, including Dr. Joseph L. White, who created new professional pathways. Personally, I would like to thank my husband, Dr. Debu Tewari, who has been by my side for over 35 years. Debu, I have loved navigating life with you as a second generation Indian American and am blessed to have you as a parent with me to our two young adult college children, Jaya and Sanjay as we continue to raise the next and third generation of South Asian Americans together here in the U.S. Last, I would like to thank Ulash and Devika for embarking on this book journey with me—I have appreciated making this happen with the two of you. Finally, I thank the contributing authors for taking time out of their busy academic, clinical, and family schedules to share their wisdom with us, our community and for being a part of our book. ~ Nita Tewari PhD

Editors

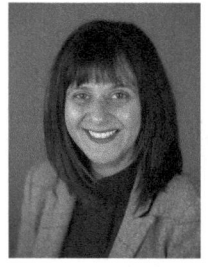 **Ulash Thakore-Dunlap** is a licensed Marriage and Family Therapist in California (CA) and resides in San Francisco. Ulash is currently full-time faculty associate professor, at the Wright Institute MA Counseling Psychology Program in Berkeley, CA. She advises and teaches students who are working towards PCC and MFT licenses, and is the past director of Diversity, Equity and Inclusion for the MA Program. Ulash maintains a private practice where she works with a wide range of clients. Ulash is also adjunct faculty at San Francisco State University, MS Counseling Program. In addition, Ulash is a current doctoral student in the Educational Leadership (EdD) program at San Francisco State University and is anticipated to graduate in 2023. Her current dissertation study explores the lived experiences of students of color in graduate counseling education and the implications for educators and leaders. Ulash's clinical experiences and area of interests includes school-based mental health, South Asian mental health, higher education, and supporting BIPOC emerging leaders. Ulash is active within her community and currently serves as Training Advisory Committee Member for the American Psychological Association (APA) Minority Fellowship Program. Ulash was also the past Commissioner for the San Francisco Behavioral Health Commission and board member at the Asian-American Psychological Association. In addition, Ulash has published articles and books on motherhood, South Asian immigrant girls, and has written a children's book. Ulash has provided many media interviews to local and national newspapers, magazines, and television networks on mental health.

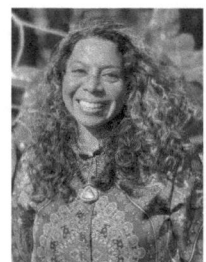 **Dr. Devika Srivastava** is a licensed Psychologist in private practice in Texas and Florida. She identifies as a second-generation Indian American woman. Dr. Srivastava received her B.S. in Psychology from University of Houston, M.S. coursework in Clinical/Counseling Psychology from Columbia University, and received her Ph.D. in Counseling Psychology from Fordham University. She completed her Doctoral Internship at the DeBakey VA Medical Center serving diverse populations of veterans, her Post-Doctoral Fellowship at the Harris Center where she conducted clinical program analysis focused on program/policy mental health needs of BIPOC individuals. Dr. Srivastava was a Doctoral Fellow at the American Psychological Association in the Office of Governmental Relations where she helped advocate federal policy in Congress for marginalized populations. Dr. Srivastava served as an Assistant Professor in the Menninger Department of Psychiatry at Baylor College of Medicine and provided psychological services to diverse populations at Ben Taub Hospital, supervised Post-doctoral Psychology Fellows, lectured medical students,

and behavioral health therapists. Also, she was Coordinator for the Social and Health Equity Course for Psychiatry Residents for issues related to inequality and diversity. Dr. Srivastava was Financial Officer in the Asian American Psychological Association and was Chair, Co-Chair, and Chair Elect in the Division on South Asian Americans (DoSAA) and helped to organize a conference focused on South Asian American mental health. Dr. Srivastava's research focuses on different issues and disorders impacting people of color. Currently, she is in private practice helping diverse intergenerational populations, including South Asian Americans.

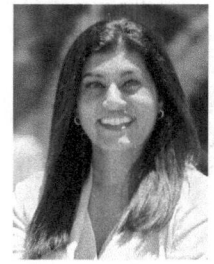

Dr. Nita Tewari works with young adults on leadership and life planning, is a consultant for social media impression management, and provides mental health education to South Asian, Asian American students, and university organizations. Throughout her career, she has dedicated, her time to improving the psychological and physical wellbeing of diverse individuals and women by serving as the Commissioner for the Orange County Behavioral Health Advisory Board, Board Member at the University of California Irvine (UCI) School of BioSci Dean's Leadership Circle, Inaugural Board Member for UCI's Black Thriving Initiative and as a Member of Beauty In Grace for MemorialCare Saddleback Medical Center. As a former Staff Psychologist and teaching faculty at UCI, she has provided clinical services and published works on mentoring, Indian Americans, South Asian and Asian Americans, and is the Senior Editor of *Asian American Psychology: Current Perspectives (*2009) and Co-editor of a second book, *South Asian American Counseling and Clinical Implications (In Progress)*. She served as Co-Chair for the Division on Women (DoW) of the Asian American Psychological Association (AAPA), Chaired Southern California Regional AAPA Conferences, was a Co-Founder of South Asian Psychological Networking Association (SAPNA) in 2001 and AAPA's first ethnic division, Division on South Asian Americans (DoSAA) in 2008 as AAPA Vice President. In 2021, she was given the AAPA Distinguished Contributions to Leadership/Service Award. Dr. Tewari has also volunteered her time in the Newport-Mesa Unified School District and was given the 2021 Corona Del Mar High School Parent Teacher Association Honorary Service Award for dedication to students, faculty and staff in public schools.

Contributors

Alif Ahmed is an associate research scientist at Global TIES for Children, New York University. His research interests broadly explore how policies and programs related to immigration impact the health and mental health of unauthorized immigrants and their families. Ahmed holds a B.S. degree in Applied Psychology from New York University and a M.S. degree in Social Work from Columbia University.

Saumya Arora is an aspiring Counseling Psychologist working towards the liberation of queer Black, Indigenous, and other People of Color (BIPOC). As a queer (bi+) Indian woman, Saumya aims to fill the research gaps that exist on this group and increase the representation of queer BIPOC therapists. Her research interests lie in the mental health and well-being of queer BIPOC folks, South Asian mental health, and advocacy through research. Clinically, Saumya has a desire to help clients work through identity-related trauma. In the future, she hopes to use her work to support queer BIPOC individuals through research, counseling practice, and community advocacy.

Dr. Jude Bergkamp is the program Chair of the clinical psychology program at Antioch University Seattle, as well as clinical faculty in the Department of Psychiatry and Behavioral Sciences at the University of Washington. He serves as the Chair of the Ethnic and Racial Diversity Committee within the National Council of Schools and Programs of Professional Psychology (NCSPP). In addition, he serves on the APA's BEA/BPA Task Force on Doctoral Competencies in Health Service Psychology. He was trained in forensic and neuropsychology and has worked in the Washington State Department of Corrections, and currently as a forensic evaluator at the Center for Forensic Services at Western State Hospital. His current research interests include the decolonization of psychology, the exploration of social privilege as the flip side of oppression, and the role social privilege plays in psychotherapy.

Dr. Lavanya Devdas is a licensed psychologist in PA and NY and received her doctorate in counseling psychology in 2015 from Lehigh University. Currently, as a private practitioner in Doylestown, PA, she believes in an integrative approach to treat mental health and relational challenges within the cultural and familial contexts and lived experiences of adults. Drawing from her own experiences to inform therapy, she helps individuals contextualize and cope with acculturation and navigate two or more cultures. She is also an advocate for addressing mental health needs and coping at the group and communal levels. She currently runs a mindfulness group for adults. She served as a mentor through the Pennsylvania Psychological Association and the Division on South Asian Americans. She also presents at conferences and panels on topics including intersecting identities, addressing mental health concerns from a cultural perspective, and intersecting feminism and culture, and stress management.

Munisa Haque MS, LMFT was born and raised in India and emigrated to the US in the 1990's. She obtained her bachelors and masters degree in counseling from the California State University, East Bay. Munisa has worked for several years in the community mental health field, with at-risk youth as well as their caregivers, providing intensive behavioral health services both at home as well as school settings. Currently Munisa works at a university counseling services center, providing brief counseling to a diverse student body, including those who identify as South Asian, Middle eastern, North African.

Sheharyar Hussain is currently enrolled in an APA accredited Clinical Psychology doctoral program at John Jay College of Criminal Justice. Prior to starting his PhD program, he graduated *magna cum laude* from John Jay College with a BA in Forensic Psychology and earned his MA in Clinical Psychology from Teachers College, Columbia University. As a Pakistani-American Muslim who has little representation in the clinical psychology field in general, Sheharyar is interested in addressing diversity related concerns within the field and making the psychology curricula more inclusive to include the narratives of people of color. Under the supervision of distinguished professor Dr. Kevin Nadal at John Jay, Sheharyar is currently leading a qualitative research project focused on understanding the types of microaggressions South Asian folx experience and the impact these experiences have on their physical and emotional well-being.

Dr. Puni Kalra has a PhD in Clinical Psychology with specialization in cross-cultural trauma. For three decades, she has been working with children, women, families, and communities of color who have faced traumatic events. She founded the Sikh Healing Collective, a mental health relief effort that stabilized the Sikh community after a mass shooting took place in their temple. She has co-founded a national division that supports the education and professional training needs of South Asian psychologists. Additionally, Dr. Kalra provides leadership development to clients across various industries. She supports them in understanding the root of their leadership challenges so they may become more effective business and community leaders. She specializes in executive leader assessment and development, team building, emotional intelligence, organizational and cultural change, strategic planning, and crisis management. Her clients come from cultures that span across five continents and more than twenty countries. Dr. Kalra resides near Denver, Colorado.

Shanta Nishi Kanukollu (a.k.a "Dr. K") has over a decade of clinical experience working with clients of culturally diverse backgrounds in the forensic and medical settings. She has also taught courses related to diversity and gender at The Chicago School of Professional Psychology and Northwestern University. Shanta was a recipient of the Minority Fellowship Award during her graduate career at The University of Michigan, where she obtained her doctorate in Clinical Psychology and Women's Studies. She currently has her own private practice in downtown Chicago where she provides psychotherapy to adults from various backgrounds, with a focus on South Asian mental health. Shanta provides education and outreach regarding mental health outcomes in ethnic minority communities through her writing and professional speaking engagements across the country.

Dr. Nina Kaur, Psy.D. is a licensed psychologist at the Sullivan Center for Children in Fresno, California. She earned her B.A. in Psychology with Honors from the University of California, Davis. She earned her doctoral degree in clinical psychology with an emphasis on social justice from the California School of Professional Psychology in San Francisco, CA. She has experience providing psychological services to underserved, diverse communities in school-based programs and community mental health settings. Her practicum sites have allowed her to provide psychological services to the South Asian community in her native language, Punjabi. Her interests include South Asian mental health, trauma, community resilience, social justice, mental health stigmas, and mental health specifically in the Punjabi Sikh community. She is currently the co-founder of South Asian Mental Health Consortium, which is a grassroots organization working to bring together those interested in mental health awareness in the South Asian community.

Dr. Preet Kaur Sabharwal is a licensed clinical psychologist based out of the Bay Area, CA. Preet has been providing clinical services at The Hume Center for the past 8 years, in their South Asian program. Preet's interests in psychology are focused on breaking stigmas of mental health and increasing utilization of services in the South Asian community. Preet is also the founder of the South Asian Mental Health Consortium which hosts the annual South Asian Mental Health Conference. Preet has presented at conferences all across the US and is considered to be one of the frontrunners of South Asian Mental Health Advocacy. In October 2019 Preet was recognized by the Asian American Psychological Association for her outstanding work, receiving the AAPA Early Career Award for Distinguished Contributions to Service. She is also a proud mother of a vibrant and sassy 5-year-old who keeps her busy in her free time.

Anastasia Khan is a doctoral student at Antioch University's Clinical Psychology program in Seattle, Washington. She has experience working with children and adults with intellectual and developmental disabilities, and refugee families in need of psychological and social support in Germany, Scotland, and the U.S. Currently, her studies at Antioch are augmented through membership in the Decoloniality and Social Privilege Awareness Institute (DSPAI), where issues of social privilege and the consequences of past and current coloniality are explored to identify and address inequities and oppressive power dynamics within the field of psychology. The inspiration for her work on this book is her husband, who is South Asian, and her son, who is a second-generation American of Indian origin.

Dr. Razia F. Kosi is the Coordinator of Culturally Responsive Practices and Anti-Racism Development, in a highly diverse Maryland public school system where she leads DEI initiatives. Dr. Kosi is also a mental health professional working to end stigma surrounding mental health in the South Asian (SA) community and was the founder of Counselors Helping (South) Asians, Inc.(CHAI). Additionally, Dr. Kosi is an adjunct professor in the doctoral program at the School of Education at the Johns Hopkins University. Advocating for both mental health and education, she has served on executive boards for both national and local organizations serving the SA and AAPI communities, including DoSAA and AAPA. She also co-founded the Asian American Educators of Howard County, currently serving on the executive board. Dr. Kosi sees clients in a small private practice primarily serving SA, and Muslim clients from varying racial and ethnic backgrounds.

Dr. Snehal Kumar, PhD is an Indian-born US educated psychologist based in New York City, where she offers individual counseling and supervision services. As both clinician and supervisor, she centers and explores how folks' identities and their experiences navigating systems of privilege and oppression impact their well-being. In her work, she leans heavily on psychodynamic, multicultural, and mindfulness-based theories. Snehal enjoys taking psychology outside of the therapy room through writing guest blogs and leading workshops. She is also a co-creator and co-facilitator of the Owning Your Power webinar series which addresses dynamics within Asian/Asian-American communities. She believes healing, learning, and liberation occurs through intentional connection, action, and rest, and is forever learning and unlearning through formal and informal ways.

Aishwarya Lonikar is a Clinical Psychology PsyD student at Antioch University Seattle. She earned her Master of Arts in Clinical Psychology from Antioch University Santa Barbara and her Bachelor of Arts in Psychology from Michigan State University. Prior to this, she grew up in India and has traveled widely across Asia allowing her the exposure to the diversity of cultures within the continent. Aishwarya's research interests are social justice and decoloniality, studying trauma from a cultural lens, and somatization of emotions in Indian cultures. At present, she is involved in research projects related to reproductive justice and decolonizing gender, resilience in trauma, and a decolonized theoretical model that looks at the historical perspective of clients in clinical work. Aishwarya is currently a fellow at her university and works as a student-therapist at her university's community counseling clinic. She aspires to bring decolonized theoretical perspectives of psychotherapy to South Asians cultures across the globe.

Dr. Harpreet Malla is a registered psychologist who is currently practicing at Shanti Orange County in Laguna Hills, CA. She identifies as a 1.5 generation Indian-American feminist and enjoys navigating the cultural nuances those experiences have brought her. Dr. Malla has a passion for working with identity development as it pertains to LGBTQ and bicultural or immigrant populations, and recently has seen a rise in couples navigating arranged or other nontraditional marital practices in her work such as poly constellations, those who practice kink, or are in interracial relationships. In addition to her clinical work, she has also taught at the university and graduate level, and hosted a variety of mental health workshops for corporate, university, and community events. She is also the Diversity Chair for the Los Angeles County Psychological Association, where she advocates for marginalized groups and seeks to promote understanding through education.

Dr. Bindu Methikalam is an Associate Professor and the Assistant Director of Clinical Training at Chestnut Hill College in Philadelphia, PA. Her clinical interests include working with grief, trauma, adjustment, anxiety, depression, family and relationship concerns as well as diversity related issues. Her research interests are in perfectionism, family expectations, multicultural issues, particularly, immigrant experiences, acculturation, and intersectionality of cultural identities.

Dr. Neha Navsaria (PhD) is an Associate Professor of Psychiatry at the Washington University School of Medicine in St. Louis. As a clinical psychologist, she has interests in parenting, parent-child relationships, and early social and emotional development. She has expertise in ethnic minority and immigrant mental health and ethnic and racial socialization in families. She has been an advocate for mental health and wellness in Asian-American communities as an active member of the Asian American Psychological Association (AAPA) elected as chair for the AAPA Division on South Asian Americans. Building upon her interests in parenting and Asian American psychology she was the co-recipient of the 2011 AAPA/American Psychological Foundation Okura Grant to fund a national parenting initiative culminating in the creation of a resource book for South Asian parents of which she is co-editor. She believes that parents are the greatest social and emotional architects of childhood and enjoys helping parents navigate this role with their children.

Ankita Nikalje is a Dalit counseling psychology researcher, practitioner, and educator. She has her Ph.D. in Counseling Psychology from Purdue University (U.S.A.), her M.Sc. in Cross-Cultural Psychology from Brunel University (U.K.), and her B.Sc. in Psychology from the University of Melbourne (Australia). Her research focuses on systemic issues within the South Asian diaspora and their impact on lived experiences and mental health. She is particularly passionate about the issue of casteism in the diaspora and how caste discrimination continues to be experienced on an institutional, interpersonal, and internalized level outside of South Asia. She has theorized Caste Critical Race Theory (CasteCRIT) and developed measures to assess the impact of caste in the diaspora.

Dr. Kinjal Panchal, Psy.D is a Clinical psychologist, artist, and co-author of the chapter on Religion and South Asian mental health. She received her doctorate degree from the Illinois School of Professional Psychology. She is currently an adjunct professor of multicultural psychology and psychological assessment. Dr. Panchal has a deep love and interest in spirituality, Vedic literature, and yoga. She specializes in the connection between spirituality, religion, and an individual's identity. Additionally, she works with individuals, couples, and families addressing issues of identity, depression and, complex trauma. When she is not in session or teaching, Dr. Panchal spends most of her time with her children, family, and friends. She is an avid reader, enjoys dancing, traveling the world, and deep-diving into her own artwork. With a love for food and culinary innovation, she explores new dishes, recipes, and restaurants with her husband.

Dr. Sarika Persaud, Psy.D. is a supervising psychologist and Coordinator of Diversity, Inclusion, and Social Justice Initiatives at Fordham University (Lincoln Center), and an adjunct professor in the psychology graduate program at City University of New York, John Jay College. Dr. Persaud's research focuses on community-based youth suicide prevention in Guyana, and has been published in International Journal of Psychology, School Psychology International. Dr. Persaud's community work focuses on relationship, sexuality, and body image issues for the South Asian diaspora. She works with numerous gender justice and arts organizations on mental health outreach in New York and the United Kingdom. Dr. Persaud identifies as a bisexual Indo-Caribbean woman, and was recently published in an anthology of South Asian LGBTQAI+ essays, "I Hope You'll Still Love Me." Dr. Persaud has also published a collection of poetry, "Poems About a Song," and she is a professional Kathak dancer and classical dance teacher.

Dr. Sheetal Shah is a licensed clinical psychologist in Sacramento, CA. Sheetal's work as a psychologist largely centers on culturally responsive therapy with a social justice lens. In her current job, Sheetal provides clinical services and well-being support physicians in training. Through her private practice, Sheetal provides long-term therapy as well as diversity consultation to various groups and organizations. Throughout her career, Sheetal focused much of her work on the South Asian community. She held a job that explicitly focused on reducing stigma about mental health within the South Asian community. She participates in scholarly effort from her dissertation which examined acculturation and intergenerational conflict for South Asians to book chapters that focused on counseling South Asian Americans to work on a project that understands aging amongst the South Asian community in the US. Sheetal earned her doctoral degrees in Counseling Psychology at Southern Illinois University at Carbondale.

Himadhari Sharma identifies as a second-generation bilingual (Hindi/Urdu-English) cisgender South Asian American woman and daughter of Asian Indian immigrants. She is currently a 5th-year doctoral candidate in the Department of Counseling,

Clinical, and School Psychology with an emphasis in Counseling Psychology at the University of California, Santa Barbara. She has a variety of professional experiences, including a previous career in business, and has worked internationally both in business and psychology. Her current work focuses on serving minoritized groups, with an emphasis on South Asian and South Asian American communities. She is passionate to continue developing a career, both as a researcher and clinician, centered in decolonization and social justice. Her current interests include access and utilization of mental health services by minoritized communities (especially South Asian and South Asian American communities), culturally salient and indigenous mental health support and psychological treatment methods, cross-cultural/international psychology, as well as bilingual psychological services.

Dr. Rahul Sharma is a DEI consultant, psychologist, musician, & keynote speaker. He is former Associate Professor at the Illinois School of Professional Psychology. He is founder of Strategic Inclusion Consulting, providing consulting, speaking, coaching, and training services. Dr. Sharma is also founder of Funkadesi, a music group which includes diverse musicians, activists, educators, and healers. In 2021, Funkadesi celebrated its 25th Anniversary. Dr. Sharma often integrates experiential multicultural music programs in conjunction with the band at conferences and trainings. Recently, Dr. Sharma led a guided visualization with live improvised music for TEDx Chicago, followed by a Funkadesi performance. In addition to all these pursuits, Dr. Sharma maintains a small private practice.

Anneliese Singh, PhD, LPC (she/they) serves as Chief Diversity Officer/Associate Provost for Diversity and Faculty Development at Tulane University and is a Professor in the School of Social Work with a joint appointment in the Department of Psychology. Trained as a counseling psychologist and counselor educator, her scholarship and community organizing explores liberation, racial healing and racial justice, as well as NIH-funded work with trans and nonbinary people and South Asian resilience, traumatology, and migration. She has written extensively on multicultural and social justice competency development in the helping professions. Dr. Singh is the author of *The Racial Healing Handbook* and *Queer and Trans Resilience Workbook.*

Lakshmi Sridaran is the Executive Director of South Asian Americans Leading Together (SAALT), a national South Asian movement strategy and advocacy organization. From 2014 to 2019, she was SAALT's Director of National Policy and Advocacy where she developed SAALT's policy agenda, which focuses on immigration, racial profiling, and hate violence. Prior to joining SAALT she served as the Policy Director for The Praxis Project, a national movement support organization focused on health justice in communities of color. Lakshmi's social justice approach is grounded in her experiences organizing in the South. Before moving to D.C., Lakshmi lived in New Orleans where she worked in Black-led organizations immediately following Hurricane Katrina. Since 2009, Lakshmi has served on the Board of the Southern Initiative of the Algebra Project. She holds a Masters degree in City Planning from Massachusetts Institute of Technology and a B.A. in Ethnic Studies from The University of California, Berkeley.

Dr. Sruthi Swami is a nationally certified school psychologist and educator of school psychologists in training. She received her degree in Counseling, Clinical, and School Psychology from the University of California, Santa Barbara. In her research, clinical work, and teaching, she focuses on promoting equity for youths and families from marginalized backgrounds, with a particular focus on social justice and dismantling racism and discrimination within K–12 school systems. Her training is also in special education assessment and intervention and, as such, she teaches courses related to the assessment of intellectual abilities and best practices for assessing individuals from diverse backgrounds. She also engages in research related to the mental health and wellbeing of Asian and Asian American individuals, with a focus on understanding experiences of racism and discrimination that contribute to the identity development of Asian Americans.

Dr. Asha Unni, Ph.D. is a licensed psychologist living in Austin, Texas. Dr. Unni provides therapy, consultation, and psychological evaluations for children, adolescents, families, and young adults. Dr. Unni received her Ph.D. in School Psychology from Texas A&M University. She previously served as the chair-elect for the Asian American Psychological Association's Division on South Asian Americans from 2019–2020. Dr. Unni identifies as a South Asian American woman and is passionate about advocating for children and families with diverse backgrounds and identities. Her research and clinical interests include trauma-informed services, race and ethnic identity, discrimination, and issues of social justice. Her doctoral dissertation, titled "Experiences Of Perceived Discrimination Among Asian Indian Youth: A Mixed-Methods Study" was completed in effort to amplify the voices of young South Asian American youth living within the US In her free time, Dr. Unni enjoys hiking with her puppy Nori, photography, reading, and attending concerts.

1 South Asian American Counseling and Psychology

Ulash Thakore-Dunlap, Devika Srivastava, and Nita Tewari

Case Overview

Ulash identifies as Asian Indian and was born in London, United Kingdom (UK). Her father was raised in Uganda, Africa who moved to London, UK before the expulsion of Asian Indians during the Ida Amin regime and her mother was born in Burundi (Africa). Raised in a working class, immigrant family, Ulash realized at an early age that she wanted to be in a career where she could improve access to resources for others. As a first generation student and professional, in the UK, Ulash worked as a teacher in schools and colleges. Ulash moved to San Francisco in 2002 to be with her husband, Oliver. Challenged to start a new life in the United States (U.S.), Ulash started a new career and has been working as a counselor, educator, and therapist in the San Francisco Bay Area. Ulash's experiences have led her to exploring the gaps and providing mental health and educational resources for communities of color. Ulash currently resides in San Francisco, U.S. with her husband Oliver, and their multiracial son Ezra.

Devika Srivastava was born in Patna, Bihar, India and was raised in Houston, Texas. Her father had come to the U.S. in the early 1960s for graduate school and her mother arrived after her Ph.D. in Psychology in the 1970s. Growing up, she did not see many faces like hers, and she felt like an outsider at times. Initially, Devika was surrounded by white children and on "show and tell" days, she talked about trips to India where she had family, but this was met with unrelatable stares. After the "white Flight" of the 1980s/1990s, she was exposed to other bipoc and second-generation individuals. In college, Devika was immersed into a large population of South Asian Americans. As she later grew into her passions, Devika then connected with other progressive South Asian Americans and she found kinship and a "home" of people. Devika has dedicated her life to serving all people of color with intersectionality, especially her intergenerational diasporic community of South Asian Americans as she has seen the gaps in mental health, health disparities, and systemic injustice and her work has focused on addressing these issues from macro and micro system levels. She currently has a private practice in Texas and Florida.

Nita Tewari is a California born second generation, Hindu Indian American married female with two young adult children. She was born in Los Angeles County (Little India area), moved to Orange County, California at 8 years of age. Her parents had an arranged marriage, her father immigrated to the US in 1968 to pursue an education as an engineer, and her mother joined later to live the "American dream." Growing up, she was very aware of her brown skin, not being the majority racial group in her Orange County neighborhood. Being raised as bicultural, she describes her biculturality as both a protective support factor and acculturative pressure simultaneously. Being inclined toward understanding people, years spent as a cultural broker, witnessing mental health struggles, and being a minority female contributed to her pursuit of becoming a psychologist. Her

DOI: 10.4324/9781003081548-1

personal and professional identity development is inclusive of racially defining herself as Asian American, ethnically defining herself as Indian American, geographically defining herself as South Asian American and regionally defining herself as North Indian American with ancestry in Uttar Pradesh and Madhya Pradesh when asked "Where are you from?".

Introduction

As editors of this book, we are case examples of our diverse South Asian American communities with intersectional identities, ages, immigration histories, and varied geographical lived experiences to illustrate the diversity and complexity of who is South Asian American. Our identities, education, and counseling training, have served as foundations to guide our clinical work, have shaped who we are, and strongly contributed to our commitment to publish this book. We (Ulash, Devika, and Nita) are thrilled to contribute to the lacking mental health literature in our field which has limited publications focused on the counseling and clinical needs of South Asian Americans (SAAs). Over 10 years ago, the three of us came together to share our professional experiences and how it intersects with our personal ethnic identities, identifying a gap and need to create a book that focuses on the South Asian American mental health and psychological issues of our rapidly growing population in the U.S. (Pew Research Center, 2017).

In this first chapter, we present the defination and identification of South Asian Americans, the influences on South Asian American Counseling and Psychology and provide a definition of this field of study. We also discuss cultural and clinical factors for consideration in working with South Asian Americans who are racially categorized as Asian Americans due to the geography of the Asian continent and the U.S. Census Bureau labeling. This is worthy to note since Asian American Ethnic Studies and Psychology both served as an impetus to the developing South Asian American Counseling and Psychology discipline.

Who Are South Asian Americans?

However, South Asian Americans are described as individuals in the U.S. with ethnic heritage from Pakistan, Nepal, India, Sri Lanka, Bangladesh, Bhutan, Afghanistan, and/or the Maldives (South Asian Americans Leading Together, 2019). This label also includes individuals from various African countries, the Caribbean, Canada, Europe, Middle East, and other countries within Asia with ancestors who immigrated from South Asian countries. The South Asian American (SAA) community also pertains to individuals who have ancestry and can trace their heritage to Maldives and to other countries of the South Asian diaspora including Trinidad/Tobago, Guyana, Fiji, Tanzania, and Kenya as well.

SAAs have a deep-rooted history of immigration to the U.S., including early immigration in the 1800s and 1900s to the most recent and largest wave in the past 30 to 40 years (López et al., 2017). Additionally, the SAA community was reportedly one of the fastest growing groups in the 2010 Census (United States Census Bureau, 2010). Indian Americans made up the largest ethnicity of the SAA population, with 80% and 5.4 million of the total U.S. population, followed by Pakistanis, Bangladeshis, Nepali, Sri Lankans, and Bhutanese (United States Census Bureau, 2010). Not only was the South Asian American population the fastest growing major ethnic group in the United States from 2000 to 2010 that grew roughly 40% between 2010 and 2017 (Pew Research Center, 2017); according to the 2020 U.S. Census Bureau, of the 20 million who identified as Asian American, Indian Americans are the second largest Asian American subgroup.

By 2065, it is projected that Asian Americans will be the largest immigrant population in the U.S. (Pew Research Center, 2017). While we acknowledge that Asian Indian Americans are the largest subgroup in the Asian and Pacific Islander American racial population (United States Census Bureau, 2010) and with respect to all South Asian and South Asian American individuals, much of the psychological research and clinical data that we encountered represented the experiences and practices of Asian Indian Americans. Nevertheless, we strove for inclusivity, invited diverse contributing authors, included unique chapter topics, and provided a counter narrative that SAAs include more than Asian Indian Americans wherever possible. Furthermore, we value research findings with disaggregated data identifying specific South Asian American regional groups and attempted to reflect the diversity of South Asian subpopulations, subregions, and experiences in chapters following ours much of the research and clinical recommendations in the Asian American psychological literature has mostly focused on East Asian populations in their subject samples and case studies.

Among those who identify as South Asian and South Asian American, there is an understanding of the shared history, culture, and experiences from those cultures of origin. With the shared cultural commonalities of SAAs, not only is there great diversity between South Asian subgroups, rich diversity exists within each subgroup population as well with regard to religious affiliation, language, immigration history, socioeconomic status, and education (Inman & Tewari, 2003). These differences include variations in religion, level of traditionalism, clothing, customs, food, and linguistics (over 30+ distinct languages are spoken in South Asia) and dating and arranged marriage practices. According to 2010 estimates (Pew Research Center, 2012), the majority of South Asians practice Hinduism or Islam, but there is also a significant number of South Asians and South Asian Americans who practice Buddhism (the majority religion in Bhutan and Sri Lanka), Christianity, Jainism or other religions.

Given the diversity of South Asian American population, we hope to give our readers a foundation of where to begin in gaining a further understanding of who South Asian Americans are, why we need our field of study, and considerations in working with South Asian Americans. Before defining what South Asian American Counseling and Psychology is, we begin by discussing how this field evolved.

Influences on South Asian American Counseling and Psychology

The field of SAA counseling and psychology has been influenced by historical counseling, psychology theories, and frameworks, as well as movements that increased the visibility and needs of communities of color. Additionally, racism post 9/11 toward SAA populations, and increased intergenerational cultural and family issues coupled with racial and ethnic identity development require further understanding to provide clinical care. The following section will briefly provide the various influences on South Asian American Counseling and Psychology.

Broadly defined, counseling and psychology are scientific fields of social science encompassing several branches of research (cognitive, experimental, lifespan developmental, personality, social), applied psychology (clinical, counseling psychology, industrial/organizational, school and educational, human factors, health, social, neuropsychology), and key clinical based therapeutic orientations (psychodynamic, cognitive behavioral therapy, acceptance commitment therapy, biofeedback, gestalt, adlerian, behavioral, etc.). The practice of counseling and psychology involves the use of psychological knowledge to: understand and treat mental, emotional, physical, and social dysfunction in individuals; understand and enhance behavior in various settings, including clinical settings, businesses, schools, universities, medical schools; and in research development, consultation, and in policy work. The main mission of counseling and psychology is to increase awareness of issues and internal processes related to individuals and communities in an attempt to improve well-being for all individuals. Culturally responsive care is an essential element in effectively practicing counseling and psychology.

Until now, counseling, psychology, and mental health has been developed with a Eurocentric worldview and Western perspective. The earliest theories in psychology emerged from philosophy around structuralism, free will, and nurture versus nature. However, as our American society has become more representative of its actual citizens, such as women, people with diverse sexualities, disabilities, and people of color, there has been an expansion of thought to better serve all individuals. In the 1930s, Vygotsky introduced the importance of culture into the understanding of psychology, and this gave rise to the true importance of how social and cultural situations influence attitudes, thinking, and behavior. This process is vitally important in understanding others but also how to help people on macro and microlevels, which include clinical care.

In challenging the White normativity in psychology, in 1968, at the American Psychological Association Convention, Black psychologists formed the first national organization to challenge traditional frameworks of psychology. They challenged the existing psychological paradigms that conceptualized Black individuals as deficient, racially inferior, having lesser IQs, and higher pathological diagnoses. They dismantled theories of Eugenics, questioned standardized, educational, and psychological testing practices with regard to unfair evaluations and applications normed and validated on upper to middle class, mostly male, White populations. This served as the impetus for the beginning of the fourth force of psychology, also known as multicultural psychology.

Simultaneously, the development of ethnic studies paralleled the need for greater minority representation and cultural competency in the field of mental health, with scholars and activists turning their focus toward providing culturally appropriate and relevant education to diverse student and community populations. The rise of the ethnic studies movement occurred due to the continuous racial and ethnic marginalization of people of color. Ethnic studies required the "community" in research to serve as a vehicle for representation, and that Asian American scholars need to conduct action-oriented research that would influence and better the lives of Asian Americans (Leong & Okazaki, 2009). Activism and the emphasis on the third world struggle may not be the current focus of present-day Asian American psychology in all domains, but it is important to note that Asian American psychology rose from the era of the Asian American movement and the needs of those times.

Asian American studies helped to increase the need and visibility of many Asian American subpopulations, including South Asian American communities. The origins of Asian American studies can be traced back to the late 1960s as part of a larger social and political movement to challenge the marginalization of Asians in the United States (Leong & Okazaki, 2009). Interestingly, this was during the time when the U.S. Immigration and Nationality Act of 1965 lifted restrictive quotas after 40 years, prioritizing immigration for highly skilled immigrants and those with family living in the U.S., many of whom were Asian American. As Asian American Ethnic Studies formed, the field of Asian American Psychology soon thereafter followed the formation of The Association of Black Psychologists that also emerged from the 1960s Civil Rights Movement and born out of decades of violence, inequality, racial tension, discrimination, and political unrest. The late 1960s and early 1970s spawned a time where racial and ethnic minorities were establishing their place in America, stronger than ever. Psychology historically relied upon Eurocentric worldviews and perspectives to conceptualize and treat Asian American and Pacific Islander Americans was challenged to shift its theories, research, conceptualization, and clinical standards in providing multiculturally sensitive and competent mental health care.

The Brown Asian movement has also been instrumental in increasing the inclusion and visibility of South Asian Americans in counseling and psychology. Since the inception of the Asian American Movement, Filipino Americans, South Asian Americans, and Southeast Asian Americans have consistently vocalized feelings of marginalization and exclusion within the pan-ethnic group (Nadal, 2019). The struggles of Brown Asians, such as South Asian Americans, within the Asian American community also include clinicians and researchers in the field of counseling and psychology and within ethnic and Asian psychological associations (Nadal, 2019). Therefore, as Asian American counseling and psychology continues to emphasize the needs of Asian American populations, this is still a growing field that needs further attention, resources, programs and policies, and visibility devoted to Brown Asian Americans that includes South Asian Americans in the Asian American umbrella.

Defining South Asian American Counseling and Psychology

In the psychological, sociological and anthropological fields, there are limited research articles and books on South Asian Americans. Few publications specifically address counseling, psychology, and clinical care pertaining to South Asian Americans. Additionally, the term "South Asian American Counseling and Psychology" has not been defined by scholars or practitioners in the field of counseling, psychology, and mental health. Therefore, we first present Dr. Nita Tewari's definition of Asian American Psychology as a framework to help us as authors formulate a working definition of South Asian American Counseling and Psychology:

> The focused study of psychology that incorporates Asian American racial and ethnic identity, cultural values, communication patterns, emotional expression, acculturation levels, generational status, socioeconomic status educational background and immigration histories, differing diasporic experiences, and intersectional identities of Asian American Pacific Islander populations.
>
> (Tewari, 2019)

In attempting to define the developing South Asian Counseling and Psychology field, since it has not been defined and believe it is important to bring attention to this term, we define South Asian American Counseling and Psychology as:

> The psychological study of individuals who identify as South Asian Americans. South Asian American Counseling and Psychology explores the cultural, behavioral, emotional, psychological, and social factors that impact South Asian American individuals given the context and environment they live in. South Asian American Counseling and Psychology aims to better inform individuals to understand the mental health and clinical needs of South Asian Americans to improve mental health and wellbeing and provide culturally appropriate resources to support the individual and system in which they function and are part of.
>
> (Thakore-Dunlap, Srivastava & Tewari, 2023)

Similarly, as Asian American Counseling and Psychology, South Asian American Counseling and Psychology will further focus on the mental health needs of intergenerational individuals of South Asian heritage and historically associated with the SAA diaspora. Our book, Counseling and Psychotherapy for South Asian Americans: **Identity, Psychology, and Clinical Implications** serves as a primer for practitioners, educators, and scholars conducting research on SAAs, gaining knowledge in providing culturally competent care and for clinical use when working with intergenerational SAA populations.

Brief Overview of South Asian American Mental Health Research

As mentioned earlier, South Asian Americans have not been studied by social scientists to an appreciable degree (Holman, 2010). Resources, research data, and mental health care have been scarce in exploring the psychology and clinical needs of South Asians and South Asian Americans. Existing research on South Asian and South Asian American individuals and counseling suggests that South Asian Americans have neutral or positive perceptions of mental health care, but infrequently use mental health services (Panganamala & Plummer, 1998; Sue & Sue, 2008). Additionally, many SAAs may not know how to connect with mental health services (Fraga et al., 2004). Furthermore, there are also significant barriers related to seeking services, including culture, language, or fear of confidentiality breaches (Fraga et al., 2004). A limited number of mental health clinics in the U.S. have practitioners that provide clinical services in Hindi, Bengali, Farsi, or other South Asian regional native languages. Another reason for this infrequent use of mental health services or connectivity may be due to the stigma related to disclosing mental problems, mental illness, creating vulnerability, and potentially bringing shame to the family (Fraga et al., 2004). Increasing evidence indicates that South Asian populations experience high rates of mental distress and suffer from psychological issues and disorders without help (Karasz et al., 2019).

South Asian American mental health is often researched under the broad category of Asian Americans. Asian Americans have a high incidence of mental distress, which is a significant concern since Indian Americans are included as a subgroup in this racial category (Lin & Cheung, 1999). The 2010 U.S. Census estimated a total of 17,320, 856 Asian Americans comprising 5.6% of the total U.S. population. For example, some of the mental health concerns affecting Asian Americans include depression, anxiety, and suicide and U.S.-born Asian American women had a higher lifetime rate of suicidal thoughts than that of the general U.S. population (Duldulao et al., 2009). Asian Americans college students were more likely than White American students to have had suicidal thoughts and to attempt suicide (Kisch et al., 2005). Asian Americans may also experience culture-bound syndromes such as neurasthenia, a condition characterized by fatigue, anxiety, headache, neuralgia, and depressed mood, and hwa-byung, which is a somatization disorder characterized by symptoms of anxiety, depression, obsessive-compulsiveness, anorexia, paranoia or fearfulness, absent-mindedness, irritability, and a heavy feeling in the chest (Sue & Sue, 1999). Additionally, older Asian American women, of which SAAs are included, have the highest suicide rate of all women over age 65 in the U.S. (Xu et al., 2010). Finally, other information has highlighted high rates of addiction, gambling, and family violence as areas of concern for some groups of Asian Americans compared to the general American population (Sue & Sue, 1999). Existing research on South Asian individuals and counseling suggests that South Asian Americans have neutral or positive perceptions of mental health care, but infrequently use mental health services (Panganamala & Plummer, 1998; Sue & Sue, 2008). Additionally, many SAAs may not know how to connect with mental health services (Gim et al., 2004). There are also significant barriers related to culture, language, or fear of confidentiality breaches (Gim et al., 2004). Another reason for this infrequent use of mental health services or connectivity may be because of stigma related to disclosing mental problems or mental illness and that it involves vulnerability or may bring shame and stigma to the entire family (Gim et al., 2004). As we encourage readers to deepen their knowledge of South Asian American Counseling and Psychology, we thought it would be important to address some of the researched and perceived similarities and differences between South Asian American and Asian American subgroups for comparison in understanding this field.

South Asian American and Asian American Population Similarities and Differences

In stimulating new theories and concepts in South Asian American Counseling and Psychology, we encourage readers to consider possible similarities and differences comparing South Asian Americans to Asian American subpopulations based on information that has emerged through research, clinical data, discussions, social media, and collective experiences of South Asian Americans living as generational Asian Americans in the U.S.

Similarities with South Asian Americans and Asian Americans

Considering that many Asian Americans have immigrated to America, the first similarity is acculturation. Cross-cultural researchers have used the concept of acculturation when studying the impact and influences of being in and adjusting to a new culture different than one's own, as is the case with many Asian Americans (Berry, 1980). Second and generally speaking, many but not all subgroups, of first generation South Asian Americans and Asian Americans immigrants value degrees of discipline, self-control, strong work ethics, higher education (often science-based careers, such as engineering or medicine among educated Asian subgroups) and have a sense of commitment to family, the Asian community and desire to preserve their culture of origin. Additionally, there is a tendency toward humility and desire to respect the wisdom and decisions of elders. Furthermore, it is not uncommon among traditional Asian cultures for elders to emphasize their desires for younger generations to marry within the culture, (i.e., marry someone from the same country or region, of the same religion, socioeconomic status, educational level, and value system) or be familiar with the practice and understanding of arranged marriages in their communities.

A third discussed similarity has been the traditional patriarchal family structure in South Asian American and Asian American families where women are the primary child caregivers, respecting the wishes of husbands, sacrificing careers for family, caretaking for family members, in-laws and are the carriers of cultural customs. Many traditional or religious first-generation women immigrants are seen wearing clothing customary to their culture more frequently than men and men have been expected to be the primary breadwinners of the family. Additionally, with several Asian American subgroups, sons have been more generally valued than daughters as evidenced in Asian laws, land ownership, religious language, and with marriage rights.

Fourth, living in a society where racism exists, many South Asian Americans and Asian Americans have faced different forms of discrimination—overt, covert, and institutional—and have been stereotyped as "Model Minorities" and are clumped together demographically, racially and culturally on U.S. Census and other self-check form categories. Also, South Asians share experiences of historical animosities between people of differing South Asian countries, similar to Asian countries; historical tension between Koreans and Japanese has existed, just as tension exists between Indians and Pakistanis. While this is not highly relevant to all SAAs, or perhaps not to those born in the U.S.

clinicians should explore negative feelings when relevant among older immigrants (Mio et al., 2007).

A fifth similarity between South Asian Americans and Asian Americans is the stigma toward mental health seeking and receiving psychological counseling due to fear bringing shame to oneself or the family. Many South Asian Americans and Asian Americans are resistant to using therapy, lack knowledge of the counseling process or distrust mental health practitioners (Tewari, 2009). Though awareness and familiarity with receiving therapy services is increasing, there continues to be hesitation toward contacting mental health providers in comparison to medical health providers.

Although there is common ground with South Asian Americans and Asian Americans as illustrated by the discussion of possible similarities, it is important to recognize that the concerns, pressures, and experiences of these groups were spoken of broadly and immigration history, acculturation, ethnic identity, and generational levels of each Asian American subgroup must be considered when researching and working with these diverse populations (Tewari et al., 2003).

Differences with South Asian Americans and Asian Americans

While Asians in Asia as a whole may share similar cultural values and experiences, Asians in the U.S. are quite distinct from each other. First, Asian Americans in the U.S. have experienced differing historical relationships between their home countries and the U.S. For example, importation of Chinese laborers to build railroads, colonization of the Philippines by the U.S., the Japanese attack on Pearl Harbor and the resultant internment camps for the Japanese Americans, Sikh farmers working in agricultural and denied land ownership, serving as indentured servants, and the U.S. involvement in the Vietnam and Korean Wars are some of the different historical experiences of Asian subgroups. In contrast, there has been no comparable military action associated with Indians and many South Asians as part of their political relationships impacting immigration post 1965.

Second, differences in immigration experiences of South Asians Americans in comparison to Asian Americans. A majority of South Asian Americans immigrated to the U.S. by free will, own choice, or to join family in America. Several Asian groups (e.g., Southeast Asians) endured refugee experiences or other notable differences in immigration patterns (i.e., necessity for survival, fleeing from their country where trauma has occurred, or forced immigration for labor in earlier times) compared to most South Asians. Many South Asian Americans arrived in the U.S. during the 1960s on an H1 visa as an international student and more came after the Immigration Act of 1965 under fairly decent financial conditions with good mental and physical health, seeking higher education, and wanting to live the "American Dream."

Third, there are many economic and educational differences among Asian subgroups. Pew Research reported that 75% of Indians are the highest group to have at least a Bachelor's degree and had the highest household income in comparison to their Asian counterparts (Pew Research, 2021). Historically, the impact of this pattern includes categorically limiting or excluding South Asians from any "underrepresented" or "minority" category for need-based financial support or affirmative action support in assuming these averages apply to all South Asians resulting in unacknowledging impoverished South Asian American populations.

A fourth difference is the British influence in India and other parts of South Asia. This influence has familiarized South Asians with English as a language since many of the schools were forced to teach English in addition to native South Asian languages (Hindi, etc.). British rule exposed South Asians to a culture different than their own, leaving many middle- to upper-class individuals to adjust to a European way of life pre-exposing South

Asians to pre-immigration and post immigration adjustment in America and ability to speak the U.S. language.

Fifth, as mentioned earlier, despite being a significantly growing ethnic group within the Asian American group, South Asian Americans have been neglected in the American and Asian American mental health literature and excluded in the Asian American studies literature (Durvasula & Mylvaganam, 1994).

Sixth, physical differences have led to South Asian Americans not being recognized as Asian American. Durvasula and Mylvaganam (1994) noted that most Asian Indians (and one could generalize that most South Asians) agree that they are distinct from other Asian migrant groups as the old racist term "Oriental," or the even the current term "Asian," is not frequently used to describe South Asian Americans. This distinction between East Asian, Southeast Asian, and South Asian populations has been one of phenotype differences as many South Asian Americans do not look physically similar to their other Asian counterparts. For example, Asian Indians as a race have been categorized as Caucasian with their facial features being viewed as "Anglo-Saxon or Caucasian," whereas other Asians (e.g., Japanese, Chinese, etc.) have been described as having Mongoloid features and are labeled as Mongoloid by race (Gupta, 1999; Lott 1998). Differences in physical appearances, skin color and facial features have impacted whether South Asians are perceived as Asian American despite the shared geographical continent. Finally, there are many other differences between South Asian and other Asian American subgroups but these were a few to explain how people think about South Asian Americans and Asian Americans. The next section more specifically addresses cultural values and experiences shared by South Asian Americans.

South Asian American Cultural Values and Experiences

South Asian American (SAAs) represent a unique subset of Asian Americans that share the vast continent of Asia. Among those who identify as South Asian and SAAs, there is an understanding of the shared history, culture, and experiences from those cultures of origin. However, along with the shared cultural commonalities of SAAs, there are regional differences based upon South Asian country of origin and interregional differences that make for a rich and varied South Asian population that differs in its expressions of culture. These differences include variations in religious, socioeconomic, education, level of traditionalism, clothing, customs, food, and linguistics (over 30+ distinct languages are spoken in South Asia) and dating and arranged marriage practices. The SAA population holds many different ethnicities with many variances including class, resources, religion, cultural beliefs even when observing the same religion, food, clothing, views on gender. Rajiva & D'Sylva (2014) also identifies that the term South Asian is primarily used by people not of the ethnicity, but often identify individuals from India. Many SAAs self-label and associate their identity based on the ancestral home of their culture of origin (i.e., state, territory, etc.) and tie that to their identity (Rajiva & D'Sylva, 2014). Knowing how SAAs label themselves from their ethnic and cultural region is important to consider when trying to conceptualize the uniqueness and differences when trying to understand the complexity of their SAA identity. Research publications in the psychological literature have found a number of values and experiences to be relevant for SAA ethnic groups. This chapter briefly presents what some of these are when working with SAA clients, families and communities.

Worldviews, Values, and Beliefs

The worldview and beliefs of the South Asian and South Asian American value system are critical to understanding the psychology, struggle, and needs of this population. Examining the significance of one's worldviews, values, and beliefs is the foundation for understanding the psychological development of first, second, and third generation individuals, developing conceptualizations, providing counseling strategies and treatment implications. Ramisetty-Mikler (1993) in her overview on sociocultural issues in counseling with Indian Americans, discussed important factors distinguishing Eastern (i.e., Indian) and Western (i.e., American) cultures. She focused on the cultural orientations that create conflicts in the process of adjustment. She noted that Asians in their "Perception of Time" tend to stress the past and future—the present is seen as a transitory period. In contrast, individuals with a more Western or Americanized worldview, may value the present and look forward to the future. Spirituality and religion are believed to be influential in a client's attitudes and beliefs. The notion of destiny or fate (pre-deterministic view, fatalistic thinking) will likely influence the degree to which a client feels control over their thoughts and behaviors. Knowing the degree to which clients adhere to culture of origin values plays an important role in developing culturally relevant psychological services (Inman et al., 1999; Kim 1998).

Acculturation

In addition to understanding a client's adherence to cultural values, an important aspect of adjustment within an emigrational context is the extent to which a client's cultural values might differ from the host culture. Acculturation is a bi-directional change process that occurs when an individual simultaneously encounters two or more distinct cultures firsthand (Berry, 1980). In acculturating within a pluralistic society such as the U.S., one is likely to be confronted with social as well as psychological adjustment difficulties. Several authors (Prathikanti, 1997; Ramisetty-Mikler, 1993; Sodowsky & Carey, 1987; 1988) have identified factors that mitigate and/or create stress for South Asian immigrant groups in their adjustment process. The struggle for many South Asian Americans to understand, incorporate, and "fit" into the American culture while still maintaining their South Asian values, traditions, attitudes, and beliefs can create different choices for parents and their children, resulting in conflict and tension for both parties. Therefore, assessing your client's acculturation level will provide clinicians with a baseline understanding of their process of adaptation in their South Asian American experience.

Network System

Sodowsky and Carey (1987; 1988) and Ramisetty-Mikler (1993) discuss the importance of a strong ethnic network within the South Asian and South Asian American community. Specifically, they note that ethnic social support established by Indians in the community have offered a strong moral and resource support for many of these immigrants in the U.S. However, while such groups provide support by organizing religious and cultural activities, Ramisetty-Mikler (1993) argued that Asian Indians' "strong sense of group identity might, in turn, hinder a person from completely assimilating and adapting to the host culture" (p. 41). In our clinical experiences, we have found the SAA extended family and community support to be both a source of support and stress, both in providing cultural validation and invalidation depending on our client's behaviors and others perceptions of mental health issues and concerns. Covert and overt expectations, whether expressed verbally or not, are often felt by SAA individuals who come from traditional families and strong ethnic communities where SAAs are the primary sources of contact, socialization and support. Practitioners would benefit from learning the ethnic composition, level of acculturation, and the amount of contact with SAA communities and level of traditionalism in client family networks.

Families

Knowing SAA family structures are critical to working with SAA individuals within the counseling profession as awareness of contextual variables such as culture, race, ethnicity, sexual orientation, socioeconomic status, religion, and gender have known influences on individual (Inman & Tewari, 2003). SAA family members are a blend of collectivistic and individualistic values based on their level of acculturation and individual identities. Intergenerationally, second-generation and proceeding SAA generations may be more acculturated than their parents and this may cause conflict associated with career, educational goals, family, marriage, parenting, and caretaking toward older adults.

With regard to intimate relationships, dating has been shown to be a major source of conflict linked to intergenerational conflict for second-generation Asian Americans, including South Asian American individuals (Srivastava, 2012; Sue & Sue, 1999). Additionally, South Asian culture holds a view that different generations of family often live together in the same household both in one's home countries or the U.S. Such views may be based on traditionalism, economic factors, filial piety, and/or respect toward elders. For example, in family unions, when a son is married, in Hindu and Muslim households, wives may move into the parent's home and often there are grandparents, parents, and children of multiple generations residing as part of one household. Also, if not in the same house, family members often live in close proximity. This view of family and household may be passed on to individuals in the SAA diaspora with SAAs living with their parents during college, returning to live with their parents after college or do not leave home until marriage. Younger generations oftentimes take care of older generations, and older generations often help with childcare. When practitioners work with older adults, it would be worthwhile to consider the multiple identities and roles when (i.e., grandmother, mother, daughter-in-law, wife, daughter) living in an intergenerational family or when caring for others (Tewari & Inman, 2012). Varying social family structures are dictated by level of adherence to culture and customs and may serve as a source of emotional and physical support for many family members.

Parenting is also impacted by SAA cultural factors and identity. There are differences in child rearing connected to individual and family values ranging from co-sleeping to choices of childhood socialization experiences in raising children. Depending on a client's acculturation level and values, SAA parents may or may not hold SAA norms central. Depending on the time of grandparental or parental immigration, children may be allowed more freedom in the U.S. than if they were in India due to the cultural values and norms of the host culture influencing parents, but there may also be a fear of children becoming more "Americanized" by these (Dasgupta Maglin 1996; Sodowsky & Carey, 1988). Decisions to raise children in an "Americanized" way or whether to foster a strong SAA identity in a child will likely influence parent and child friendships with other SAAs or non-SAA's. Second-generation American born parents also tend to be faced with determining "how South Asian" they want to raise their third-generation child or may struggle with how much effort they should place in teach their children about their SAA culture; as opposed to many first-generation parents who may have believed raising their children in the U.S. in the "most South Asian way" was the "best way." Food and holidays of importance are also transmitted by the family system, and typically conveyed through parenting as a means of maintaining tradition, family customs, and cultural socialization for families (i.e.,: Holi, Eid, Diwali, Durga Puja, etc.) with many SAAs describing food as a "language of love" in their homes and while in the presence of extended family members.

Families can be another resiliency factor; SAAs are described as being family oriented, formal with respect to elders, dependent, and responsible toward parents, older siblings, and other family members. Although the South Asian American family system is considered a form of security and the core source of support for family members as mentioned earlier, family role adaptations and conflicts can also be major sources of stress given the interdependent nature of the family system.

Intergenerational Conflicts

Sodowsky & Carey (1987), Ramisetty-Mikler (1993), and Prathikanti (1997) discuss intergenerational conflicts as significant stressors. Prathikanti (1997) discusses the notion of selective acculturation as an important acculturative experience among South Asians. She notes that Asian Indians respond variably to the challenges of acculturation in that individuals selectively adapt to some sociocultural norms (e.g., speaking the English language, career goals, etc.) of the U.S. culture while holding on to other cultural values (e.g., family relations, marriage, etc.) to facilitate their goal attainment. Ramisetty-Mikler (1993) notes that most immigrant families try to maintain their traditional patterns but may change in gender role expectations and assignments based on their length of stay in North America. Such changes may include families becoming more egalitarian, with couples sharing decisions, domestic duties, prioritize dual income and share child labor responsibilities. Given frequent generational differences, the generations may face cultural conflicts in issues such as sex-role development, associations with members of the opposite sex, dating, and marriage just to name a few with intergenerational conflicts being worthwhile areas to assess in working with SAA clients as the SA population continue to expand (Inman et al., 1999).

Discrimination

As with most ethnic and racial minority groups, discriminatory experiences have played a significant role among South Asian Americans. Differences in clothing style (women wearing burkas, sari's, bindi's, sindoor (red powder symbolizing being a married woman), Sikh men wearing turbans, facial beard's language accents, physical appearances, perceived negative stereotyping, non-majority status, and racism against immigrants have led to economic hardship, social, emotional, and physical stress among SAAs. In the past two decades, the continued growth in immigration of South Asians has caused SAAs to experience further discrimination and racism in the U.S., especially post 9/11. The terrorist attacks of September 11th, 2001 led to a spike in prejudice against South Asian Americans increasing living in fear and negatively impacting mental health, wellbeing, and experiencing traumatic stressors and anxiety.

Duration of Stay

Sandhu et al. (1999) discuss that Asian and Pacific Islanders who choose to permanently stay in the U.S., often experience greater acculturative stress than those who come to America for a short period of time and intend on returning to their homeland (i.e., international students who after a few years sojourn home upon completion of their academic plans). Length of stay, adjustment experiences, and other factors discussed above become important variables in understanding the South Asian American experience. Again, it is important to note that some of the factors that create resiliency and help in the adjustment process might also negatively impact the immigrant process. For example, Sodowsky and Carey (1987) suggest that many Indians may have had an easier time assimilating into America due to their voluntary immigration status, their levels of education, and the fact that many were from middle class backgrounds in India, although Indian women were shown to indicate poorer assimilation than their male counterparts. Therefore, it is essential that social scientists, clinicians, and researchers consider that there is no "one" South Asian American personality in understanding this growing minority group.

Why We Need Diversity in the Counseling and Psychology Workforce

Though America is becoming increasingly diverse, discrimination and bias remains pervasive, as do disparities in wealth, health, poverty among different racial and ethnic groups. The field of counseling and psychology is not immune to similar inequities. In 2016, the American Community Survey found that the active mental health/psychology work force is estimated to be approximately 84% White identified which is an over-representation as the average national population, which is 76% White (Luona et al., 2018). Mental health research continues to be focused on White, western, and wealthier samples of individuals compared to the total global population. Of this research, there is an additionally disparate focus on American society (Arnett, 2008). Therefore, clinical providers are not truly representative of the populations they consistently serve. For example, when observing the racial make-up of psychologists, as of 2015, 86% of psychologists in the U.S. were White. 5% of U.S. psychologists were Asian, 5% were Hispanic, and only 4% of psychologists were Black (Lin et al., 2018). The health service psychology workforce is also compromised as it is approximately 88% White and 12% nonWhite (Hamp et al., 2016). There is some change in early career psychologists entering the field. In 2015, 66% early career psychologists were White and 34% identified as people of color (National Center for Science and Engineering Statistics, 2015). Additionally, in 2016, 68% of doctoral degrees in psychology were awarded to Whites and 32% were to people of color (Department of Education, National Center for Education Statistics, 2015).

The lack of racial representation in the mental health field and focus on racially and ethnically different populations as well as resources to enable culturally responsive care, does impact how these individuals get the mental health treatment they may require. The American Psychological Association reported that half of Asian Americans, which includes South Asian Americans, do not get treatment for mental health issues due to a language barrier (APA Commission of Ethnic Minority Recruitment, Retention, and Training, 2017). Additionally, only a little over 2% of doctorate psychologists are Asian (APA Commission of Ethnic Minority Recruitment, Retention, and Training, 2017). Therefore, there is a real need to diversify the counseling and psychology workforce to serve the needs of diverse cultural groups to include South Asian Americans.

Understanding South Asian American Counseling and Psychology: Being a Culturally Responsive Provider

As it stands, there is not a truly representative set of clinicians, behavioral health providers, and psychologists in the workforce, therefore it is essential for existing mental health providers to be trained in cultural competence and minority mental health issues. When clinicians understand the unique issues and history faced by people of color, they can provide better treatment and overall health outcome. This also becomes more layered when including different intersectional social identities, such as gender, sexual identity, disabilities along with ethnic and racial identity. In order for mental health professionals to provide effective and culturally sensitive interventions to South Asian Americans, it is essential for practitioners to understand multiple aspects that contribute to the formation of one's South Asian American identity (Shah & Tewari, 2019). This systemic view to understanding individuals in different groups is enhanced by further understanding the meaning of different cultural elements as well as family structure to truly allow someone to provide effective mental health treatment and serve as a culturally competent practitioner.

Given the diversity within South Asia between countries and within group differences among the populations, mental health education and treatment needs to consider specific cultural factors such as immigration histories, acculturative experiences, identity issues, religious views, family values, and other salient topics relevant to these ethnic groups. South Asian Americans live with numerous intersectional identities that include race, age, social class, geographical location, immigration experiences, level of education, and so much more as the reader continues to immerse themselves in the chapter topics presented in this book. We hope our chapter emphasizes the importance of honoring and understanding the complexity of South Asian American identities and ways it shapes people's experiences and clinical needs as we worked toward providing a valuable text for anyone working with South Asian American clients looking to gain an understanding and increased knowledge to provide culturally competent care when working with intergenerational and diasporic populations of South Asian Americans.

Summary

Chapter 1 of "Counseling and Psychotherapy for South Asian Americans: Identity, Psychology, and Clinical Implications" highlights the evolution of the field with respect to the Black Civil Rights movement, Ethnic studies, Asian American studies, and Brown Asian movements that have shaped and paved the way for the development of South Asian and South Asian American Counseling and Psychology. This chapter introduces a brief overview of research, explored how South Asian Americans are similar and dissimilar to Asian American subgroups, discussed culturally specific values, and emphasized the importance of diversifying the workforce and the criticalness of being a culturally responsive provider to underserved and South Asian American communities in behavioral and mental health as well. In the following chapters, this book delves into other important topics that are personally and professionally meaningful to each of our contributing authors. We also hope that you gain a deeper understanding of topic areas relevant to you and that you find our content valuable as you continue to immerse yourself in understanding South Asian Americans. Finally, we hope that you find this book to be normalizing, validating, inspiring, and informative as you continue to serve our population and make a positive difference in the mental health and psychology of our people.

References

Arnett, J.J. (2008). The neglected 95%: Why American psychology needs to become less American. *American Psychologist, 63*(7), 602–614. 10.1037/0003-066X.63.7.602

American Psychological Association (2016). *2015 Survey of Psychology Health Service Providers.* www.apa.org/workforce/publications/15-health-service-providers/index.aspx

American Psychological Association (APA) Commission on Ethnic Minority Recruitment, Retention, and Training in Psychology Task Force (CEMRRAT2) (2017). *Asian Americans need culturally competent mental health care.* https://www.apa.org/advocacy/civil-rights/diversity/asian-american-health

Berry, J. (1980). Acculturation as varieties of adaptation. In A. M. Padilla (Ed.), *Acculturation: Theory, models and some new finding* (pp. 9–24). Boulder, CO: Westview.

Budiman, A. & Ruiz, N.G. (2021). Key facts about asian americans, a diverse and growing population. *Pew Research Center.* pewrsr.ch/2JGh5Pu

Crary, D. (2012). Gallup study: 3.4 percent of US adults are LGBT. *WTOP*. Associated Press. https://news.gallup.com/poll/158066/special-report-adults-identify-lgbt.aspx

Dasgupta, S.D., & Dasgupta, S. (1996). Public face, private space: Asian indian women and sexuality. In N. B. Maglin & D. Perry (Eds.), *Bad girls, good girls: Women, sex, and power in the nineties* (pp. 226–243). New Brunswick, NJ: Rutgers University.

DeNavas-Walt, C., Proctor B.D., & Lee, C.H. (2006). Income, poverty, and health insurance coverage in the United states: 2005. *U.S. Census Bureau, Current Population Reports, P60-231*. Washington DC: Government Printing Office.

Duldulao, A.A., Takeuchi, D.T., & Hong, S. (2009). Correlates of suicidal behaviors among Asian Americans. *Archives of Suicide Research, 13*, 277–290.

Durvasula, R.S., & Mylvaganam, G.A. (1994). Mental health of Asian Indians: Relevant issues and community implications. *Journal of Community Psychology, 22*, 97–108.

Fraga, E.D., Atkinson, D.R., & Wampold, B.E. (2004). Ethnic group preferences for multicultural counseling competencies. *Cultural Diversity and Ethnic Minority Psychology, 10*(1), 53–65.

Gates, G., & Newport, F. (2012). Gallup poll: *Special report: 3.4% of U.S. Adults Identify as LGBT* https://news.gallup.com/poll/158066/special-report-adults-identify-lgbt.aspx

Gim, R.H., Atkinson, D.R., & Whiteley, S.M. (2004). Asian-American Acculturation, Severity of Concerns, and Willingness to See a Counselor.

Gupta, S. (1999). *Emerging voices: South Asian American women redefine self, family and community*. New Delhi, India: Sage.

Hamp, A., Stamm, K., Lin, L., & Christidis, P. (2016). *2015 APA Survey of psychology health service providers*. APA Center for Workforce Studies.

Holman, S. (2010). The unique challenges faced by south Asian American social work graduate students: Campus communities, academics, and field: A project based upon an independent investigation (2010). Masters Thesis, Smith College, Northampton, MA. https://scholarworks.smith.edu/theses/480

Hune, S. (2002). Demographics and diversity of Asian American college students. *New Directions for Student Services, 2002*(97): 11–20. 10.1002/ss.35

Inman, A.G., Constantine, M.G., & Ladany, N. (1999). Cultural value conflict: An examination of asian Indian women's bicultural experience. In D. S. Sandhu (Ed.), *Asian and Pacific Islander Americans: Issues and concerns for counseling and psychotherapy* (pp. 31–41). Commack, NY: Nova Science Publishers.

Inman, A.G., & Tewari, N. (2003). The power of context: Counseling South Asians within a family context. In G. Roysircar, D. S. Sandhu, & V. E. Bibbins (Eds.), *Multicultural Competencies Guidebook: A Guidebook of Practices* (pp. 97–107). Alexandria, VA: ACA.

Joo, N., Reeves, R., & Rodrigue, R. (2016). *Asian-American success and the pitfalls of generalization*. Brookings: Social Mobility Papers. https://www.brookings.edu/research/asian-american-success-and-the-pitfalls-of-generalization/

Karasz, A., Gany, F., Escobar, J., Flores, C., Prasad L., Inman, A., Kalasapudi V., Kosi, R., Murthy, M., Leng, J., & Diwan, S. (2019). Mental health and stress among South Asians. *Journal of Immigrant and Minority Health, 21*(supplement 1), 7–14.

Kim, B.S. (1998). *Kim Asian Values Adherence Scale (KAVAS): Development and Psychometric Properties*. Paper presented at the 106th Annual Meeting of the American Psychological Association Conference, San Francisco, CA.

Kisch, J., Leino, E.V., & Silverman, M.M. (2005). Aspects of suicidal behavior, depression and treatment in college students: Results from the spring 2000 National college health assessment survey. *Suicide and Life-Threatening Behavior, 35*, 3–13.

Luona L., Stamm, K., & Christidis, P. (2018). How diverse is the psychology workforce? *News from APA's Center for Workforce Studies, 49*(2), 19.

Leong, F.T.L., & Okazaki, S. (2009). History of Asian American psychology. *Cultural Diversity and Ethnic Minority Psychology, 15*(4), 352–362.

Lin, K.-M., & Cheung, F. (1999). Mental health issues for Asian Americans. *Psychiatric Services, 50*(4), 774–780. 10.1176/ps.50.6.774

Lin, L., Stamm, K., & Christidis, P. (2018). How diverse is the psychology workforce? *Monitor on Psychology*, *49*(2). http://www.apa.org/monitor/2018/02/datapoint

López, G., Ruiz, N.G., & Patten, E. (2017). Key facts about Asian Americans. Pew Research.

Lott, J.T. (1998). *Asian Americans: From racial category to multiple identities*. Walnut Creek, CA: Altmira.

Lott, J.T., & Tamayo, J. (2004). *Asian-American children are members of a diverse and urban population*. Population Reference Bureau.

Lugo, L., Stencel, S., Green, J., Smith. G., Cox, D., Pond, A., Miller, T., Podrebarac, E., & Ralston, M. (2008). U.S. religious landscape survey: Religious affiliation: Diverse and dynamic. *Pew Forum on Religion & Public Life*. Pew Research Center.

Mio, J., Nagata, D., Lin, A., & Tewari. N. (2007). Racism against Asians. In F. Leong., A. G. Inman, L. Kinoshita, L. Yang, & M. Fu (Eds.), *Handbook of Asian American psychology*, 2nd Ed. Sage Publications.

Nadal, K.L. (2019). The brown Asian American movement: Advocating for South Asian, Southeast Asian, and Filipino American communities. *Asian American Policy Review*. 2019; *29*, 2–11, 95. https://aapr.hkspublications.org/2020/02/02/the-brown-asian-american-movement-advocating-for-south-asian-southeast-asian-and-filipino-american-communities/

National Science Foundation (NSF), National Center for Science and Engineering Statistics. (2013). https://ncsesdata.nsf.gov/doctoratework/2013

National Science Foundation. (2015). National center for science and engineering statistics. *National Survey of College Graduates Public Use Microdata File and Codebook*. https://ncsesdata.nsf.gov/datadownload

Ng, F. (1998). *The history and immigration of Asian Americans*. Taylor & Francis. (p. 211).

Panganamala, D.R., & Plummer, D.L. (1998). Attitudes toward counseling among Asian Indians in the United States. *Cultural Diversity and Mental Health*, *4*(1), 55–63. 10.1037/1099-9809.4.1.55

Pew Research Center (2021a). Key facts about Asian origin groups in the U.S.

Pew Research Center (2021b). Key facts about Asian Americans, a diverse and growing population pewrsr.ch/2JGh5Pu.

Pew Research Center (2017). Future immigration will change the face of America by 2065. pewrsr.ch/1ja3uON.

Pew Research Center (2012). Portrait of Asian Americans: The rise of Asian Americans report.

Prathikanti, S. (1997). East indian american families. In E. Lee (Ed.), *Working with Asian Americans: A guide for clinicians* (pp. 79–100). New York: Guilford.

Rajiva, M., & D'Sylva, A. (2014). "I am goan [not] Indian": Postcolonial ruptures in the South Asian diaspora. *Canadian Ethnic Studies 46*(1): 145–167.

Ramisetty-Mikler, S. (1993). Asian Indian immigrants in America and sociocultural issues in counseling. *Journal of Multicultural Counseling*, *21*, 36–49.

Rumbaut, R.G., & Komaie, G. (2010). Immigration and adult transitions. *The Future of Children*, *20*(1): 43–66.

SAALT (2019). Demographic information. https://saalt.org/south-asians-in-the-us/demographic-information/

Sandhu, D.S., Kaur, K.P., & Tewari, N. (1999). Acculturative experiences of Asian and pacific Islander Americans: Considerations for counseling and psychotherapy. In D. S. Sandhu (Ed.), *Asian and Pacific Islander Americans: Issues and concerns for counseling and psychotherapy*. (pp. 3–19). New York: Nova Science Publishers.

Shah, S., & Tewari, N. (2019), Cognitive behavioral therapy with South Asian Americans. In P. A. Hays & G. Y. Iwamasa (Eds.), *Culturally Responsive Cognitive-Behavioral Therapy*, 2nd Ed. (pp. 161–182). American Psychological Association.

Sodowsky, G.R., & Carey, J.C. (1987). Asian indian immigrants in America: Factors relating to adjustment. *Journal of Multicultural Counseling and Development*, *15*, 129–141.

Sodowsky, G.R., & Carey. J.C. (1988). Relationship between acculturation-related demographics and cultural attitudes of an Asian Indian immigrant group. *Journal of Multicultural Counseling and Development*, *16*, 117–136.

Srivastava, D. (2012). The effects of ethnic identity, family conflict, and acculturation on racial discrimination and mental distress of second generation Asian Americans. *Fordham University Dissertations*.

Stoops, N. (2004). Educational attainment in the United States: 2003. *United States Census Bureau*. United States Department of Commerce.

Sue, D.W., & Sue, D. (1999). *Counseling the culturally different: Theory and practice* (3rd ed.). John Wiley & Sons.

Sue, W.D., & Sue, D. (2008). *Counseling the culturally diverse: Theory and practice* (5th ed.). John Wiley & Sons.

Tewari, N. (2009). Seeking, receiving and providing culturally competent mental health services: A focus on Asian Americans. In N. Tewari & A. Alvarez (Eds.) (2009), *Asian American psychology: Perspectives*. (pp. 575–606). New York: Taylor & Francis.

Tewari, N. Alvarez, A., & Cheng, J. (Oct. 2019). The state of Asian American psychology: White normativity, invisibility, and microaggressions. Invited Presentation Fuller Theological Seminary, Pasadena, CA.

Tewari, N., & Inman, A. (2012). Case illustration: Culturally adaptive model of counseling: Using a multicultural skills-based perspective in working with a first-generation Asian Indian American elderly female. In M. E. Gallardo, C. Yeh, J. Trimble, & T. A. Parham (Eds.), *Culturally adaptive counseling skills: Demonstrations of evidence-based practices* (pp. 155–166). Thousand Oaks, CA: Sage Publications.

Tewari, N., Inman, A.G., & Sandhu, D.S. (2003). South asian americans: Culture, concerns and therapeutic strategies. InJ. Mio & G. Iwamasa (Eds.), *Culturally diverse mental health: The challenges of research and resistance*. (pp. 191–209). New York: Brunner-Routledge.

United States Department of Education, National Center for Education Statistics, Integrated Postsecondary Education Data System. (2015). *Completions Surveys*. http://nces.ed.gov/ipeds/datacenter/DataFiles.aspx

United States Census Bureau (2006–2010). American community survey. https://www.census.gov/programs-surveys/acs

United States Census Bureau. (2010). U.S. demographic census: Total population: Asian alone or in combination with one or more other races. Census Summary File 2. http://www.census.gov/2010census/data/

United States Census Bureau (2015). *American Community Survey 1-Year PUMS File*. www.census.gov/programs-surveys/acs/data/pums.html

United States Census Bureau (2017). American community survey 1-year estimates "Asian alone by selected groups". bit.ly/2CHSr

United States Census Bureau (2017). National population projections tables: Main series. https://www.census.gov/data/tables/2017/demo/popproj/2017-summary-tables.html

United States Census Bureau (2018). Asian-American and pacific Islander heritage month: May 2018. https://www.census.gov/newsroom/facts-for-features/2018/asian-american.html

United States Census Bureau (2020). 2020 Census illuminates racial and ethnic composition of the country. https://www.census.gov/library/stories/2021/08/improved-race-ethnicity-measures-reveal-united-states-population-much-more-multiracial.html#:~:text=The%20White%20and%20Black%20or,people%2C%20a%20230%25%20change

Weingarten, L., & Smith, R.A. (2009). Asian American immigration status. *Majority Rule and Minority Rights Issue Briefs*. Columbia University.

Xie, Y., & Goyette, K.A. (2005). *A demographic portrait of Asian Americans*. Russell Sage Foundation.

Xu, J., Kochanek, K.D., Murphy, S.L., & Tejada-Vera, B. (2010). Deaths: Final data for 2007. *National Vital Statistics Reports, 58*, 10.

Xue, L.R., & Preissle, J. (2008). *Educating immigrant students in the 21st century: What educators need to know*. SAGE Publications.

2 Casteism, Colonization, and Colorism

Ankita Nikalje and Snehal Kumar

Case Overview

Rupali, a single, heterosexual, Dalit woman in her mid-30s, is seeking therapy for the first time. She is an Indian national who immigrated to the U.S. 8 years ago. She recently experienced a breakup, which is what motivated her to seek therapy. Rupali described feeling isolated, fearful of talking to others, experiencing anxiety in social situations, and is experiencing physical symptoms of muscle aches and tension, rapid heart rate, and light-headedness. She reported her counseling goals as wanting to process her breakup, be less fearful and anxious in social situations, and feel connected to others.

Introduction

This chapter discusses the ways in which casteism, colonization, and colorism can impact the mental health experiences of South Asian Americans (SAA). Relevant theories and research are briefly discussed to provide a framework about these systems of oppression. Using a case study, we discuss how these systems can impact a client's experience, clinical distress, stressors, resilience, treatment, and goals. Two other clinical stories are provided along with discussion questions to help readers integrate important concepts. We also briefly introduce Rupali and later return to her case to demonstrate how these systems can impact a client's distress and needs from therapy. Two clinical stories about other clients provide a snapshot of how clients with similar demographics might need a different therapeutic approach. Suggested clinical interventions identify opportunities for growth, healing, and liberation from these intersecting systems of oppression. Finally, we provide discussion questions to help integrate the material.

As authors, we want to acknowledge and celebrate the wide range of experiences within the South Asian diaspora, where there is so much diversity in nationality, language, class, caste, reason for immigration, as well as geographic location. In terms of our identities, Ankita Nikalje identifies as Dalit and Snehal Kumar identifies as mixed caste, patriarchally Thiyya (categorized as other backward class in India) and matriarchally Brahman. Furthermore, we are both of Indian descent, and as a result hold privilege within the SAA diaspora. Due to the wide range of experiences within the diaspora as well as the context and limitations of our own worldviews and experiences, we will likely not do justice in capturing the nuanced experiences of the diaspora.

This chapter offers a sociohistorical framework that takes into consideration the impact of hierarchical and oppressive systems. This framework is essential in understanding the experiences of SAA. Casteism, colonization, and colorism are three systems that impact the psychological landscape of SAA, affecting their relationships with themselves, with each other, and the larger U.S. context (Inman et al., 2015; Nikalje & Çiftçi, 2021; Nikalje, 2022).

DOI: 10.4324/9781003081548-2

While some might argue that these systems are "in the past" or only applicable to some ethnic subpopulations, it is important to recognize that the trauma and legacy of the trauma continues to live on as evidenced in recent research and other narratives (Zwick-Maitreyi et al., 2018; Nikalje & Çiftçi, 2021; Frayer, 2020) that document the presence of these dynamics through both intentional discriminatory practices as well as unconscious acts that might be taught as "cultural." As a result, even if individuals remain geographically and generationally far away from their countries of origin, this legacy of oppression can be unfortunately enacted and passed down generations under the guise of "culture" if the practices, beliefs, and values are not critically examined.

Given the wide range of experiences and identities within this large group, SAA will understandably have differing interests and abilities to name and outline the lineage of their experiences within the context of casteism, colorism, and colonization. For some, this lineage might be painful and very apparent, for others, amorphous, hidden under their parents' silence, fears, and rage (Ahammed, 2019). As a result, it is important to attend and assess clients' readiness to name these important systems, as well as how privilege, shame, and trauma may impact their readiness. Some factors that might impact this interest and ability include one's own relationship to privilege and oppression, family narratives about oppression and privilege, family and community response to trauma or difficult experiences (e.g., avoiding talking about the traumatic past, parents working multiple jobs and not having time to share history, linguistic barriers between generations), and level of access to multiple SAA narratives.

Systems and Frameworks to Consider when Working with South Asian Americans

A liberation psychology framework (Martín-Baró, 1994) encourages understanding history through raising critical consciousness and cultivating an accurate and appropriate understanding of history (termed recovering historical memory) by listening to perspectives of those whose histories have not been heard. Irrespective of their specific SAA identities, clients can learn to engage in a critical examination of their everyday experiences to help them attend to how casteism, colonization, and colorism shaped and continue to shape their world. This process of recovering historical memory and contextualizing experience can help cultivate awareness and liberation from dehumanizing beliefs and ideas that consciously or unconsciously shape intrapersonal, interpersonal, and systemic interactions.

Many clients may present with symptoms like depression and anxiety, as they navigate confusing and often unnamed dynamics within their communities that are further confused by the often unnamed power dynamics within the U.S. While mental health providers have developed techniques to help reduce client distress, providers have historically had less training to attend to systemic dynamics that contribute to distress such as racism, heterosexism, sexism, and other oppressive dynamics that impact clients experience outside and within the therapy room (Sue & Sue, 2012). Typical skill-building (e.g., shifting cognitive distortions, mindfulness) and mood-regulation techniques (e.g., wise mind, opposite action) can help contain stress but may not address the root cause or shed light on ways to address these structural dynamics. For example, a client may come in for panic attacks because of casteism in the workplace and their clinician might help them build breathing techniques to help manage and reduce panic attacks. However, if the underlying trauma of casteism is unaddressed, we would be treating the symptoms rather than the root cause.

By ignoring the impact of the systems of colonization, casteism, and colorism on SAA clients' experiences, it is likely that existing systems of oppression and power will remain unnamed, unexamined, and intact. Thus, a clinical approach that does not take into consideration the impact of these systems may feel more like treating the symptoms of pain rather than liberation from the pain of oppression and internalized oppression. It is important to consider intrapersonal, interpersonal, and systemic dynamics.

Intrapersonal

There are many ways in which dynamics relating to casteism, colorism, and colonization can impact clients' relationship with themselves. For example, a client may come to treatment due to depression, mentioning struggles with self-worth. The client might, with further gentle exploration, name a deep fixation on their skin tone or features, with an appreciation for lighter skin and light eyes, features stereotypically associated with Europeans and dominant castes. A body-positive approach that addresses racism but ignores casteism and colorism might prove ineffective, particularly if the approach ignores the power offered to those with specific features, from the larger U.S. culture as well as within the SAA diaspora.

Interpersonal and Systemic

The systems of oppression relating to casteism, colonization, and colorism shape interpersonal dynamics as well, within families, communities, and friends. For example, a client may discuss the emphasis his family placed on speaking English "properly," and a norm of making fun of others from his community who spoke English in non-American or non-European accents. If unexplored, there might be a missed opportunity to offer curiosity about what these dynamics mean for this client and their family, in terms of possible internalized colonial mentality and possible shame and internalized inferiority toward one's own culture.

Key Definitions, History, and Evidence

Casteism

The caste system is one of the longest systems of oppression in the world. While the caste system is often noted as archaic and something "in the past" that no longer exists or affects people, this 3,000-year-old system continues to be pervasive in Hindu Indian culture (Jodhka, 2018; Thorat & Attewal, 2007; Vaid, 2014; Zwick-Maitreyi et al., 2018). For example, roughly half of Hindu Indian Americans identify with a caste group (Badrinathan et al., 2021).

Casteism is the discrimination based on one's caste identity where caste-marginalized groups are considered as inferior, unclean, and immoral. The caste system is defined by its classifications and subcategories, such as varnas and jatis. The hierarchical caste system is based in Hindu mythology and asserts that Brahmans (priests, knowledge keepers) are at the top (i.e., they are considered superior, pure, and most moral) followed by Kshatriyas (soldiers and warriors), then Vaishyas (merchants), and at the bottom are the Shudras (peasants). Considered falling outside of this hierarchy are Dalits (formerly known as untouchables) and Adivasis (indigenous people).

Discrimination based on caste has been illegal for several years in India. Both in contemporary India and the global Indian diaspora evidence shows that caste discrimination is prevalent in employment, education, and interpersonal relationships (Jodhka, 2018; Thorat & Attewal, 2007; Vaid, 2014; Zwick-Maitreyi et al., 2018). Therefore, like any other form of oppression, despite the criminalization of caste discrimination, there are systemic ways in which caste continues to exist and caste inequities remain.

While the caste system is typically associated with India, there is evidence that similar systems of hierarchy exist in other South Asian countries. For example, evidence for discrimination on the basis of caste has been found in Bangladesh, Pakistan, and Sri Lanka (Jodhka & Shah, 2010) as well as in the diaspora in other countries. Similarly, despite being rooted in Hinduism, the caste system is also evident in other religions. Research shows that caste oppressed people have experienced discrimination in places of worship like churches, gurudwaras, and mosques (Zwick-Maitreyi et al., 2018).

Several theories about the persistence of caste exist (e.g., Jaspal, 2011). One recent theory, Caste Critical Theory (CasteCRIT), based in Critical Race Theory, states that casteism is endemic, transnational, and deeply ingrained in the Hindu Indian diaspora (Nikalje, 2022). The transnational nature of casteism is seen through the evidence of casteism in other countries with large Indian diaspora such as the UK (Metcalf & Rolfe, 2010) and the U.S. (Zwick-Maitreyi et al., 2018). In the U.S, roughly half of all Hindu Indian Americans identify with a caste group and three quarters of all Indian Americans identify religion as playing a central role in their life (Badrinathan et al., 2021), highlighting how caste practices continue to inform cultural norms within the Hindu Indian American community. Evidence also shows that in a large national survey of caste-oppressed immigrants and citizens in the U.S. two out of three have experienced being treated unfairly at work, 60% reported experiencing caste-based derogatory jokes or comments, 20% reported discrimination at a place of business, one in three caste-oppressed people expressed fear of their caste identity being "outed," and over 40% of respondents reported being rejected in a romantic partnership because of their caste (Zwick-Maitreyi et al., 2018).

U.S. immigration policies have shaped and reinforced caste-based hierarchies in the U.S. Immigration post the Civils Rights Era led to the influx of "highly skilled" employees from India to the U.S. (Bhatia & Ram, 2018). These immigrants were majority caste-privileged groups who have benefitted from caste-based inequities in their access to education and careers in India (Zwick-Maitreyi et al., 2018). Ultimately, this Hindu Indian, caste-privileged diaspora shaped "Indian culture" in the U.S. and accrued significant political, cultural, and economic power. The opening of the U.S. to H1-B workers in the 1990s has facilitated the immigration of a more diverse group of Indians (Bhatia & Ram, 2018), especially those from caste-oppressed groups who have benefited from Affirmative Action policies. This relatively new group of immigrants does not hold as much cultural, political, and social power as their caste-privileged counterparts who had the privilege to immigrate earlier and shape the narrative about Indians in the U.S. (Zwick-Maitreyi et al., 2018).

This transnational nature of casteism is captured in the words of Dr. B. R. Ambedkar (1916), a Dalit civil rights leader and author of India's constitution, "If Hindus migrate to other regions on earth, Caste would become a world problem." While there is evidence of this transnational nature of casteism, the experience and violence of caste discrimination is often rendered invisible because of opposition from well-established Hindu groups in this U.S. that deny the existence of caste-discrimination and make claims of "Hinduphobia" (Soundararajan, 2016). Caste remains a complex and deeply contested issue, nonetheless, the needs of those most marginalized by casteism ought to be centered when conceptualizing SAA mental health.

Colonization

Almost 90% of the world has been colonized by the British and other imperialist powers (Tharoor, 2016). Colonization is a complex, systemic form of oppression that has a long historical legacy of denigration and subjugation of people in the South Asian subcontinent.

While colonization has been formerly "over" and South Asian nations have gained independence, the legacy of colonization continues to persist on the internalized, interpersonal, and systemic/institutional level (David & Okazaki, 2006a). For SAAs, there might be multiple systems of colonial dynamics they need to navigate—values and histories shaped by the impact of colonization in South Asia that might be generationally passed down, as well as the values and histories shaped by the impact of colonization in North America.

On the institutional and systemic level, the impact of colonization in South Asia is evident such as in the education system with English as the first language of instruction or government systems that continue to mirror and replicate archaic British imperialist laws (Tharoor, 2016). Similarly, there are many ways in which the legacy of colonization may affect people interpersonally. For example, when considering those who speak English without an accent and those who are more Westernized as superior/better than less Westernized counter-parts (Bhatia, 2018). The most insidious and damaging way in which colonization continues to persist is through colonial mentality (Fanon, 1965; Freire, 1970; Memmi, 1965). Some ways in which colonization manifest on this internalized level include feeling ashamed and inferior because of one's ethnic culture and background, discriminating against less-Westernized diasporic others, desiring to have a lighter skin tone and finding lighter skin more attractive than darker skin tones, and feeling indebted for being colonized (David & Okazaki, 2006a).

A large body of research has explored the manifestation of colonial mentality among Filipino-Americans (e.g., David & Okazaki, 2006a, 2006b; Felipe, 2016), however, there is limited research in this area for SAA. One study with Asian Indians in the U.S., found that a third of the sample of Asian Indians endorsed some form of colonial mentality (Nikalje & Çiftçi, 2021). While the impact of colonization is known for some South Asian countries (e.g., India, Pakistan), the impact of colonization and its contemporary consequences are invisible and less known for other diasporic South Asians. For example, today's Indo-Carribean population draws its roots to the colonial legacy of indentured servitude of Indians who were brought to the Carribean to "work" after the abolishment of slavery ("Our History", 2021). More research needs to be undertaken to understand the Indo-Caribbean experience of colonization, immigration to the U.S., and resilience to inform clinical practice with Indo-Caribbeans in the U.S. Similarly, a lot remains unknown about the consequences of colonization among SAA groups (e.g., Sri Lankan Civil War, Bangladesh Liberation War) and how genocide and forced migration may have affected and continues to affect intergenerational trauma among SAA families. One example of this is the Partition of India and Pakistan, the result of British colonial rule and policies such as "divide and rule" led to the largest forced migration in the 20th century and with over a million people killed (Zamindar, 2013). Therefore, the true trauma of colonization remains unknown and invisible. The invisibility of the violence of colonization and its impact intergenerationally remains a critical area for inclusion within SAA scholarship and clinical practice.

Colorism

Colorism has been defined as the "prejudicial or preferential treatment of same-race people based solely on the color of their skin" (Walker, 1983). Colorism has been documented across the globe, highlighting the prevalence of this framework internationally. For many racial minorities in the U.S., preference for lighter skin is often attributed to internalized racism (David et al., 2019). However, colorism in the context of the SAA diaspora intersects with dynamics relating to casteism and colonization as well and is the preference for a lighter skin-tone over a darker skin-tone and physical features that are stereotypically considered European or dominant caste in appearance (Prameswaran & Cardoza, 2009).

The prevalence of skin-lightening products, media portrayals of lighter skin as the ideal as well as believing that darker skin indicates one's caste status (Prameswaran & Cardoza, 2009) are some examples of how colorism is pervasive for SAA.

Colorism is evident in the caste system through its illustration of the skin color to indicate where groups sit on the hierarchy, moving from lighter skin caste-privileged to darker-skin Dalits and Adivasis. Brahmans are stereotyped as having white/fair or lighter skin and Dalits and Adivasis are stereotypically considered "black" (Prameswaran & Cardoza, 2009). The color of one's skin is an assumed marker for one's caste status (Mahalingam, 2003; 2007a; 2007b; Vaid, 2014), however, this is a myth with significant variation in skin color across caste groups. This relation between skin color and casteism is borne out of the colonial theory of "Aryan Invasion," where upper-caste Hindus claim a common Aryan ancestor with Europeans who colonized the "dark natives" of the South Asian subcontinent (Mazumdar, 1989). This endorsement of the theory of "Aryan Invasion" of the South Asian subcontinent serves two purposes. One, it serves as a legitimizing, scientific notion of the superiority of the Brahmans over caste-oppressed people by claiming a common European ancestor (Thapar, 1996). Two, it supports the myth that the color of one's skin-tone reflects their caste status.

Colorism is also tied to colonization and can be traced to colonial racist and white supremacist narratives of the "dark native" (Prameswaran & Cardoza, 2009). Postcolonial theorists explain that the desire for a lighter skin-tone highlights the desire to be more like colonizers because of assumed inferiority because of one's darker skin tone. The "dark native" tropes facilitated the subjugation and denigration of natives and as such internalizing the preference for lighter skin can be seen as a remnant of colonization.

Contemporarily, lighter skin is cultural capital to mobilize toward social and economic capital within societal contexts that show preference for lighter skin (Hunter, 2002), so it is likely that lighter skin color is also a cultural capital for SAA. Nikalje and Çiftçi, (2021) in their study on colonial mentality found that Asian Indians in the U.S. endorsed a preference for lighter skin tone both for themselves as well as their children. Importantly, those who endorsed a greater preference for lighter skin also appeared to endorse more depressive symptoms related to racism-related stress. In this case, it is likely that skin color is the cultural capital for SAA to evade racism in the U.S. context. Similarly, Harpalani (2013) theorizes in DesiCrit (Desi Critical Race Theory) that SAA are oftentimes seen as racially ambiguous, which can affect their social positioning in the U.S. racial hierarchy. Specifically, SAA racial ambiguity facilitates the active agency of some SAAs to claim "honorary whiteness" or the ascription of "whiteness" to SAAs by other non-SAAs (Harpalani, 2013). Therefore, it is likely that the preference for lighter skin color may also serve as a mechanism of coping or protective factor. Ultimately, the preference and cultivation of lighter skin may afford power both within the SAA community and the larger U.S. racial context, however, it also results in colonial mentality and internalized casteism.

Case Study Discussion

Background Information and Presenting Issues

Rupali is a 39-year-old, South Asian, Dalit, cisgender, heterosexual, single, Buddhist woman. She described herself as passionate, independent, and said she has typically enjoyed her work at a multinational technology company. She was promoted and transferred to work at the Chicago office 8 years ago because of her positive performance in Mumbai, India. She was promoted again 2 years ago, which led to her relocating to New York City.

She oversees a department and manages a mixed-race group of individuals, including several other South Asian and SAA coworkers.

Rupali let her therapist know that she feels homesick and lonely. She had a difficult breakup with a serious partner and said her partner's family would not accept her as "suitable" to marry their son because of differing caste status and her darker skin color. She expressed anger, disappointment, and surprise that her partner was not willing to fight for them even though he said he did not care about caste. Rupali is not looking to date at this time and has been frustrated with the discrimination she has experienced in dating throughout life, both in India and in the U.S. Rupali also reported symptoms of social anxiety and physical symptoms of aches and pains.

Rupali said there are other South Asian and SAA people at work, but that she does not feel very connected with them. She reported that though she is a manager, she has felt excluded by her South Asian colleagues, including those who directly report to her. She stated that at the very first social event with her SA colleagues in New York she was asked about her family background, what region of India she is from, and specifically asked her about her last name. Rupali expressed that she felt pressured to answer these questions and later felt ignored for the remainder of the event. Rupali also reported that when she tried to make friendly conversations with her coworkers during lunch, they seemed to notice her food and become uncomfortable. They now keep distance and often find ways to report to her boss, rather than to her directly. Rupali also stated that in her first year in NYC she thinks she heard a coworker mutter "yeh kaali hey" (she is black in Hindi) and when she asked the person to repeat what they said, they denied saying anything.

Rupali said that her non-SAA colleagues in the Chicago office as well as the New York office have been overall friendly and interested in her background, though has heard one or two comments about immigrants, and "jobs being stolen." She said non-SAA white Americans seem confused and enamored by her physical appearance and she often gets asked where she's from and complimented on her skin tone. She said that some people assume she's an African immigrant or African American and she laughs this ignorance off, saying that she knows that most Americans aren't familiar with the diversity of South Asian physical features.

Rupali explained that she initially believed her caste identity would not be a concern or an issue in the U.S. She expressed frustration and hopelessness about experiencing caste-based discrimination and colorism in the U.S., especially in a city like New York. Rupali added that she does not feel stressed about the comments from her non-SAA coworkers because she feels grateful to be in the U.S.

Background in India

Rupali described her experiences in India as generally positive because of the strong support of her parents. She expressed that her parents' inculcated pride about their Dalit identity and taught her their history and lineage. She reported that she lived in a community that was primarily other Dalit families; however, she experienced a lot of discrimination in school as a young child. She reported that she was reprimanded excessively by her teachers, other students made fun of her, and she often ate her lunch separately because other students did not want to sit with her because she ate meat. Rupali shared that her parents and others in her community strongly encouraged her to learn English to move out of her rural town to an urban city, Mumbai, for better educational and financial opportunities and to improve her quality of life. She noted that her ability to learn English and go to english-medium schools in India is what determined her success in a big way.

Rupali reported that she was able to secure college admission in Mumbai and move out of her rural town. She added that she expected less discrimination when she moved to an urban area, however, she reported she still experienced significant caste discrimination. She mentioned that because of her accent when speaking English, she was teased and bullied and other students used caste-based slurs to belittle her. She also added that some professors "accused" her of taking advantage of reservation (affirmative action policies) to gain acceptance into college. Rupali said they judged her ability, competence, and intelligence. She also added that she was unable to find roommates and had difficulty securing housing because others wanted "vegetarian only" roommates. She reported similar concerns when she got her first job, however, she reported that being close to family and friends who were a strong source of support helped her cope. Rupali explained that she was ecstatic when she received the promotion and was given the opportunity to immigrate to the U.S.

CASE CONCEPTUALIZATION

Rupali appears to have multiple strengths—resilience based in identity within the context of India, pride in her own history, and closeness with family and strong support network of other Dalits in India. She appears to be confident in her work ethic and skills. She also shows an ability to adapt to new contexts and be flexible, as evidenced by her ability to relocate to new places, multilingual abilities, and willingness to consider new forms of support (including seeking therapy). She has reported a history of strong leadership qualities, which shows an ability to navigate oppressive dynamics relating to casteism and colorism in India and use the protective support of her family and Dalit community.

Rupali has experienced multiple shifts to her support system: distance with her family, loss of a romantic relationship, and feeling discrimination and undermined at work. Her current distress appears to be caused and amplified by the loss of an important romantic relationship and navigating discrimination within the relatively newer context of being a manager in the New York office. It is possible that the loss of connection and experiences of discrimination, both in a romantic relationship as well as work, was particularly distressing because Rupali was not expecting to face caste-discrimination and colorism in the U.S. The recent rejection from her partner who was unwilling to stand up for them may impact how Rupali sees herself, her future in regard to romantic relationships, as well as expectations for future partners.

Rupali's experiences of casteism in the U.S. appear to mirror her experience of casteism in India. CasteCRIT theorizes that due to large immigration of Asian Indians to the U.S., systems of oppression from India have been exported to the U.S. (Nikalje, 2022). Within Rupali's context, her workplace and relationship are microcosms where caste-based practices and norms are exercised by those in power (i.e., caste-privileged groups). Rupali's rejection as a "suitable" partner highlights how endogamy as perpetuated by the caste system may be uncritically accepted as part of Indian culture in the diaspora and appears to highlight how deeply ingrained caste is found to be within the Indian culture. For Rupali, her feelings of hopelessness may be explained because of not being able to escape this deeply ingrained system of oppression despite being miles away from India.

Additionally, Rupali appears to be experiencing microaggressions related to her caste status in her workplace. Microaggressions are brief and commonplace daily verbal, behavioral, and environmental indignities, that can communicate hostile, derogatory, or negative slights and insults to the target person or group (Pierce et al., 1978; Sue et al., 2007). Microaggressions can be intentional or unintentional (Sue et al., 2007), highlighting how these behaviors still have impact irrespective of intent. While microaggressions were initially defined within the context of race, the concept has been extended to other identities such as sexual orientation, gender, ethnicity, religion, immigration status, and age. Rupali's coworkers' insistence on knowing her family background, what region in India she is from, and her last name, are examples of microaggressions in Rupali's case. While these questions may seem harmless, caste-oppressed people are often asked these questions by caste-privileged people to determine their caste identity. Similarly, her coworkers becoming uncomfortable with her food indicates the difference in dietary preference of caste groups. Specifically, eating meat is associated with caste-oppressed groups and caste-privileged groups who practice vegetarianism believe that eating meat is associated with being unhygienic, unclean, and impure. These beliefs of cleanliness, hygiene, and purity are also rooted in caste-based beliefs (Mahalingam, 2007a).

The impact of British colonization in India is also evident in Rupali's experiences both pre- and post-immigration. Colonial debt is a feeling of gratefulness and indebtedness for colonization, where negative treatment is accepted as a natural cost of civilization (David & Okazaki, 2006a, 2006b). Rupali appears to feel indebted for having had the opportunity to learn English and improve her educational and employment opportunities. Learning English is seen as a benefit of colonization and valued as cultural capital (Bhatia, 2018). This feeling of indebtedness is also evident in how Rupali does *not* appraise and downplays the racism she is experiencing from non-SAA in her workplace as stressful. Downplaying the racism and xenophobia she is experiencing may serve to somewhat protect her well-being, especially when she is already confronting casteist abuse from her SAA coworkers. Therefore, Rupali is experiencing both racism and casteism, however, it is likely too painful for Rupali to name and acknowledge her marginalization across two intersecting systems of oppression within which she exists.

Rupali's experiences of colorism also intersect with both casteism and colonization within the U.S. racial hierarchy. Rupali's rejection by her ex-partner's family for the darker color of her skin and its intersection with her caste identity appears to be a particularly painful reminder of her vulnerability as a darker-skinned Dalit woman. With her caste identity as a Dalit person and the darker color of skin, she has been ascribed a lower status (twice) within the microcosm of SAA. Among non-SAA she does not have the agency to claim "honorary whiteness" or have "passing privilege" within the U.S. racial hierarchy. Rupali's breakup appears to have made salient how systems of oppression are deeply woven into the SAA diaspora that can be dominated by Indian dominant caste narratives.

Therefore, Rupali's distress and symptoms may be explained by the intersecting systems of casteism, colonization, and colorism in the U.S. She appears to hold varying levels of power in her personal and professional life contexts that is further complicated by her positionality in SAA and non-SAA microcosms. She may benefit from having space to name and address these nuances in her connection with Americans of all races, including those of South Asian background.

INTERVIEW/ASSESSMENT QUESTIONS AND INTERVENTION STRATEGIES

We have outlined specific interventions that would be beneficial working with Rupali. While these interventions are numbered, they are not linear and might be recursive and overlapping in nature.

Intervention 1: Therapist Invests in Cultivating Self-Awareness A therapist's worldview, defined as the lens through which we see the world (Ivey et al., 1997) shapes the ways in which we can see or not see our client's perspectives. Worldviews represent our core values, beliefs, and assumptions about people, relationships, nature, time, and activity (Ibrahim & Kahn, 1987). In a very tangible way, our worldview can widen or limit the empathy we have as well as solutions we can co-create with our clients. A therapist's own unresolved emotions and biases relating to systemic oppression can have a deep impact on clinical work, where we unconsciously shift where conversations go or might even ask our clients to take care of our own unprocessed feelings. As a result, we encourage clinicians to be curious and process their awareness and narrative about caste, colonization, and colorism.

Issues that may come up for therapists include grief or shock about the presence of bias in the diaspora, validation in seeing these dynamics being named, discomfort with owning one's own privilege, as well as guilt in participating in practices that perpetuate oppression such as caste-based discrimination, colorism, or colonial mentality. For therapists of South Asian heritage, there might be a wide range of responses that may come up. Some of these responses might be difficult to name and process, especially since some SAA spaces encourage avoidance of these issues. Therapists of South Asian heritage may feel anger at the ways in which trusted elders or institutions perpetuate oppression, guilt about participating in these discriminatory systems, resentment at feeling reduced to an "oppressor," validation or relief in naming dynamics that have caused harm, and strong desire to shift these dynamics. Identity development is a process and we encourage therapists to seek consultation, connect with, or create spaces where they can invest in their own growth and awareness so that they are better able to serve *all* SAA clients, particularly those whose identities are marginalized within the SAA community.

Intervention 2: Intake—Centering the Working Alliance While Naming Identity. When interviewing or assessing a client, it is always helpful to tailor questions to the client's presentation and comfort. A strong working alliance has been shown to have a consistent positive impact on change within the context of therapy. Bordin (1979) defined three components of the working alliance: agreement of the tasks of therapy, agreement of the goals of therapy, and the affective bond between therapist and client.

A strong working alliance is essential for someone like Rupali, who holds multiple marginalized identities, and has likely learned to move in spaces where she cannot expect trust, respect, safety, or understanding. As a Dalit woman in the U.S., this experience of marginalization might be heightened because she is a minority within a minority and there is additional invisibility around Dalit experiences in the U.S. due to the tendency to homogenize South Asian experiences and the dominant narrative of Hindu Indian culture. For these reasons, it will be important to engage in verbal and non-verbal interventions that are attentive to Rupali's goals, identities, sense of safety and comfort during and after the intake so that a strong working alliance can be built. Rupali's concerns are focused on the impact of caste discrimination and colorism on her well-being. As a result, intake questions need to focus on exploring these concerns directly and offering empathy to her felt experiences, while also cultivating space to name appropriate goals.

For clients of South Asian descent who do not name these dynamics, we recommend that one or two curious, open-ended questions about caste, colorism, and colonization be included when discussing identity-dynamics. A client's answers and affective responses to these questions can shed light on their own awareness and identity development regarding these issues, perceived relevance to primary concerns, and their openness to considering these dynamics in their healing process.

Example 1. "What aspects or parts of your South-Asian culture or values are important to maintain or nourish?"

Clients' answers may help assess where the client is in terms of understanding and connecting with their SAA heritage, as well as awareness of privileges and hierarchies within SAA culture. For some clients, they might talk about retaining practices that they have coded as "cultural" when they might also be caste-based, for example, "wanting to marry someone in the community," or "wanting to be with someone with similar religious practices," without awareness that casteist dynamics shift access to and practice of religion. As clinicians, we can attend to themes of closeness, distance, dissonance, oppression, and privilege in how a client answers this question, and build on them in further sessions.

Example 2. "I know in some spaces in the South Asian community there are systems of hierarchy, such as sexism, colorism, and casteism, how much have you had to deal with these issues?"

A client's answer will indicate how much they have needed to be aware of these dynamics and provide some insight on how they understand these dynamics. Some clients might make jokes about these issues, stating it is "part of the culture," or deny their presence, while others may have different emotional reactions to specific systems due to being hurt by them or witnessing others being hurt by them.

Example 3. "How much did your family talk about issues like colorism, caste, and colonization growing up?"

A client's answer and non-verbal cues will provide some insight into their own and their familial messaging about these issues. Depending on their response, this question can offer an opportunity for follow-up questions about the client's perspective. For example, a family that says "Casteism is archaic" may have a very different worldview from a family that says, "We left India because reservations made it difficult to get jobs."

Intervention 3: Assessment of Symptoms and Strengths   In the case of Rupali, it would be important to ask how these stressors are impacting her daily functioning and mood. For example, gentle inquiry into her symptoms of how she experiences social anxiety would be beneficial. Given her report of hopelessness, it might be important to assess what this hopelessness means to her, in terms of her hope for her future, her career, and her romantic life. Though Rupali did not mention depression, further assessment of possible depressive symptoms such as reduced motivation, disrupted sleep, or increased self-blame would be beneficial. It would also be important to assess for risk of self-harm including suicide, while also attending to the ways in which stigma might lead to possible underreporting.

Many clients, especially those attending therapy for the first time, may not recognize all the protective strategies they engage in. Therefore, it would be helpful to inquire how Rupali has processed difficult experiences in the past and what she finds beneficial now. Exploration about how and why these strategies are helpful, might reinforce their utilization, as well as address barriers to access. For example, Rupali may report that she built a support system in Chicago through finding other Dalit and non-Dalit Buddhist practitioners who were open and interested in her history and practice of Buddhism. She may state that the move to NYC and the stress of her newer role, and the ongoing discrimination made it difficult to explore similar supports in a new city. In addition, interventions that help identify and underline past and current strengths might be particularly important, given the impact trauma and relational loss can have on self-image.

Intervention 4: Here and Now Processing   Given the invisibility and violence of casteism, colorism, and colonization, here and now questions assessing both Rupali's comfort with talking about these topics as well as any concerns about a therapist understanding them can help determine fit as well as provide opportunity to strengthen the alliance. Here and now processing can be a wonderful way to model to clients' multiple relational experiences that could be corrective and healing. In the case of Rupali, where she has experienced both nonverbal and verbal discrimination, it might be very beneficial to disclose therapist's own identity and worldview relating to these systems of oppression so that these dynamics can be named and addressed directly. This kind of disclosure can be a way to honor similarities and differences, as well as model ways of making connections through similarities and across differences.

Examples of ways to process how Rupali might be experiencing session:

Example 1. "We have some shared similarities and some differences in our own identities and background, for example, I am _____. I wonder what comes up for you as you hear about my own background and worldview."
   This example is specifically bringing the relational aspects of identity into the room for Rupali and her clinician. Clinicians tend to hold a lot of power in the room and by naming their humanity and biases, it can be a way to explicitly recognize how both individuals in the dynamic bring histories that shape perception and experience.

Depending on the therapist's identity, Rupali may respond differently, and her responses might be shaped by her past experiences with others. For example, Rupali might be initially more cautious with a South Asian therapist as she waits to see if her South Asian therapist has the capacity to earn her trust because she has been let down by well-meaning South Asian folk who are caste-unaware or claiming to be "liberal." She might be more guarded or reserved with a South Asian therapist with a dominant caste last name, because of past experiences of overt discrimination. Rupali might find herself more comfortable in working with a non-SAA therapist because she may be more comfortable with the idea of "explaining" her perspective to an outsider rather than feeling invalidated by someone who on the surface shares identities with her. Since she experienced non-SAA coworkers as friendly and curious, she may assume that a non-South Asian therapist would be more likely to offer curiosity. She may possibly be more comfortable with a Black therapist because of some shared history between the Civil Rights Movement and Dalit liberation. For example, she knows that the Dalit Panther movement in India was inspired by the Black Panther movement in the U.S. and may have assumptions about a Black therapist's own racial identity development and worldview.
   These scenarios highlight how Rupali's own assumptions, past experiences, hopes, and concerns about the efficacy of therapy may change based on who she is working with and how they respond to her. As a result, it would be very beneficial to name and explore this dynamic with her. It is essential that if a therapist chooses to use a here-and-now intervention like this, that the therapist has the emotional capacity to hear and respond empathetically to the client's response.

Example 2. "I know that therapy is less familiar to you. We've had a chance to talk for a bit and get a sense of my approach and style. How has this session felt for you?"

Rupali may have some understandable reservation about the benefits of therapy for her concerns. Most minorities have learned to expect to be not understood and may also associate therapy with the idea of "western" healing. This intervention might be helpful to ask Rupali how this session is feeling and notice her comfort with checking in with her emotions and sharing them directly with the therapist. Some clients might be more prone to identify what feels good and some might be more prone to point out their reservations. For those who lean toward attending to others' emotions, they might not name what makes them uncomfortable and might focus on what feels good. In these circumstances, it can be helpful to follow up with a statement like this,

> Thank you, this is really helpful to hear, and we can continue incorporating the parts that you've found helpful. In addition to what's helpful, I wonder if you listen to yourself and see if you might have any reservations about us working together.

Thereby continuing to invite the client and normalizing sharing their concerns.

Intervention 5: Ways to Assess and Treat Trauma   In assessing experiences that might be traumatic, it is beneficial to model consent, cocreation of focus, and tailor language to the interpersonal needs of the client. It is also important to remember that many SAA folk have experiences within their lives and their familial history that relate to war, genocide, domestic violence, forced migration, and other forms of violence that may skew what they view as "traumatic." For some SAA folk, there might be a sense of survivor guilt or desire to be grateful for what they have, which may then make it difficult for them to name or own any experiences of their own as traumatic. We recommend when assessing for difficult experiences, to move beyond the word trauma because of SAA folks' tendency to underplay trauma.

In Rupali's case, she appears able to name and access her emotions and internal world easily. She also appears to have supportive friends and parents, suggesting a certain level of interpersonal skills in negotiating space and boundaries. For clients who have a history of being consistently overpowered by authority figures including parents, we might encourage a lighter touch where we consistently model consent and check in with the client about format and focus.

EXAMPLE OF AN INTRODUCTION SENTENCE

> I realize we've already talked about some difficult experiences of harassment. I'm going to ask about other experiences that might be difficult. Please listen to your instinct in terms of how much you might want to share. It is important that you feel comfortable, and we respect a pace that works for you.

> Example 1: "Have you ever felt bullied or harassed?"
> Example 2: "Have you ever had any experiences of unwanted sexual contact?"
> Example 3: "Have you ever had any experiences of unwanted physical contact?"
> Example 4: "Have you or your family ever felt persecuted because of group identity or how people perceive you?"

The clinician can listen to clients' verbal and non-verbal cues to help determine how much to delve into trauma assessment questions and how to best shape them. Example 4 is a particularly broad question that can be taken in multiple directions based on a client's response. In Rupali's case, she may outline generational trauma relating to caste violence and how it impacted decision-making and choice for herself and her ancestors. She may say "they went through a lot" but may not label these experiences as trauma. For others, experiences relating to genocides, forced migration, civil wars, or discrimination after relocating to the U.S. might come up.

It will be important to offer a framework of treatment that attends to treating the impact of daily systemic trauma. For a client like Rupali, it might also be helpful to name how violence and microaggressions relating to casteism, colonization, and colorism are traumatic and can cause symptoms that look like depression and anxiety. In addition to psychoeducation about how trauma can impact the nervous system, it would be beneficial to collaboratively identify strategies to regulate the nervous system and build internal and external practices to heal trauma (e.g., shifting internalizing beliefs, naming, and connecting emotions with body sensations, connecting with others who center her identities).

Intervention 6: Identifying and Building Goals It will be important to make space for Rupali to articulate her goals and hopes for therapy. In early conversations, Rupali articulated a desire to process her breakup, feel more connected, and be less anxious in social situations.

It is likely that as work continues, goals for Rupali may evolve and change, especially as a more systems-level approach is taken. As a result, it will be important to reassess, tweak, or change goals based on Rupali's evolving needs and perspective of her experience. For example, over time, Rupali may reshape the original goal of "less anxiety" that implies a focus on self to include other language like "discrimination," "solidarity," "microaggressions," or "triggers." By broadening this language, she would then be more able to identify and build multi-levels of support and solutions that address the interplay within herself and oppressive behaviors and systems.

Process her breakup: Interventions can focus on helping Rupali name and process her grief about this loss, as well as the experience of discrimination that relate to this loss. Furthermore, making space for what she may want for herself in her future might be very beneficial. For example, Rupali might say she wants to find a partner soon, or might say she is done with "looking" but is open. Questions about the future may offer space to identify and clarify her hopes for her future, her own perception about the importance and possibility of romantic relationships, as well as clarifying her own values and needs in romantic relationships.

In clarifying her hopes for romantic relationships, it will be important to help Rupali articulate and center the identities that matter most to her. Through processing her grief and the betrayal, Rupali may realize she wants to find a partner who similarly centers her Dalit identify and experiences relating to caste and colorism, rather than just someone who claims "I don't care" but does not challenge discriminatory beliefs. Work may then also help her learn to identify whom she can be more able to trust in being aligned in values and behaviors.

Be less fearful and anxious in social situations: Given the level of discrimination Rupali has felt, her anxiety and fear in social situations is understandable. It would be beneficial to frame any anxiety-reducing interventions within the context of her experiences of systemic discrimination, as a way to shift blame from a purely self-focused language onto recognizing the interplay between Rupali and oppressive systems that place immense pressure on Rupali.

Some possible ways to address this goal include identifying and naming situational and internal factors that increase her anxiety, developing strategies that facilitate healing from relational and systemic trauma, and reconnecting with healing experiences that have been helpful in the past. Through these conversations, Rupali may choose to engage in spaces that celebrate Dalit identity in India as well as the U.S., she may choose to prioritize

Table 2.1 Moane's Approach (2003)

Levels	Aim	Possible Ways to Envision Practice
Personal	Build strengths	Self-validation of strengths (anxiety, breakup) Notice and shift self-blame patterns that are encouraged by systems of oppression(anxiety, breakup) Increase awareness of adaptive ways to heal from systemic oppression or discrimination (anxiety, connection)
Interpersonal	Make connections	Seek groups that celebrate and support Dalit identity and causes (anxiety, connection) Identify ways to use existing supports (anxiety, connection, breakup) Choose to either purposefully engage in or disengage from SAA spaces that are inherently casteist (anxiety, connection) Provide and receive mentoring with folks who support and understand Rupali's experience (anxiety, connection)
Political	Take action	Seek support from organizations relating to her experience of workplace discrimination (anxiety, connection) Create mentoring spaces for Dalits in the U.S. (anxiety, connection)

talking with her friends at home, and she may consider filing a report about the discrimination she experiences in the workplace.

Feel connected to others: Rupali's sense of isolation is understandable, given her recent breakup and ongoing experiences of discrimination at work. Framing her experience of isolation within the context of casteism, colorism, and colonization can help validate her experience and help her identify the kind of connection she might be truly looking for. In an effort to meet this overall goal, Rupali and her clinician may together clarify values she looks for in meaningful social connection, explore current support systems and ways in which she is or isn't using them and why, as well as identify new support systems that she can connect with that fit values and needs.

SUMMARY OF GOALS USING A STRUCTURAL FRAMEWORK

Moane (2003) provides a table (see Table 2.1) to help recognize the structural levels of change and healing that can occur for a client through a liberation psychology lens. While the above section is written more like a typical outline of goals, we would like to use Moane's approach to identify how these interventions fall naturally into these three categories.

Clinical Stories

Two individual SAA clients present to therapy due to generalized anxiety and social anxiety. Their demographics on the surface look very similar: they are both male, raised Hindu, in their 20s, and are of Indo-Guyanese descent. Though in so many ways these two clients are similar, they demonstrate how their clinical needs and arc of treatment are very different.

Clinical Story One

Ganesh came in with much more ability to name his inner world in a nuanced way and experience and tolerate difficult emotions. He also brought in an awareness of systems of oppression in terms of gender, colonization, and race, and appeared more able to name ways these systems impact his experience. For example, he reported loving his family and also at times being frustrated by them, and needing to seek support for certain things from friends instead. He was able to name how his parents worked hard, offered a lot to him and his sister, and "were not good with emotions." On prompting, he reported that his family went through a lot in Guyana in the 1960s, which led to their immigration to the U.S. and said they did not talk about it, but he knew "it was bad." He said that though he appreciated his family, he noticed how his parents treated him better than his sister which he attributed to his lighter skin tone and being male. When discussing race, Ganesh reported noticing anti-blackness within some of his extended family, which he said made him uncomfortable since "he knew it was wrong," and he also said that he has at times been rejected by Indian Hindu girls because "their family wouldn't approve of him." In the session, Ganesh appeared able to emotionally hold a multiplicity of experiences and emotions without getting too over-whelmed or shut down in the therapy room. For example, naming his privilege as a male and noticing ways he feels invisible as an Indo-Guyanese man.

Due to his framework coming in as well as his ability to experience emotions in session without being too overwhelmed, early interventions that focused on queries about identity and history worked well for him as these questions matched his worldview and helped him process his experience.

Clinical Story Two

Mohan came in both eager to reduce his distress, and afraid and cautious about being in therapy. His descriptions of his world and his family tended to be more superficial, he seemed status-oriented, and he tended to focus on ways in which others negatively im-pacted him rather than the interplay between individuals. He denied any family mental health issue though when asked about substance use history, he stated that both his grandfather and uncle struggled with alcoholism. He spoke highly of his father who he said was very strict and demanding and appeared to show anger and distaste toward his re-latives with substance use issues. A liberation psychology framework can offer nuanced hypotheses about his experience. For example, Mohan may have been raised in a family where some male family members coped with difficult or traumatic experiences with substance use, while others learned that staying in control and avoiding emotions and vulnerability helped maintain power and control. His family may have also encouraged gaining power through avoiding certain behaviors that may involve losing status (e.g., being vulnerable, making mistakes, taking responsibility for mistakes) and by moving up systems rather than dismantling them (e.g., going to Ivy Leagues, not worrying about or critiquing systems like caste or race).

While conceptually helpful, early interventions that excessively focused on caste, colo-nization, or colorism would have most likely ruptured the alliance, given Mohan's goal to reduce distress, avoidance of emotion, and skepticism of therapy. As a result, early in-terventions focused on building the alliance, offering support, and reducing the stigma and unnamed shame that seemed to impact the way he told his story. Over time, work focused on allowing for multiplicity of experiences without shame, which then also helped Mohan name his role in relational dynamics, to help him find agency. For example, he was able to name both his admiration for his father and his frustration at him for punishing him every time he made a mistake. We were also able to name the anger he experienced at work when he felt pressure to be more "Americanized," and ways in which he and his family also exhibited colonial mentality by making fun of "FOBS."

Reflection Questions

We encourage you to take time to answer these questions and go at a pace that works for you.

1   **Countertransference:** What would come up for you if you were assigned to work with Rupali, Ganesh, and Mohan? Who would you feel most comfortable working with and why? What would be most difficult for you to attend to?
2   **Knowledge:** What is your current understanding about Dalit experiences and caste dynamics? What is your understanding of how colonization has impacted various SAA communities? What is your understanding of how colorism impacts SAA clients' experiences?
3   **Self-disclosure:** How might it be for you to disclose your identities to a client? What factors may make it easier or more difficult to disclose your identities to a client? What client factors are you paying attention toward to help you decide if a disclosure would be clinically beneficial?
4   **Supports:** What spaces or supports might you need to help you broaden your ability to work with clients who are navigating various systems of oppression?

Summary

Through this chapter, we outline the ways in which casteism, colorism, and colonization can continue to shape and impact the lived experiences of SAA clients. While it might be easy for some to name these systems as "archaic" or in the past, the legacy of old trauma as well as ongoing trauma can continue to have an impact on clients today. As SAAs advocate for greater wellness, it is important for us to consider what healing might look like for SAAs who are experiencing systems of oppression from both outside and within the community. Like Rupali, we may need to begin to have tough conversations with ourselves and with others so that we can begin to build true solidarity, agency, and coalitions that serve a deeper level of psychological and physical liberation. As clinicians, we may need to consider the ways in which we can invest in research, education, practice, and teaching so that we and future generations of clinicians are better equipped with the knowledge, skills, awareness, and humility needed to show up for our SAA clients as they navigate and heal from these systems of oppression.

Suggested Resources

For further learning (i.e., articles, books, films, websites, educational resources).

1   Annihilation of Caste
2   Ants Among Elephants
3   Hindu Nation and its Queers
4   Equality Lab's Caste in U.S. Survey
5   30-minute NPR podcast: How to be anti-casteist https://www.npr.org/transcripts/915299467
6   Caste is a Queer Issue- Webinar
7   Caste Reading List: https://www.equalitylabs.org/castereadinglist

References

Ahammed, S. (2019). Caste-based oppression, trauma and collective victimhood in erstwhile south india: The collective therapeutic potential of Theyyam. *Psychology and Developing Societies, 31*(1), 88–105. 10.1177/0971333618825051

Ambedkar, B.R. (1916, May 9). *Castes in India: Their Mechanism, Genesis and Development* [Paper presented at an Anthropology Seminar taught by Dr. A. A. Goldenweiser at Columbia University].

Badrinathan, S., Kapur, D., Kay, J., & Vaishnav, M. (2021, June 9). *Social Realities of Indian Americans: Results From the 2020 Indian American Attitudes Survey.* Carnegie Endowment for International Peace. https://carnegieendowment.org/2021/06/09/social-realities-of-indian-americans-results-from-2020-indian-american-attitudes-survey-pub-84667

Bhatia, S. (2018). *Decolonizing psychology?: Globalization, social justice, and Indian youth identities.* Oxford University Press.

Bordin, E.S. (1979). The generalizability of the psychoanalytic concept of the working alliance. *Psychotherapy: Theory, Research, and Practice, 16*, 252–260.

Bhatia, S., & Ram, A. (2018). South Asian immigration to United States: A brief history within the context of race, politics, and identity. In M. J., Perera , & Chang, E. C. (Eds.), *Biopsychosocial approaches to understanding health in South Asian Americans.* (pp. 15–32). Cham, Switzerland: Springer.

David, E.J.R., & Okazaki, S. (2006a). Colonial mentality: A review and recommendation for filipino american Psychology. *Cultural Diversity and Ethnic Minority Psychology, 12*(1), 1–16. 10.1037/1099-9809.12.1.1

David, E.J.R., & Okazaki, S. (2006b). The colonial mentality scale (CMS) for Filipino Americans: Scale construction and psychological implications. *Journal of Counseling Psychology, 53*(2), 241–252. 10.1037/0022-0167.53.2.241

David, E.J., Schroeder, T.M., & Fernandez, J. (2019). Internalized racism: A systematic review of the psychological literature on racism's most insidious consequence. *Journal of Social Issues, 75*(4), 1057–1086. 10.1111/josi.12350

Fanon, F. (1965). *The wretched of the earth.* New York: Grove.

Felipe, L. C. S. (2016). The relationship of colonial mentality with Filipina American experiences with racism and sexism. *Asian American Journal of Psychology, 7*(1) , 25–30. 10.1037/aap0000033.

Frayer, L. (Host) (2020, October 13). What does caste privilege mean for south asians in the U.S.? [Audio podcast episode]. In *All things considered.* Northern Public Radio. https://www.northernpublicradio.org/2020-10-13/what-does-caste-privilege-mean-for-south-asians-in-the-u-s

Freire, P. (1970). *Pedagogy of the oppressed.* New York: Continuum.

Harpalani, V. (2013). DesiCRIT: Theorizing the racial ambiguity of south asian americans. *Annual Survey of American Law, 69*(1), 77.

Hunter, M.L. (2002). "If you're light you're Alright": Light skin color as social capital for women of color. *Gender & Society, 16*(2), 175–193. 10.1177/0891243202016002003

Ibrahim, F.A., & Kahn, H. (1987). Assessment of worldviews. *Psychological Reports, 60*, 163–176.

Inman, A.G., Tummala-Narra, P., Kaduvettoor-Davidson, A., Alvarez, A.N., & Yeh, C.J. (2015). Perceptions of race-based discrimination among first-generation Asian Indians in the United States. *The Counseling Psychologist, 43*(2), 217–247. 10.1177/0011000014566992

Ivey, A.E., Ivey, M.B., & Simek-Morgan, L. (1997). *Counseling and psychotherapy: A multicultural perspective.* Boston: Allyn & Bacon.

Jaspal, R. (2011). Caste, social stigma and identity processes. *Psychology and Developing Societies, 23*(1), 27–62. 10.1177/097133361002300102

Jodhka, S.S. (2018). *Caste in contemporary India.* London: Routledge.

Jodhka, S. S., & Shah, G. (2010). Comparative contexts of discrimination: Caste and untouchability in South Asia. *Economic and Political Weekly, 45*(48), 99–106.

Mahalingam, R. (2003). Essentialism, culture, and power: Representations of social class. *Journal of Social Issues, 59*(4), 733–749. 10.1046/j.0022-4537.2003.00087.x

Mahalingam, R. (2007a). Essentialism, power, and the representation of social categories: A folk sociology perspective. *Human Development, 50*(6), 300–319. 10.1159/000109832

Mahalingam, R. (2007b). Beliefs about chastity, machismo, and caste identity: A cultural Psychology of gender. *Sex Roles, 56*(3-4), 239–249. 10.1007/s11199-006-9168-y

Martin-Baró, I. (1994). *Writings for a liberation psychology.* Cambridge, MA: Harvard University Press.

Mazumdar, S. (1989). Racist responses to racism: The aryan myth and south asians in the United states. *Comparative Studies of South Asia, Africa and the Middle East, 9*(1), 47–55. 10.1215/07323 867-9-1-47

Memmi, A. (1965). *The colonizer and the colonized.* Boston, MA: Beacon.

Metcalf, H., & Rolfe, H. (2010). *Caste discrimination and harassment in Great Britain* (Rep.). Retrieved 2020, from National Institute of Economic and Social Research website: https://www.gov.uk/government/publications/caste-discrimination-and-harassment-in-great-britain

Moane, G. (2003). Bridging the personal and the political: Practices for a liberation Psychology. *American Journal of Community Psychology, 31*(1–2), 91–101. 10.1023/a:1023026704576

Nikalje, A., & Çiftçi, A. (2021). Colonial mentality, racism, and depressive symptoms: Asian indians in the United states. *Asian American Journal of Psychology.* 10.1037/aap0000262

Nikalje, A. (2022). Caste Critical Theory (CasteCRIT): Theorizing and Scale Development Measuring Caste Beliefs in the United States. Purdue University Graduate School. Thesis. 10.253 94/PGS.20303214.v1

Pierce, C., Carew, J., Pierce-Gonzalez, D., & Willis, D. (1978). An experiment in racism: TV commercials. In C. Pierce (Ed.), *Television and education* (pp. 62–88). Beverly Hills: Sage.

Prameswaran, R., & Cardoza, K. (2009). Melanin on the margins: Advertising and the cultural politics of fair/light/white beauty in india. *Journalism & Communication Monographs, 11*(3), 213–274. 10.1177/152263790901100302

Sue, D.W., Capodilupo, C.M., Torino, G.C., Bucceri, J.M., Holder, A.M., Nadal, K.L., & Esquilin, M. (2007). Racial microaggressions in everyday life: Implications for clinical practice. *American Psychologist, 62*(4), 271–286. 10.1037/0003-066x.62.4.271

Sue, D.W., & Sue, D. (2012). *Counseling the culturally diverse: Theory and practice.* Hoboken, NJ: John Wiley & Sons.

Soundararajan, T. (2016). Erasing caste: The battle over California textbooks and caste apartheid. *Huffington Post.* Retrieved 2020. https://www.huffpost.com/entry/erasing-caste-the-battle_b_9817862

Tharoor, S. (2016). *An era of darkness: The British empire In India.* New Delhi: Aleph.

Thapar, R. (1996). The theory of Aryan race and India: History and politics. *Social Scientist, 24*(1/3), 3–29.

Thorat, S., & Attewal, P. (2007). The legacy of social exclusion: A correspondence study of job discrimination in India. *Economic and Political Weekly, 42*(41), 41–45.

Vaid, D. (2014). Caste in contemporary india: Flexibility and persistence. *Annual Review of Sociology, 40*(1), 391–410. 10.1146/annurev-soc-071913-043303

Walker, A. (1983). *In search of our mothers' gardens?: Womanist proser.* Harcourt Brace Jovanovich.

Zamindar, V. F.-Y. (2013). India–Pakistan Partition 1947 and forced migration. In I. Ness (Ed.), *The Encyclopedia of Global Human Migration.* 10.1002/9781444351071.wbeghm285.

Zwick-Maitreyi, M., Soundararajan, T., Dar, N., Bheel, R.F., & Balakrishnan, P. (2018). Caste survey. Retrieved from https://www.equalitylabs.org/caste-survey-read

3 Implications of Immigration, Racism, and the Current Sociopolitical Climate

Asha Unni and Puni Kalra

Case Overview

On August 5, 2012, a mass shooting took place at a Sikh Temple in Oak Creek, Wisconsin. Gunman Wade Michael Page fatally shot six members of the congregation and wounded many others just before taking his own life on that fateful Sunday morning. Page was an avowed white supremacist who had been radicalized in the army, immersed himself in the neo-Nazi rock music world, and was a member of Hammerskin Nation, one of the most violent and dominant skinhead groups in the United States (U.S.)(Elias, 2012). At the time, the massacre was deemed the largest act of violence on a faith community since the 1963 church bombings in Birmingham, Alabama. It was only the latest domestic terrorist attack in a wave that began in late 2008 with the election of Barack Hussein Obama, the first Black President in U.S. history.

After the Sikh Temple shooting, 12-year-old Sahara, an only child, was referred for child therapy and counseling due to defiance, difficulty with attention, and difficulty with completing schoolwork. She was born in the U.S. and her mother, Priya, is Indian and her father, Adesh is Sri Lankan. Priya was born in the U.S. as well, but Adesh was born in Sri Lanka and is undocumented. About 4 years ago, the U.S. Immigration and Customs Enforcement (ICE) came to the family's house with guns drawn and was verbally aggressive toward the family. They were looking to pick up Adesh due to him not having papers. He was detained for a total of 18 months across two detention camps, where he reportedly had little communication with the family and was maltreated at the facility in which he was detained. After 18 months of detention, Adesh was deported back to Sri Lanka and has not been able to see his family since, though he keeps in touch with them via phone and video calls.

Introduction

This chapter will focus on South Asian American (SAA) experiences with immigrating to and living within the U.S. Specifically, the chapter will discuss the shifts in immigration, how these movements have influenced the sociopolitical climate, and the nature of discrimination that SAAs have experienced as a result of these changes. The psychological impact of discrimination experiences will also be discussed. Additionally, the chapter will include two case studies, including Oak Creek's community needs after a hate crime and the case of a 12-year-old girl named Sahara, to illustrate clinical practices and therapeutic interventions to consider when working with SAAs who have experienced ethnic and racial discrimination while living in the U.S.

DOI: 10.4324/9781003081548-3

Patterns of South Asian Immigration

The SAA population in the U.S. has significantly increased by 40% between 2010 and 2017, from 3.5 million to 5.4 million. The most significant growth was within the Nepali community of 206.6% followed by Indian, Bhutanese, Pakistani, Bangladeshi, and Sri Lankan populations. By 2065, Asian Americans are predicted to be the largest immigrant population residing in the U.S. (SAALT, 2019a). It is likely that a portion of this exponential growth can be attributed to the employment and educational opportunities available within the U.S. (Inman et al., 2015).

SAAs experiences with immigrating to the U.S. have not always been straightforward, however (Ibrahim et al., 1997; SAALT, 2015). Institutional barriers such as the Barred Zone Act of 1917 and the Asian Exclusion Act of 1924 specifically targeted immigrants arriving from countries including those in South Asia. When South Asians (along with other Asians) were finally allowed into the U.S. in 1946 when the Exclusion Act was repealed, it was still entry by quota. This caused South Asian immigrants to be viewed as "outsiders," a category not ascribed to other marginalized communities in the U.S. (Ibrahim et al., 1997). The perception of South Asians and SAAs as outsiders and the general xenophobia continued to be reinforced with media publishing stories about the "threat" of Indians "spreading diseases and backwards culture and superstitions" (Hess, 1969). As SAAs continued to immigrate into communities that were previously mostly White, acts of overt discrimination began to rise steadily. One group, the "Dot Busters," was responsible for a number of deadly assaults against Asian Indians living in New Jersey due to their intent to "remove" South Asians living in the area (Inman et al., 2015; Tewary, 2005).

Over the years, the continued growth in immigration has caused tension among the communities in which SAAs live. It was the terrorist attacks of September 11, 2001, however, that led to a spike in prejudice against SAAs (Inman et al., 2015; Livengood & Stodolska, 2004). SAAs began to be seen as "terrorists" because of observable traits and practices, such as skin color and the use of religious headscarves. This also was reflected in Islamophobic and anti-immigrant language and discriminatory acts used against SAAs in several settings including schools, places of employment, and communities (Inman et al., 2015). Trends in anti-Muslim hate crimes have risen exponentially since the 9/11 attacks and it is hypothesized that these numbers will only continue to increase considering the current sociopolitical climate that fosters "xenophobic rhetoric" (SAALT, 2017, p. 5). These trends are alarming, so it is imperative to understand how South Asian immigrants are conceptualizing these discrimination experiences. One of the first steps in this understanding is to explore how South Asian immigrants experience the process of acculturation while living in the U.S.

Acculturation

Acculturation is defined as the process during which a person may experience changes in their beliefs, language, lifestyle, and values to accommodate a foreign host culture (Londhe, 2014). Berry's (1997) model is well known for describing how individuals experience acculturation. It is a process of navigating political, demographic, economic, and social contexts of two separate cultures (the host and the origin), moderated by individual factors such as age, gender, education, and personality. Individuals can experience acculturative stress, which is the psychological and somatic response to the process of acculturation and adjustment (Berry, 1997). Acculturative stress is an important factor in the SAA experience within the U.S. Berry's (1997) model suggests that a person living in a host society will eventually adapt, even though it may not be with the best adjustment.

Acculturative stress is something that both first- and second-generation immigrants experience, though bicultural stress may be best conceptualized from the perspective of second-generation immigrants specifically (Roysircar & Maestas, 2002). This is because second-generation immigrants must navigate between their family and host cultures. The value systems of families and host cultures are most at conflict when involving concerns such as coping skills, relationships, the value of family, and the emphasis of cultural practices. These conflicting value systems can cause conflict in an individual's sense of ethnic identity, or cultural alienation, when a person experiences a sense of discontinuity in their identity. SAAs may experience this cultural alienation if they are confronted with racial/ethnic stereotypes about themselves in the course of discrimination. This experience can potentially make it difficult for a SAA to identify with either of the cultural value systems and, in turn, experience cultural conflict. When a South Asian American believes the family and host cultural norms are incompatible, this can result in marginalization from both groups and feelings of anger and guilt (Roysircar & Maestas, 2002). Identity conflict may continue to arise among SAAs when navigating cultural values between generations in the family as well (e.g., between child, parent, and grandparent's value systems).

Nature of Discrimination Experiences

Generally, there is a discrepany in information about the discrimination South Asians experience (Gee et al., 2009). This is partially due the "Model Minority Myth," a stereotype that first developed in the 1960s when Asian American immigrants were seen as highly successful, high-achieving individuals who contributed to society (Osajima, 1988, as cited in Wong et al., 1998). The media perpetuated an image of Asian Americans demonstrating resilience with their high academic performance and economic success, which also suggested that they could overcome adversities caused by racial tensions (Lee et al., 2009, as cited by Gupta & Leong, 2011). The perception that Asian Americans are immune to negative effects of discrimination can unfortunately lead to an incomplete understanding of their lived experiences (Kaduvettoor-Davidson & Inman, 2013; Lee et al., 2009; Mahmud, 2001). This is especially concerning, considering the available research indicates that Asian Americans are experiencing discrimination in comparable levels to Latinx and Native American individuals (Alvarez et al., 2006; National Public Radio, Robert Wood Johnson Foundation, & Harvard T. H. Chan School of Public Health, 2017a–c). It is important for practitioners to understand the nature of discrimination that SAAs experience in a variety of contexts and settings.

Types of Discrimination

Some of the most common discrimination experiences of SAAs involve racial and ethnic discrimination (Inman et al., 2015; Nadimpalli et al., 2016; Poolokasingham et al., 2014; Yoshihama et al., 2012). Across studies, individuals have reported personal interactions based on racial and ethnic prejudice with statements such as, "go back to your country!" or being told that they "sound Indian" with the request to speak with someone else who was not SAA (Inman et al., 2015). Others have felt "singled out" with airport security searches or being called a "terrorist"; sentiments that echo the tension for SAAs after 9/11 (Tummala-Narra et al., 2016). These experiences reflect biases in both ethnic and racial judgments. However, one of the challenges with documenting discrimination experiences of SAAs is that South Asian Americans and practitioners tend to utilize the terms "ethnic" and "racial" interchangeably when describing discrimination (Rivas-Drake et al., 2014). This becomes problematic because there may be nuances in the nature of discrimination that are important for practitioners to understand for case conceptualization. Ethnic discrimination can be conceptualized as discrimination based on the recipient's beliefs, values, and practices; this is different when considering racial discrimination is based on skin color alone (Jackson, 2011).

Another important question to consider with SAAs' discrimination experiences is the role that generation/immigration status may play (Inman et al., 2015; Kaduvettoor-Davidson & Inman, 2013; Tummala-Narra et al., 2011). South Asians have a long history of experiencing British imperialism, which initiated the idea that lighter or white skin and British values and cultural practices (e.g., speaking English) was equivalent to supremacy and higher class. The continued reinforcement of these values may lead to first-generation immigrant South Asians, or those who immigrated to the U.S. as adults, being more likely to experience ethnic discrimination (Kaduvettoor-Davidson & Inman, 2013). This may be due to more readily observable cultural and ethnic practices such as the use of a *bindi*, cultural clothing, and accents and language (Kaduvettoor-Davidson & Inman, 2013). They may also experience race-based discrimination due to the sociopolitical implications of skin color (Inman, 2006). On the other hand, second-generation South Asian Americans may mostly experience race-based discrimination since they may not express cultural or ethnic markers as often (for example, they may not have accents). In this sense, it is possible that first-generation South Asian Americans may feel safer assimilating to American culture to avoid situations that lend them to the potential of experiencing discrimination (e.g., using English to avoid ethnic discrimination based on language differences). This is another reason to establish clear distinction between ethnic and racial discrimination among South Asian Americans of different generations.

While South Asian Americans often experience overt racial and ethnic discrimination at the individual level, research indicates discrimination experiences may also be more subtle in the form of microaggressions (Poolokasingham et al., 2014). Racial microaggressions are subtle negative racial insults or slights that can be communicated with body language, facial expression, gestures, and speech (Sue et al., 2007). These behaviors can further be understood as microinvalidations, microinsults, and microassaults (Sue et al., 2007). Microinvalidations are comments that potentially negate or undervalue the person of color's experiences. An example of this type of microaggression in therapy can be an interaction where a clinician remarks to a SAA client that they "speak English well" for an immigrant or individual of South Asian descent. On the other hand, microinsults may include comments that are rude or insensitive of the person's background. An example of this category of microaggression could include a South Asian American student being overlooked in a class among predominantly white students. While microinvalidations and microinsults might include more implicit discrimination, microassaults are more explicit attacks involving racial slurs or other discriminatory actions (Sue et al., 2007). An example of a microassault could be a professor using Islamophobic language when there is a Muslim student in class. Poolokasingham et al. (2014) found support for these patterns in their study that examined South Asian Canadian students, a population that shares some similarities with South Asian Americans. For example, students reported others talked to them slowly with the expectation that they would not understand English, or have a line of questioning that assumed cultural expertise (e.g., asking "you're allowed to drink? I thought you couldn't because of your religion" to someone who does not practice). Outside of this study, other possible examples of microaggressions within the clinical setting include individuals feeling targeted for being "exotic," receiving feedback about their "Whiteness," and assumptions about cultural and religious practices. Importantly, because of the subtle nature of microaggressions, it is possible that SAAs are underreporting and underestimating the extent of discrimination they face.

Discrimination can also be experienced at the institutional level for SAAs (Inman et al., 2015). These experiences can span across healthcare, immigration, employment, and housing outcomes (Inman et al., 2015). For example, SAAs may be subject to immigration quotas and the many hurdles that come with visa applications. Additionally, there may be confrontation with the perception of South Asian Americans "stealing jobs" from Americans (Inman et al., 2015). Similar to microaggressions, these systemic and institutional examples are illustrative of the more subtle nature of discrimination that SAAs face, which may contribute to under-reporting and invalidation of discriminatory experiences.

Detention Centers

One form of institutional discrimination that affects a large portion of South Asian immigrants is detention centers. More than 34,000 South Asians have been arrested along the U.S. borders since 2008 for immigration-related problems (SAALT, 2019b). The rates of migrants being apprehended have only risen since then, with the largest number of migrants originating from India, Nepal, and Bangladesh. Aside from the individuals apprehended at the borders, it is estimated that there are more than 630,000 undocumented Indians alone; a 72% increase for undocumented Indians between 2010 and 2017. Most of these undocumented cases are due to migrants overstaying their visas (SAALT, 2019b). With these arrests, there have been patterns of abuse and harmful behaviors observed at detention facilities. This includes a lack of access to legal resources due to language barriers and denial of religious accommodations (e.g., being forced to cut their hair or banned from wearing turbans, or not being provided with vegan/vegetarian meals). Other indications of detention center abuse include the "use of solitary confinement as a form of retaliation, gross medical neglect, and high bond amounts" (SAALT, 2019b). Under these extreme conditions South Asian migrants have retaliated with hunger strikes to raise awareness of their abusive and discriminatory experiences.

The experience of being detained in an immigration detention center likely has profound effects on South Asian migrants. A large systematic review of studies assessed the experience of individuals in detention centers and found profound mental health outcomes (von Werthern et al., 2018). Migrants in detention centers were more likely to report symptoms of Post-Traumatic Stress Disorder (PTSD), including anxiety, depression, and poor quality of life (von Werthern et al., 2018). Some of the studies controlled for previous mental health conditions, suggesting that the experience of being detained in a detention center alone can cause poor mental health outcomes. Additionally, there was a relationship between duration of detention and worsening mental health conditions. Understanding these outcomes in conjunction with the racially and ethnically based barriers presented in detention centers for South Asians is significant for providers to consider in treatment.

Unfortunately, detention and deportations also have a profound impact on the families of those who are detained. It is likely that many South Asian families in the U.S. are experiencing family separation (SAALT, 2019b). Deportation and detention can be incredibly stressful and traumatizing for individuals and families involved due to the separation event itself, maltreatment at the detention centers, and how individuals and families cope with the separation (Bustamante et al., 2018; SAALT, 2019b). There is research to suggest that parental deportation can have significant negative impacts on the children left behind (Allen et al., 2015; Zayas et al., 2015). In particular, the research indicates children with deported parents are more likely to experience clinically significant internalizing and externalizing difficulties, including symptoms of depression and anxiety, aggression, and conduct problems (Allen et al. 2015; Zayas et al., 2015).

EFFECTS OF DISCRIMINATION

SAAs are experiencing significant effects as a result of discrimination. Individuals report heightened anxiety and hypervigilance, stress, lower self-esteem, depression, and feelings of isolation (Frey & Roysircar, 2006; Kaduvettoor-Davidson & Inman, 2013; Nadimpalli et al., 2016; Tummala-Narra et al., 2011; Yoshihama et al., 2012). In addition to the effects on mental health, SAAs may experience physical health concerns related to discrimination experiences (Gee & Ponce, 2010; Gee et al., 2009, Yoshihama et al., 2012). There is research to suggest that Asian Americans may be more likely to abuse substances, have cardiovascular problems, and experience higher mortality rates, with mortality being linked in part to hate crimes (Gee et al., 2009). If a clinician encounters a SAA client, before addressing mental health concerns, it is important to assess the underlying cultural context and possible racial/ethnic discrimination that may be occurring for the individual. It may also be beneficial for physical healthcare providers to consider these somatic symptoms as possible mental health indicators of discrimination tied to hate crimes. While ethnic and racial discrimination is correlated with a range of mental health concerns, the impact of hate crimes is particularly profound.

Hate Crimes

Paramjit Kaur was one of six killed at the Sikh Temple in Oak Creek and she was the only female victim. She was a 41-year-old mother of two young sons who had immigrated to the U.S. eight years prior with her family. Her son recounts in a CNN news interview (Kaye et al., 2012) that when his mother was in the temple praying, "My aunt told her that there was a shooting going on outside, we need to get up and leave," said 20-year-old son Kamal Saini. "Rather than just getting up and leaving, she wanted to just bow down and pray for the last time and then get up and leave. She was just getting up. She was shot in the back."

Kaur's other son, Harpreet Singh Saini, testified before the Senate Judiciary Committee after his mother was killed and asked that she be given "the dignity of being a statistic" (Associated Press, 2012). He further stated, "I'm here because my mother was murdered in an act of hate 45 days ago. I'm here on behalf of all the children who lost parents or grandparents during the massacre in Oak Creek, Wisconsin. This was not supposed to be our American story, this was not my mother's dream." Three years later in 2015, the FBI began tracking hate crimes against Sikhs, Hindus, and Arabs. Sikh Americans had lobbied for years for such documentation, arguing it was a key step in combating violence against them and their communities.

The sociopolitical environment in the U.S. contributed to fueling a wave of hate crimes and violence against SAAs. During the Presidency of Barack Obama between 2008 and 2016, White supremacists had increased their acts of violence and spread of conspiracy theories while hate groups and antigovernment "Patriot" organizations had experienced explosive growth (Southern Poverty Law Center, 2019). As a result, South Asian communities across the country began to face an upward trend in hate crimes that has continued to the present day. From November 2015 to November 2016 during the presidential campaign of Donald J. Trump, there were 207 incidents of hate violence and xenophobic political statements targeted at South Asian, Muslim, Sikh, Hindu, Middle Eastern, and Arab communities (SAALT, 2017). Based on SAALT's, 2018 report titled "Communities on Fire," during Trump's first year of presidency from November 2016 to November 2017, these incidents increased by 45% from the previous year, with 82% of them being motivated by anti-Muslim sentiment. The report further documented that perpetrators in one out of every five of these hate violence incidents referenced "President Trump," a Trump campaign slogan, or a Trump administration policy. These trends suggest that a correlation exists between the increase in hate violence and Trump's anti-Muslim agenda. A 2017 report by the Southern Poverty Law Center showed that the highest growth in organized hate groups between 2015 and 2016 focused on anti-Muslim hate groups (Southern Poverty Law Center, 2019).

Additional evidence comes from the FBI 2014 to 2017 annual hate crimes statistic reports that showed an increase in hate crimes against South Asian communities for the third consecutive year, surpassing the surge that had occurred in 2002, the year following the 9/11 terrorist attacks (Federal Bureau of Investigation, 2014-2017). The number of hate crimes reported to the FBI in 2017 had increased by 17% from 2016, a more than triple increase from the 5% that had been reported between 2016 and 2015. From 2014 to 2015, anti-Muslim hate crimes had increased by 67%, then increased by another 19% from 2015 to 2016, and rose by 38% from 2016 to 2017, the same year that anti-Sikh hate crimes grew by 17%. During 2015, anti-Hindu hate crimes increased to 100%. When hate crimes and racist remarks primarily target the Muslim community, they also affect Hindu and Sikh communities due to cases of mistaken identity. Perpetrators of hate crimes indiscriminately target people who look different from them, speak a language they do not understand, and dress in traditional clothing. Sikhs are one of the most visible representations of that with their turbans and beards. Most Americans know little about Sikhs, so when a perpetrator sees a person wearing a turban, they may assume that they are Muslim. Hate crimes against South Asians are grossly underreported, thus these statistics represent a fraction of the violence South Asian communities experience on a regular basis.

Reasons for Underreporting

There are several reasons that most hate crime data on SAAs is underreported and unreliable. A 1990 federal law called the Hate Crime Statistics Act requires the FBI and the Justice Department to publish an annual report on hate crime statistics. Local law enforcement agencies are not required to report their data to the FBI for their annual crime report. Of the more than 18,000 agencies in the U.S., nearly 17% of them chose not to submit their hate crime statistics to the FBI in 2019 (Federal Bureau of Investigation, 2019). Of the 16,000 agencies that did provide their data, six out of seven (86%) reported zero instances of a hate crime. According to ProPublica's "Documenting Hate" project, 88% reported zero hate crimes in 2016 similar to the 87% who reported zero hate crimes in 2017. It is unlikely that there were no hate crimes committed in these years, but rather that hate crime reporting is inaccurate and inconsistent across the various law enforcement agencies.

Another reason hate crime data on SAAs is underreported and inaccurate is because victims are often reluctant to contact the police when it has occurred. It is difficult to prove the intent of the perpetrator and provide tangible evidence that the hate crime was in fact motivated by racial bias. Language or cultural barriers further prevent victims from reporting hate crimes. If the victim is not a U.S. citizen, for example, they may have a fear of repercussions for their immigration status or have a general distrust of law enforcement (SAALT, 2021).

Impact of Hate Crimes

As hate crimes have continued to steadily increase in America, they have a lasting effect on individuals and communities. Survivors of hate crimes are likely to experience more psychological distress than survivors of other violent crimes (Herek et al., 1999). More specifically, those who experience hate crimes often report greater levels of anxiety, depression, post-traumatic stress along with a general sense of anger, fear, and hopelessness (McDevitt et al., 2001; Boeckmann & Turpin-Petrosino, 2002). An attack on even one individual within a community is an attack on the entire community. Members of a community can experience these feelings regardless of whether they were directly impacted by the hate crime. When a hate crime occurs, it sends a clear message to the victim and to all members within the victim's group that they are not welcome or safe, thus negatively impacting the mental health of members of the entire community. After the terror attacks of September 11, for example, Arab-Americans living in the U.S. were more likely to report high levels of psychological distress and lower levels of happiness (Padela & Heisler, 2010).

Case Study Discussion

Oak Creek and Sahara

Oak Creek is a small town outside of Milwaukee, Wisconsin that had a population of 34,000 in August 2012 when it became the site of the deadliest attack against Sikhs on U.S. soil. The mass shooting left six members of the Sikh congregation dead in their house of worship (Gurdwara), and one later died from his injuries. They were six men and one woman ranging in age from 39 to 84 years. All six of the male victims wore turbans as part of their Sikh faith. Every victim was an immigrant from India. The Sikh community that worshiped there was a close-knit group of about 120 immigrant families that had come to America decades earlier for a brighter future.

In the days immediately following the horrific hate crime, there was understandable shock, numbness, and disbelief within the community. After the funerals had taken place and the media left town, the Sikh community returned to its new normal, which allowed for the healing process to begin. It was during this time that symptoms were being first reported to health professionals. Despite the presence of counselors and therapists in the Gurdwara, the community members preferred speaking with medical doctors. The members of the congregation disclosed that they were experiencing survivor guilt, intrusive thoughts, insomnia, and other indicators of post-traumatic stress disorder. Their initial complaints often manifested as having psychosomatic ailments such as headaches, backaches, weaknesses, dizziness, and digestive problems. Upon further probing, it was clear that their nightmares, flashbacks, difficulties with concentration, hypervigilance, and feelings of irritability, fear, and hopelessness were reactions to the trauma they had experienced.

In the case study illustrated at the start of the chapter, Priya reported that Sahara's symptoms began after the separation experience. In particular, Sahara has had nightmares, crying spells, and "mood swings" where she is irritable and verbally and physically aggressive. She is hyperactive, has difficulty paying attention, and is often defiant with Priya. Sahara also describes experiencing intrusive thoughts and memories about the separation. Priya is struggling as the sole source of income for the family after Adesh's deportation, and she believes her relationship with Sahara is very strained. Sahara often becomes sad and asks where her father is and when she can see him again. Priya reports feeling sad and hopeless about his return, feeling that they may never be reunited. She is actively working with an immigration attorney and frequently describes the difficulty in navigating the system with the paperwork and documentation to have Adesh return. Further, she feels that Adesh's Sri Lankan background and Priya's Indian background sometimes create a "clash" in their cultures with the way they see and work through the stress of the legal case.

Sahara's therapist may be inclined at first to work with Sahara's immediate symptom presentation, including her defiance, inattention, and hyperactivity. Sahara may even be assessed for commonly diagnosed mental health conditions such as Attention-Deficit/Hyperactivity Disorder, which can present similarly to Sahara's symptoms. However, it is important to assess Sahara's experience of traumatic symptoms in a culturally responsive manner. For many children, trauma can manifest in behaviors such as defiance and aggression, as they may have difficulty in regulating their emotions (The National Child Traumatic Stress Network, 2020). Considering concerns about immigration, deportation, and/or refugee status, mental health professionals should keep cultural considerations in mind while assessing for trauma. It will be most helpful to explore how the family interprets the response and whether Sahara's symptoms are related to her father's deportation, for example, and to understand how other members of the family perceive the presenting problem. This will also lead to a discussion about discipline practices and how the family perceives disciplining and the roles of children vs. caregivers. Many South Asian families are more likely to use solution-focused approaches to quickly address the concerns, which makes techniques grounded in cognitive-behavioral interventions ideal as well (Shariff, 2009). At the same time, clinicians should be careful when discussing biases and thinking traps in the context of ethnic and racial discrimination and identity, as any perception of discrimination from the client should be validated and treated as legitimate. In Sahara's case, it will be beneficial to understand the extent to which intergenerational trauma may be impacting her behaviors. Priya may need support in understanding her own background and upbringing and how that may impact Sahara's behaviors and expectations of discipline. It may also be helpful to ensure Priya has her own supports in place for coping with the loss and adjustments as well.

Clinical tools to consider administering to Sahara include the UCLA Post Traumatic Stress Disorder Reaction Index (PTSD-RI), given its adaptability within non-Western cultures. This would help the clinician to assess for the clinical significance of Sahara's traumatic stress despite potential underreporting of symptoms. Additionally, evidence-based interventions such as Trauma-Focused Cognitive Behavior Therapy (TF-CBT) are flexible in administration and can be helpful with a client like Sahara. TF-CBT provides clients with a strong foundation of coping strategies and uses gradual exposure in the form of a narrative, helping the clinician to meet Sahara's needs based on her comfort and pace. TF-CBT encourages parental involvement, which will support Sahara's needs as she navigates trauma in the context of the family and host cultures.

Clinical Implications and Best Practices

Mental health professionals were tasked with the unique challenge of providing an effective mental health intervention following a hate crime against a South Asian American immigrant community. The circumstances surrounding the mass shooting required providers to be understanding and sensitive to South Asian American cultural norms and values while setting aside their preconceived beliefs and assumptions about what actions must be taken following a tragedy. We often come with general ideas of what is effective trauma intervention, but to be successful in these types of situations, we need to be open, flexible, and willing to customize our approach every step of the way based on the community's expressed needs. The ultimate result is that a traumatized community is empowered to drive its own healing process while embracing mental health practices along the way.

Building Rapport and Trust within a Community after a Hate Crime

As with all hate crimes, the media ascended to the site of the tragedy to learn more about the events and the victims. Members of the community were in shock and disbelief. Most of the conversations were focused on understanding the sequence of events, the perpetrator's motives, and the identity of the victims. A great deal of confusion, chaos, and misinformation ensued in this initial period. As community members responded to the media's repeated questions, they continued to relive the trauma. After several weeks, the community yearned to return to its new normal and engage in the routines and traditions that were in place before the tragedy occurred. It was during this time that the healing began.

A mental health relief effort called The Sikh Healing Collective was established at this time by Puni Kalra, one of the authors of this chapter. Its mission was to bring together all trained mental health professionals to provide support to the community. There was a paucity of South Asian mental health professionals; hence, various methods were used to identify them while accounting for the community's specific cultural and linguistic needs. The result was nearly 50 mental health professionals representing ten states across the country came together to provide support to the Sikh community in their time of need. Volunteers were South Asian and non-South Asian; they were Sikhs, Hindus, Muslims, Christians, and Jews, making it a truly collective effort. The following list of best practices is based on experiential learnings from the Sikh Healing Collective:

- Learn more about the community's culture, customs, and values through observations, inquiry, and independent research. If appropriate, attend the funerals to learn and observe how the community grieves and copes after experiencing a hate crime.
- If you have a Doctorate in the mental health field, introduce yourself as a doctor as it is associated with less stigma among South Asians than "counselors" or "therapists."
- Avoid language such as counseling, therapy, or support groups as they are similarly loaded with stigma. Rather, focus on building relationships with the community in a more informal manner. This requires mental health professionals to be willing to initiate casual dialogue over a cup of *chai*, for example, rather than waiting for community members to approach them.
- When learning about others, be curious about who they are (e.g., how long they have lived there, who is part of their family, what they do for a living, etc.) rather than inquiring about their association with the tragedy (e.g., what did you see, how are you feeling about it, did you know the victims). Such questions may be retraumatizing for the individual.
- If possible, utilize mental health providers who have experience and familiarity working with South Asians. Those with language fluency are key in working with adults and immigrants for whom English is a second language.
- Mental health providers can identify and partner with key community leaders who are respected and influential. In Oak Creek, these community leaders were male medical doctors and priests.
- In building partnerships with these key leaders, providers can ask for their opinions and support rather than telling them what their community needs to do.
- Providers can also inform and share with key leaders how mental health practices can support the community's collective healing and showcase their resilience in the face of adversity. Presenting a direct correlation between mental health services and outcomes that are tied to their values can help garner greater support from these community leaders.

• Enlisting the support of these community leaders and forming a partnership is a critical component of introducing mental health services into South Asian communities. This partnership formed shortly after the funerals in Oak Creek had occurred. To publicly show their support and approval, these leaders introduced the mental health team to the Sikh congregation.

For the next six months, the Sikh Healing Collective joined the community in their healing process by focusing on building a relationship with its members, slowly and gradually, using the same small team of mental health professionals each week. Consistency in providers was key for two reasons. First, it prevented members from having to retell their stories and risk being retraumatized. Second, it allowed the congregation to become more familiar with the providers and to begin to see them as part of their community. As comfort with mental health providers increased over time, community members began to share additional familial and life stressors with them such as mental illness, suicide, drug abuse, addiction, domestic violence, and sexual abuse. Mental health has a place within South Asian communities, and it is most effective when it can be introduced in such a way that reduces cultural stigma.

Reframing Mental Health

The Sikh Healing Collective had identified that education was an important value within the Sikh community. Thus, they chose to support the community by packaging information about the grief process in educational materials. More specifically, the mental health team would listen carefully each week for what symptoms and ailments the community members were collectively presenting to them and other medical professionals. They would then compile information on that topic, convert it into simple, lay-friendly language, and produce a single-page document that would be distributed to the congregation at the following Sunday services. These information sheets were written in English on one side and translated into the Punjabi language on the other side. At the Sunday service, the mental health team would also provide a brief oral presentation in Punjabi elaborating on the information sheets, further clarifying the topic with examples and increasing the congregation's familiarity with different mental health providers. Examples of topics that were covered included symptoms of post-traumatic stress disorder, survivor guilt, intrusive thoughts, and insomnia. Understanding the community's immediate needs and addressing them in real time on a weekly basis had two advantages. First, it allowed the mental health team to build a deep level of trust with the community. Second, it helped the community to see greater value and utility of mental health ideas and practices.

During the same six-week time period that the adults were receiving psycho-education materials, the mental health needs of the community youth were addressed differently. They were placed in one of three groups of about 20 members each. Group #1 had children under the age of 11. Group #2 had only teen boys and group #3 had only teen girls. The parents would only allow for the adolescents to participate in the counseling services if they were separated by gender. For these counseling sessions, the Sikh Healing Collective partnered with non-South Asian trauma therapists from Children's Hospital of Wisconsin, providing them with language translation and cultural context. The children's teachers and school counselors also became involved, meeting with the community mental health team to learn about Sikh culture and about specific challenges Sikh children faced upon returning to school, such as bullying and increased symptoms of anxiety and PTSD.

Trauma-Informed Practices

Assessment

While the aforementioned section referenced how a community responded to a hate crime, this next section will focus on how trauma can manifest in clinical settings. Considering the potentially traumatic nature of discrimination experiences that South Asian Americans face at the individual, community, and institutional levels, it will be beneficial for clinicians to utilize culturally responsive instruments in their assessment. In particular, when working with children who may have experienced traumatic acts of discrimination, it is best practice to use an evidence-based screening tool such as The University of California at Los Angeles Posttraumatic Stress Disorder Reaction Index for DSM-5 (PTSD-RI-5), a tool developed to assess symptoms of traumatic stress among school-aged children. This assessment is in self-report format and provides the opportunity for an individual to endorse their experience of stressful/traumatic experiences as well as the option to elaborate on symptoms they may be experiencing as a result (National Center for PTSD, 2021). For adult clients, the Clinician-Administered Posttraumatic Stress Scale for DSM-5 (CAPS-5) is a widely used tool to assess for symptoms of traumatic stress (Weathers et al., 2013). Both the PTSD-RI-5 and the CAPS-5 have been assessed and normed on diverse populations, including among Asian Americans (Doric et al., 2019; Kim et al., 2019).

Though these assessments have been utilized among diverse populations, clinicians should be mindful of cultural nuances in the delivery and interpretation of items in each assessment. Specifically, it may be beneficial for clinicians to pay particular attention to somatic symptoms and the use clients' language to define how their potentially stressful experiences impacted them. It also may be helpful to modify questionnaires for use with SAA clients. For example, the Trauma History Questionnaire (THQ) has been used with diverse populations and is a self-report measure that asks about potentially traumatic experiences that an individual may have experienced through their lifetime (Hooper et al., 2011). A clinician can consider modifying the measure as needed to inquire about immigration-specific questions (e.g., asking about fears of deportation, if they witnessed a loved one being separated, if they have been a target of discrimination based on their immigration status, etc.). Of course, when a measure is modified, the results should be interpreted with caution considering psychometric properties would have also been impacted. Other interview questions that may be useful to consider can include questions about the individual's health, such as the experience of headaches, stomachaches, or tension, considering SAAs often experience somatic symptoms as indicators of mental health difficulties.

Underutilization of Mental Health

A significant challenge in the aftermath of the Oak Creek shooting was addressing the need for mental health services in the Sikh community. Most of the community did not understand the field of mental health or how it could serve to alleviate their symptoms. For this reason, South Asians suffering from mental health issues tend to delay or dismiss mental health services as a treatment option. Little research has been conducted on rates of mental health utilization within South Asian populations, but research findings can be extrapolated from Asian American communities who share similar perceptions of mental health.

Asian Americans utilize mental health services at lower rates compared to the general population, 8.6% versus 17.9% (Abe-Kim et al., 1997). They have low utilization rates for both outpatient mental health services as well as inpatient admissions to state hospitals (Lin & Cheung, 1999). Of Asian Americans with a diagnosable mental health disorder, only 28% used specialty mental health services such as those delivered by a psychiatrist, psychologist, or other mental health professional (Le Meyer et al., 2009). Similarly, one-third of Asian Americans diagnosed with any depressive disorder sought mental health treatment (Alegria et al., 2008). If they eventually seek services at all, it is after their conditions are more severe and chronic (Segal, 1998; Lin & Cheung, 1999). Level of acculturation also impacts rates of mental health utilization as Asian Americans born in the U.S. had higher rates compared with immigrants (Abe-Kim et al., 1997).

Reasons for Underutilization of Mental Health Services

The underutilization of mental health services among SAAs is due in part to societal stigma, believing that mental health problems result from lack of willpower and weakness (Kwok, 2013; Yang et al., 2013; Masuda & Boone, 2011; Golberstein et al., 2008). South Asians consider discussing personal or intimate problems with members outside the extended family as taboo, often discouraging help-seeking behavior for fear they will cause embarrassment and humiliation for themselves and their families (Leong & Lau, 2001). South Asian culture places high importance on perceived prestige, pride, privacy, and "saving face" (Khanna et al., 2009; Kwok, 2013). Those who experience mental health problems feel embarrassed and ashamed, causing them to conceal their symptoms and fail to seek treatment (Sussman et al., 1987). In fact, most individuals do not engage with physicians and clinicians until their symptoms have worsened and are quite severe (Segal, 1998; Lin & Cheung, 1999).

Other factors that contribute to the underutilization of mental health services include language barriers (e.g., English-speaking vs. non-English speaking) and generational differences (Chu et al., 2011; Kung, 2004; Jang et al., 1998). It is easier to process and express emotions in one's native language, making it preferable for South Asians to speak with mental health professionals who have some language fluency and sensitivity to cultural norms and values. This is particularly important for older, less acculturated members within the community (Abe-Kim, Takeuchi, et al., 1997).

Religion and spirituality play a key role in shaping South Asian beliefs about healing and help-seeking behaviors. Prayer is a common coping strategy among ethnic minorities facing mental distress (Sproston & Bhui, 2002). South Asian women, for example, often use prayer to cope with their depression (Gilbody et al., 2001). A strong social network is often embedded within South Asian communities who worship together, and this serves as a protective factor in recovery from mental health stressors (Heath, 1999). South Asians may also explore home remedies, herbal medicines, or traditional healers as treatments for mental health problems before being willing to seek help from outside the community.

Oak Creek Barriers to Mental Health

Based on the observations of Dr. Kalra, founder of the Sikh Healing Collective serving the Oak Creek community after the hate crime, there were many significant findings. Many of the aforementioned barriers to mental health were present in the Sikh community after the mass shooting. The cultural stigma was evident from the beginning when community members would not accept support from the American Red Cross during the funeral ceremonies. Similarly, they were unwilling to join support groups or counseling sessions that were offered to them. They were hesitant to openly accept mental health services for fear that they would be perceived as weak, emotionally vulnerable, or unable to manage their trauma on their own.

Significant language and cultural barriers were present within this community. The congregation primarily consisted of immigrant parents with first generation children and

English was the second language for most of them. Several of the victims were primary breadwinners of their families back in India. After they were killed, their wives and their children moved to America. These immigrant Sikh families had to suddenly adjust to a new country, language, and culture while grieving the loss of their husbands and fathers.

Attitudes toward mental health in this community varied based on age. Children and adolescents were more open to receiving mental health services than adults. This was especially true if the support came from counselors within the community because of language and cultural similarities. Older children were also more receptive to treatment if it was less overtly focused on emotion expression. Teenagers, for example, wanted to continue meeting with the mental health professionals as long as "they didn't have to talk about their feelings all the time."

Gender differences were more prevalent among adults. Men preferred to speak separately and privately with a mental health professional where no one could see them. Women were more comfortable speaking publicly with therapists and counselors and were less concerned about how others in the community might judge them. Both men and women responded more favorably to a male therapist than a female therapist due to South Asian cultural gender bias that men are more respected and trustworthy than their female counterparts.

Reflection Questions

1   Discuss the importance of language, culture, immigration status, and psychological adjustment for survivors of hate crimes and implications for mental health professionals.
2   How can mental health professionals be stronger advocates for South Asian Americans and proactively build partnerships within those communities (e.g., activists, law enforcement agencies)?
3   How do we assess the level of acculturation of South Asian Americans in clinical settings when a specific measure is not available?

Chapter Summary

SAAs have held a significant presence in the U.S.' immigrant history. With the U.S.' history of immigration barriers, South Asians have understandably been subjected to not only logistical challenges (such as visas) but also to the social difficulties such as discrimination. Discrimination, whether based in ethnicity or race, is something SAAs experience at individual, community, or institutional levels. These discriminatory acts can be overt (e.g., hate crimes) or covert (e.g., microaggressions and institutional barriers). These experiences of discrimination are likely to go underreported for several reasons, including cultural stigma, internalization of the Model Minority Myth, and the strained relationship that SAAs have with law enforcement entities. This becomes problematic when considering the negative mental and physical health outcomes that South Asians experience as a result of discrimination, especially hate crimes. Thus, it is beneficial for clinicians to consider utilizing trauma-informed assessments and interventions and culturally responsive techniques. These techniques may include modifying language about mental health to reduce stigma, collaborating with community leaders, providing consistency in support, and taking time to observe, research, and ask questions to learn more about the client's cultural context.

References

Abe-Kim, J., Takeuchi, D., et al. (1997). Use of mental health-related services among immigrant and U.S.-born asian americans: Results from the national latino and asian american study. *American Journal of Public Health*, *97*(1), 91–98.

Alegria, M., Canino, G., Shrout, P.E., Woo, M., Duan, N., Vila, D., et al. (2008). Prevalence of mental illness in immigrant and non-immigrant U.S. Latino groups. *Am J Psychiatry*, *165*(3), 359–369.

Allen, B., Cisneros, E.M., & Tellez, A. (2015). The children left behind: The impact of parental deportation on mental health. *Journal of Child and Family Studies*, *24*, 386–392. doi: 10.1007/s10826-013-9848-5

Alvarez, A.N., Juang, L., & Liang, C.H. (2006). Asian americans and racism: When bad things happen to "Model Minorities." *Cultural Diversity and Ethnic Minority Psychology*, *12*(3), 477–492. doi: 10.1037/1099-9809.12.3.477

Boeckmann, R.J., & Turpin-Petrosino, C. (2002). Understanding the harm of hate crime. *Journal of Social Issues*, *58*, 207–225.

Berry, J. (1997). Immigration, Acculturation, and Adaptation. *Applied Psychology*, *46*, 5–34. doi:10.1111/j.1464-0597.1997.tb01087.x

Bustamante, L.H.U., Cerqueira, R.O., Leclerc, E., & Brietzke, E. (2018). Stress, trauma, and Posttraumatic stress disorder in migrants: A comprehensive review. *Brazilian Journal of Psychiatry*, *40*, 220–225. doi: 10.1590/1516-4446-2017-2290

Chu, J.P., Hsieh, K., & Tokars, D.A. (2011). Help-seeking tendencies in Asian Americans with suicidal ideation and Attempts. *Asian Am J Psychology*, *2*(1), 25–38.

Doric, A., Stevanovic, D., Stupar, D., Vostanis, P., Atilola, O., Moreira, P., Dodig-Curkovic, K., Franic, T., Davidovic, V., Avicenna, M., Noor, M., Nussbaum, L., Thabet, A., Ubalde, D., Petrov, P., Deljkovic, A., Luis Antonio, M., Ribas, A., Oliveira, J., & Knez, R. (2019) UCLA PTSD reaction index for DSM-5 (PTSD-RI-5): A psychometric study of adolescents sampled from communities in eleven countries. *European Journal of Psychotraumatology*, *10*(1), doi: 10.1080/20008198.2019.1605282

Elias, M. (2012, November 11). *Sikh temple killer Wade Michael Page radicalized in army*. Southern Poverty Law Center. https://www.splcenter.org/fighting-hate/intelligence-report/2012/sikh-temple-killer-wade-michael-page-radicalized-army

Federal Bureau of Investigation. (2014). *Hate crimes*. Washington, DC: U. S. Department of Justice. Retrieved from https://ucr.fbi.gov/hate-crime/2014

Federal Bureau of Investigation. (2015). *Hate crimes*. Washington, DC: U. S. Department of Justice. Retrieved from https://ucr.fbi.gov/hate-crime/2015

Federal Bureau of Investigation. (2016). *Hate crimes*. Washington, DC: U. S. Department of Justice. Retrieved from https://ucr.fbi.gov/hate-crime/2016

Federal Bureau of Investigation. (2017). *Hate crimes*. Washington, DC: U. S. Department of Justice. Retrieved from https://www.fbi.gov/about-/investigate/civilrights/hate_crimes/overview

Federal Bureau of Investigation. (2019). Hate crime statistics. Retrieved from https://www.justice.gov/hatecrimes/hate-crime-statistics

Frey, L.L., & Roysircar, G. (2006). South asian and east asian international students' perceived prejudice, acculturation, and frequency of help utilization. *Journal of Multicultural Counseling and Development*, *34*, 208–222.

Gee, G.C., & Ponce, N. (2010). Associations between racial discrimination, limited english proficiency, and health-related quality of life among 6 asian ethnic groups in California. *American Journal of Public Health*, *100*(5), 888–895.

Gee, G.C., Ro, A., Shariff-Marco, S., & Chae, D. (2009). Racial discrimination and health among asian americans: Evidence, assessment, and directions for future research. *Epidemiologic Reviews*, *31*, 130–151.

Gilbody, S.M., House, A.O., & Sheldon, T.A. (2001). Routinely Administered questionnaires for depression and anxiety: Systematic review. *British Medical Journal*, *322*, 406–409.

Golberstein, E., Eisenberg, D., Gollust, S.E. (2008). Perceived stigma and mental health care seeking. *Psychiatr Serv, 59*(4), 392–399.

Gupta, S., & Leong. (2011). The "Model minority Myth": Internalized racialism of positive stereotypes as correlates of psychological distress, and attitudes toward help-seeking. *Asian American Journal of Psychology, 2*(2), 101–114.

Heath, I. (1999) Commentary: There must be limits to the medicalization of human distress. *British Medical Journal, 318*, 439–440.

Herek, G.M., Gillis, J.R., & Cogan, J.C. (1999). Psychological sequelae of hate-crime victimization among lesbian, gay, and bisexual adults. *Journal of Consulting and Clinical Psychology, 67*, 945–951.

Hess, G.R. (1969). The "Hindu" in America: Immigration and Naturalization Policies and India, 1917–1946. *Pacific Historical Review, 38*(1), 59–79. 10.2307/3636886

Hooper, L., Stockton, P., Krupnick, J., & Green, B., (2011). Development, use, and psychometric properties of the trauma history questionnaire. *Journal of Loss and Trauma, 16*, 258–283. doi: 10.1080/15325024.2011.572035

Ibrahim, F., Ohnishi, H., & Sandhu, D.S. (1997). Asian american identity development: A culture specific model for south asian americans. *Journal of Multicultural Counseling and Development, 25*(1), 34–50.

Inman, A.G. (2006). South asian women: Identities and conflicts. *Cultural Diversity and Ethnic Minority Psychology, 12*(2), 306–319. doi:10.1037/1099-9809.12.2.306

Inman, A.G., Tummala-Narra, P., Kaduvettoor-Davidson, A., Alvarez, A.N., & Yeh, C.J. (2015). Perceptions of race-based discrimination among first-generation asian indians in the United states. *The Counseling Psychologist, 42*(2), 1–31.

Jackson, L.M. (2011). Defining prejudice. In *The psychology of prejudice: From attitudes to social action* (pp. 7–28). Washington, DC: American Psychological Association. doi:10.1037/12317-001

Jang, M., Lee, E., & Woo, K. (1998). Income, language, and citizenship status: Factors affecting the health care access and utilization of chinese americans. *Health Soc Work, 23*(2), 136–145.

Kaduvettoor-Davidson, A., & Inman, A.G. (2013). South asian americans: Perceived discrimination, stress, and well-being. *Asian American Journal of Psychology, 4*(3), 155–165. doi:10.1037/a0030634

Kaye, R., Harlow, P., & Gast, P. (2012, August 7). Wisconsin city holds prayer vigil for temple shooting victims. *CNN*. https://www.cnn.com/2012/08/07/us/wisconsin-shooting-victims

Kim, W., Jung, Y., Roh, D., Kim, D., Kang, S., Jeong-Ho, C., & Park, J.E. (2019). Reliability and validity of the korean version of clinician-Administered Posttraumatic stress disorder scale for dsm-5. *Journal of Korean Medical Science, 34*. doi:10.3346/jkms.2019.34.e219

Khanna, A., Mcdowell, T., Perumbilly, S., & Titus, G. (2009). Working with Asian Indian American Families: A Delphi Study. *Journal of Systemic Therapies, 28*, 52–71. 10.1521/jsyt.2009.28.1.52

Kung, W.W. (2004). Cultural and practical barriers to seeking mental health treatment for chinese americans. *Journal of Community Psychology, 32*(1), 27–43.

Kwok, J. (2013). Factors that influence the diagnoses of asian americans in mental health: An exploration. *Perspectives in Psychiatric Care, 49*(4), 288–292.

Le Meyer, O., Zane, N., Cho, Y.I., & Takeuchi, D.T. (2009). Use of specialty mental health services by asian americans with Psychiatric disorders. *J Consult Clin Psychology, 77*(5), 1000–1005.

Lee, S.J., Wong, N.W.A., & Alvarez, A.N. (2009). The model minority foreigner: Stereotypes of asian americans. In N. Tewari & A. N. Alvarez (Eds.), *Asian American psychology: Current perspectives* (pp. 69 – 84). New York: Routledge/Taylor & Francis Group.

Leong, F. T. L., & Lau, A. S. L. (2001). *Mental Health Services Research, 3*, 201–214. 10.1023/a:1013177014788

Lin, K., & Cheung, F. (1999). Mental health issues for asian americans. *Psychiatric Services, 50*(6), 774–780.

Livengood, J.S., & Stodolska, M. (2004). The effects of discrimination and constraints negotiation on leisure Behavior of american muslims in the post-september 11 America. *Journal of Leisure Research, 36*(2), 183.

Londhe, R. (2014). Acculturation of Asian Indian parents: relationship with parent and child characteristics. *Early Child Development and Care, 185*, 528–53710.1080/03004430.2014.939650

Mahmud, T. (2001). Genealogy of a state-engineered "Model Minority": "Not quite/not White" south asian americans. *Denver University Law Review*, *78*(4), 657–686.

Masuda, A., & Boone, M.S. (2011). Mental health stigma, self-concealment, and help seeking attitudes among asian american and european american college students with no help-seeking experience. *Int J Adv Couns*, *33*(4), 266–279.

McDevitt J., Balboni J., Garcia L., & Gu J. (2001). Consequences for victims: A comparison of bias- and non-bias-motivated assaults. *American Behavioral Scientist*, *45*, 697–713. doi:10.1177/0002 764201045004010

Nadimpalli, S.B., Kanaya, A.M., McDade, T.W., & Kandula, N.R. (2016). Self-reported discrimination and mental health among asian indians: Cultural beliefs and coping style as moderators. *Asian American Journal of Psychology*, *7*(3), 185–194.

National Center for PTSD (29, March 2021). *UCLA Child/Adolescent PTSD Reaction Index for DSM-5*. Retrieved from https://www.ptsd.va.gov/professional/assessment/child/ucla_child_reaction_dsm-5.asp

National Public Radio, Robert Wood Johnson Foundation, & Harvard T. H. Chan School of Public Health. (2017a). *Discrimination in America: Experiences and views of Asian Americans*. Retrieved from https://www.npr.org/assets/news/2017/12/discriminationpoll-asian-americans.pdf.

National Public Radio, Robert Wood Johnson Foundation, & Harvard T. H. Chan School of Public Health. (2017b). *Discrimination in America: Experiences and views of Latinos*. Retrieved from https://www.npr.org/documents/2017/oct/discrimination-latinos-final.pdf

National Public Radio, Robert Wood Johnson Foundation, & Harvard T. H. Chan School of Public Health. (2017c). *Discrimination in America: Experiences and views of Native Americans*. Retrieved from https://www.npr.org/documents/2017/nov/NPR-discrimination-native-americans-final.pdf

Osajima, K. (1988). Asian americans as the model minority: An analysis of the Popular Press image in the 1960s and 1980s. In *Reflections on Shattered Windows* (pp. 165–174). Pullman, WA: Washington State University Press.

Padela, A.I., & Heisler, M. (2010). The association of perceived abuse and discrimination after september 11, 2001, with psychological distress, level of happiness, and health status among arab americans. *Am J Public Health*, *100*(2): 284–291.

Poolokasingham, G., Spanierman, L.B., Kleiman, S., & Houshmand, S. (2014). "Fresh off the boat?" racial microaggressions that target south asian canadian students. *Journal of Diversity in Higher Education*, *7*(3), 194–210.

Rivas-Drake, D., Seaton, E.K., Markstrom, C., Quintana, S., Syed, M., Lee, R.M., ... Ethnic and Racial Identity in the 21st Century Study Group. (2014). Ethnic and racial identity in Adolescence: Implications for Psychosocial, academic, and health outcomes. *Child Development*, *85*(1), 40–57. 10.1111/cdev.12200

Roysircar, G., & Maestas, M. L. (2002). Assessing Acculturation and Cultural Variables, Asian American Mental Health (pp. 77–94. 10.1007/978-1-4615-0735-2_6

Segal, U.A. (1998). The asian indian american family. In C. H. Mindel, R. W. Habenstein, & R. Wright, Jr., *Ethnic families in America: Patterns and variation* (4th ed.), Upper Saddle River, NJ: Prentice-Hall.

Shariff, A. (2009). Ethnic identity and parenting stress in south asian families: Implications for culturally sensitive Counselling. *Canadian Journal of Counselling*, *43*(1), 35–46.

South Asian Americans Leading Together (2015). *A demographic snapshot of South Asians in the United States*. Retrieved from http://saalt.org/wp-content/uploads/2016/01/Demographic-Snapshot-updated_Dec-2015.pdf

South Asian Americans Leading Together. (2017). *Power, pain, potential: South Asian Americans at the forefront of growth and hate in the 2016 election cycle*. Retrieved from http://saalt.org/wp-content/uploads/2017/01/SAALT_Power_rpt_final3_lorez.pdf

South Asian Americans Leading Together. (2018). *Communities on fire: Confronting hate violence and xenophobic political rhetoric*. Retrieved from https://saalt.org/wp-content/uploads/2018/01/Communities-on-Fire.pdf

South Asian Americans Leading Together. (2019a). *Demographic snapshot of South Asians in the United States.* Retrieved from https://saalt.org/wp-content/uploads/2019/04/SAALT-Demographic-Snapshot-2019.pdf

South Asian Americans Leading Together. (2019b). *South Asian migrants in detention.* Retrieved from https://saalt.org/wp-content/uploads/2019/08/South-Asian-Migrants-in-Detention-Factsheet.pdf.

South Asian Americans Leading Together (2021, March 27). *Racial justice.* https://saalt.org/policy-change/racial-justice/

Southern Poverty Law Center. (2019). *The year in hate and extremism 2019: A report from the Southern Poverty Law Center.* Retrieved from https://www.splcenter.org/sites/default/files/yih_2020_final.pdf.

Sproston, K., & Bhui, K. (2002). Coping mechanisms. In W. O'Connor, & J. Nazroo (Eds.), *Ethnic Differences in the Context and Experience of Psychiatric Illness: A Qualitative Study.* (pp. 41–50). London: The Stationary Office.

Sue, D.W., Capodilupo, C.M., Torino, G.C., Bucceri, J.M., Holder, A., Nadal, K.L., & Esquilin, M. (2007). Racial microaggressions in everyday life: Implications for clinical practice. *American Psychologist, 62,* 271–286. doi:10.1037/0003-066X.62.4.271

Sussman, S., Dent, C. W., Flay, B. R., Hansen, W. B., & Johnson, C. A. (1987). Chapter 2: Psychosocial predictors of cigarette smoking onset by White, Black, Hispanic, and Asian Adolescents in Southern California. *Morbidity and Mortality Weekly Report, 36*(4S), 11S–16S. http://www.jstor.org/stable/24244494

Tewary, S. (2005). Asian indian immigrant women: A theoretical perspective on mental health. *Journal of Human Behavior in the Social Environment, 11*(1), 1–22. doi:10.1300/J137v11n01_01

Tummala-Narra, P., Inman, A. G., & Ettigi, S. P. (2011). Asian Indians' responses to discrimination: A mixed-method examination of identity, coping, and self-esteem. *Asian American Journal of Psychology, 2,* 205–218. 10.1037/a0025555

Tummala-Narra, P., Deshpande, A., & Kaur, J. (2016). South Asian adolescents' experiences of cculturative stress and coping. *American Journal of Orthopsychiatry, 86*(2), 194–211.

von Werthern, M., Robjant, K., Chui, Z., Schon, R., Ottisova, L., Mason, C., & Katona, C. (2018). The impact of immigration detention on mental health: A systematic review. *BMC Psychiatry, 18,* 382. doi: 10.1186/s12888-018-1945-y

Weathers, F.W., Blake, D.D., Schnurr, P.P., Kaloupek, D.G., Marx, B.P., & Keane, T.M. (2013). The Clinician-Administered PTSD Scale for DSM-5 (CAPS-5). [Assessment] Available from www.ptsd.va.gov.

Wong, P., Lai, C. F. , Nagasawa, R., & Lin, T. (1998). Asian Americans as a Model Minority: Self-Perceptions and Perceptions by other Racial Groups. *Sociological Perspectives, 41,* 95–118. 10.2307/1389355

Yang, L.H., Purdie-Vaughns, V., Kotabe, H., Link, B.G., Saw, A., Wong, G., et al. (2013). Culture, threat, and mental illness stigma: Identifying culture-specific threat among chinese american groups. *Soc Sci Med, 88,* 56–67.

Yoshihama, M., Bybee, D., & Blazevski, J. (2012). Day-to-day discrimination and health among asian indians: A population-based study of gujarati men and women in metropolitan Detroit. *Journal of Behavioral Medicine, 35,* 471–483.

Zayas, L.H., Aguilar-Gaxiola, S., Yoon, H., & Rey, G.N. (2015). The distress of citizen-children with detained and deported parents. *Journal of Child and Family Studies.* doi: 10.1007/s10826-015-0124-8

4 South Asian American Identity

Himadhari Sharma and Sruthi Swami

Case Overview

Anjali (fictional case study) is a 26-year-old heterosexual cisgender second-generation Asian Indian American woman. She has been in a long-term relationship with Mark for approximately 2 years. Mark identifies as a 28-year-old heterosexual cisgender White American Christian man of German descent. While Anjali described that her relationship with Mark has been "going well," there seem to be cultural misunderstandings between both of them, which has been a struggle for the couple. Anjali's family identifies as "Hindu Brahmin" and expects her to marry within her caste and religion. Due to such pressures, Anjali has kept the relationship a secret from her family. However, the couple has begun talking about getting married and Anjali is worried about how her parents may react. Recently, Anjali has been having difficulty sleeping, noticing that her heart races when talking to her parents, and having ruminating thoughts of fear that her parents will disown her. In this chapter, we will take a closer look at the different aspects of Anjali's identities and experiences of trying to balance her multiple cultural identities as it relates to her presenting distress.

Introduction

This chapter aims to broadly explore what it means to be "South Asian American." However, similar to the issues created by homogenizing all Asian Americans, the South Asian American identity can be somewhat of a misnomer due to the diverse individuals and range of experiences within the community. Accordingly, this chapter will focus on reviewing various aspects of South Asian American identities that may be more common among various South Asian subgroups, and based on the opinions of the authors. Specifically, the chapter will provide a brief history of South Asian American immigration, stereotypes and labels associated with South Asian Americans, and how the community is depicted within popular culture and media. It will also provide an overview of identity theories specific to South Asian Americans, review psychological research focused on South Asian American identity and mental health, as well as provide psychotherapeutic recommendations for mental health practitioners. Additionally, to illustrate one way in which identity-related issues may manifest, we will explore the case of Anjali as it relates to the themes presented in each section.

Who are South Asian Americans?

While the South Asian American community is often grouped with other Asian communities, it, too, is highly diverse (Ibrahim et al., 1997) with unique national, religious, caste, and cultural identities that may feel more salient and representative to the individual as

DOI: 10.4324/9781003081548-4

compared to the broader South Asian American label (Bhatia & Ram, 2018; Kaduvettoor-Davidson & Weatherford, 2018). Early South Asian immigrants included farm workers, most often from Punjab (a state in northern India) to the west coast of the United States (U.S.) and Canada, as well as individuals who identified as Bengali arriving in various parts of the East Coast (Bhatia & Ram, 2018). South Asian groups who arrived in the U.S. during this time, along with other Asian groups (e.g., Chinese, Japanese, and Filipinos) were subjected to xenophobic and racist laws that specifically limited immigration and restricted pathways to citizenship for Asian immigrants. The U.S.' exclusionary policies continued until the mid-1950s when a series of laws were passed that finally relaxed immigration attitudes toward Asian groups. Consequently, there was an influx of South Asian immigrants to the U.S. between 1965 and the early 1990s who were overwhelmingly well-educated, had higher incomes, and came from backgrounds that provided them the privilege and opportunity to immigrate (such as being of higher caste). This group of immigrants embodies the stereotypical image of South Asian Americans that exists today, even though, within the community, many are aware of the diversity of socioeconomic status, caste, education, citizenship status, and professions. As such, the "South Asian American" identity is complex, given the diverse journeys and identities of Asian immigrants across time.

Additionally, the "South Asian American" identity may also be a misnomer, similar to the "Asian American" label. Older generations and recent first-generation immigrants whom we may classify as South Asians may not even identify with the label, given that South Asia as a monolith does not exist outside of Western categorizations. Outside of a western context, South Asian individuals may identify more with their national, regional, or specific ethnic identities, as they may find more similarities and homogeneity with people who identify in the same way. On the other hand, second-generation Indian American or Pakistani American individuals, for example, may identify as South Asian American in an effort to find community and camaraderie with individuals who may have some cultural similarities in the U.S. that does not have a critical mass of specific South Asian subgroups as compared to White Americans. Thus, understanding the nuances of an individual's "South Asian American" identity is complex and should be approached with care and humility.

What Impacts South Asian American Identity?

Stereotypes and Labels

South Asian Americans' history is long within the U.S., dating back to the 19th century. As the community began to grow, awareness and xenophobia toward South Asians (and immigrants in general) also took root. This was reflected in the stereotypes and racial/ethnic slurs that developed as well as in the increasing violence and discrimination targeting South Asian immigrants. Such history has likely impacted South Asian American identity development.

Notably, many of the discriminatory labels used for South Asian Americans (see Table 4.1 for common discriminatory and derogatory terms used towards South Asian Americans based on the authors' (Sharma & Swami) personal and professional experiences) by non-South Asian Americans were created without distinguishing among the various within-group communities. Such mass grouping through slurs and labels creates and perpetuates animosity and conflict among South Asian American groups, who may protectively try to distance themselves from other groups within the community and/or attempt to associate themselves with other minoritized communities (i.e., Black Americans, Latinx Americans, etc.) or with the majority community (i.e., White Americans). This is in addition to stereotypes and labels about other South American Asian groups that immigrants may have brought over with them from their country of origin. There also appears to be high levels of

Table 4.1 Common Discriminatory/Derogatory Terms Used Toward South Asian Americans

Discriminatory & Derogatory Terms	Context and Meaning
Towel head	An offensive term used for a person who wears a *pagdi* (turban) or kaffiyeh
Red Dots, Dotheads	This is in reference to individuals who identify as Hindu and/or wear a bindi
Curry Munchie, Curry Eaters	Often used in regard to South Asian identifying individuals and their traditional food/cuisine
Paki	Refers to someone who identifies as having ancestry from Pakistan or as Muslim
Terrorist	Term is often used to criminalize, promote fear, and hatred toward Brown, particularly Muslim and, at times, Sikh, identifying individuals
Smelly	This term could be used in reference to traditional South Asian food or the individual's body odor
Brownie, Darky	These terms refer the South Asian Americans' brown skin tones
ABCD (American Born Confused Desi), White-washed	Many times, South Asian immigrants will use this term for South Asian Americans born in the U.S., calling out their struggles with cultural identity or accusing them of being "too" assimilated with American culture
Coconut	This term is used to make fun of South Asian Americans who are considered as being "too" assimilated with American culture, while physically appearing South Asian

regionalism and country-to-country discrimination within the broader South Asian American community which can be seen through within-group stereotypes and labeling. For example, stereotypes centered around an individual's physical phenotypic characteristics may perpetuate questions of if the person is "South Asian enough." Offensive labels and stereotypes can also be generational. The term "FOB" or "fresh off the boat" has been used as an offensive term describing first-generation South Asian Americans or newly immigrated relatives in a discriminatory way. Children of immigrants who are born in the U.S. are sometimes called "American Born Confused Desis" (ABCDs) to make fun of their mixed cultural background by calling attention to a potentially complex relationship with immigrant/parental heritage and American culture. As such, South Asian Americans may be forced to consider how much they can express their racial and ethnic identities to the public, which may be at odds with how they feel about themselves internally. Forcing oneself to appear more or less American may cause internal conflict related to identity development and external conflict with one's family or community who may want the individual to internally and externally identify and express their cultural heritage (Dasgupta, 1998; Gupta et al., 2011; Shariff, 2009).

Model Minority Myth

Many South Asian Americans are subject to the Model Minority myth, which states that Asian individuals, as a race, perform well academically and professionally, need minimal external support, and experience low amounts of social and emotional issues (Abraham, 2002; Museus & Kiang, 2009; Yoo & Castro, 2011). The Model Minority myth can show up in a variety of settings, from workplace expectations to students struggling to receive aid from teachers in school (Chae, 2004; Cherng & Liu, 2017). It is also exhibited as individuals not speaking up to authority figures out of fear of "rocking the boat" or having an internalized need to be the "good minority" (Bablak et al., 2016; Lee 2015). The myth can perpetuate the inaccurate belief that South Asian Americans are not "affected" by racism and discrimination, and places an expectation on people within the community to thrive regardless of contextual and situational factors. However, we know that the Model Minority myth and other experiences of racism (including being stereotyped and labeled) can place high levels of pressure on Asian Americans, including South Asian Americans, leading to poor physical and mental health outcomes (Cheah et al., 2020; Hahm et al., 2010; Kim et al., 2017; Wu et al., 2020).

Perceptions and Media Representation of South Asian Americans in the U.S.

Media is one of the few direct glimpses that many non-South Asian Americans have of the South Asian American community. Labels, such as the Model Minority myth, may be a negative label but also have a powerful influence on the perception of the South Asian American identity. The same concept can be applied to other labels, stereotypes, popular media representations, and sociocultural depictions in Western society, which is why the authors chose to delve into media representations of South Asians and South Asian Americans.

One of the most prevalent stereotypes and portrayals of South Asian Americans is the Model Minority myth. This myth has been further refined, to also include stereotypes that all South Asian Americans work in technology or medicine. In the mid-2000s, popular news articles cataloged what was termed the "White flight" of middle to upper-class White folx leaving neighborhoods in the Silicon Valley in the San Francisco Bay area (commonly known as the Bay Area) due to feeling that Asian Americans, including South Asian Americans, were infiltrating their neighborhoods, increasing competition in the local schools, and "stealing" professional/career opportunities from their White children (Huang, 2005). This portrayal of Silicon Valley as an area that is densely packed with South Asian Americans, is not necessarily incorrect, as the Bay Area has one of the highest populations of South Asian Americans in the entire country. However, the transformation of the Bay Area into a technology hub has also reinforced the media stereotype of the "hyper nerdy" and competitive South Asian American engineers and "tech bros" with poor social skills (i.e., Dinesh Chugtai in *Silicon Valley* and Raj Koothrappali in *The Big Bang Theory television series*). Additionally, South Asian American "nerdy" engineers, often played by men, are frequently portrayed as feminine foils and sidekicks who help masculinize and develop the character of the often White main role (Muffuletto, 2018; Thakore, 2016). One notable role that subverts this trope is Aziz Ansari's character in the Netflix show *Master of None*. Ansari's character has a White male sidekick, and he (Ansari) becomes a chef, which is a non-stereotypical South Asian American career path. Additionally, he is darker skinned compared to other South Asian American actors typically seen in popular media and noted to be Tamil, an ethnic identity rarely made visible or distinguished when portraying South Asians. We should also acknowledge that the diverse ethnic groups within various South Asian countries are rarely talked about in popular American media.

With Aziz Ansari being Indian- American and also Muslim, a consideration that aids to address in American media is the problematic and xenophobic history of portraying Brown, Middle Eastern, and Muslim folx as terrorists and religious extremists. This stereotype villainizes individuals who identify as South Asian American, Middle Eastern, and/or are from Islamic communities, greatly impacting the ways these individuals are able to safely display their religious and cultural identities. These portrayals negatively reinforce stereotypes about Islam and also create fear within Muslim and other Brown communities (i.e., Sikhs) who are targeted by hatred and violence.

As South Asian Americans search for the best ways to express their racial, ethnic, and cultural identities, individuals, including media icons, may end up utilizing problematic behavior that appropriates other minoritized communities, particularly Black American communities. While South Asian American creatives and media personalities such as Rajakumari, Lilly Singh, and Rupi Kaur are all trailblazers in terms of the massive platforms they have amassed, all three have also been accused on social media of appropriating and exploiting Black and African American culture (i.e., saying the n-word, wearing blackface and stealing from black poets' writings; Anonymous, 2017; Balram, 2018). It should also be noted that while these three visible icons are females, there are certainly many South Asian American men in popular media who display similar behaviors. The authors of the current chapter (Sharma & Swami) suggest that there is a White supremacist expectation that racial and ethnic minorities suppress parts of their identities or act in familiar (American) culturally sanctioned ways to be accepted and understood by the majority group (i.e., White Americans). While artists, such as the three previously mentioned, exhibit pride in certain aspects of being South Asian, they also appropriate the language, art, etc. of other marginalized communities. Not only is this behavior problematic as it reinforces that South Asian Americans can achieve status or power by appropriating other People of Color, but it also simultaneously highlights some of the struggles with gaining acceptance into the broader American culture. South Asian American identity is complex not only because of the diversity within South Asia but also because of the racial politics and ways in which South Asians consciously or unconsciously navigate their own identities at the expense of other People of Color. Thus, more research is needed to better understand such racial/ethnic and cultural identity nuances.

The problem with media representations is that characters presented on screen are not representative. Often South Asian American individuals are pigeonholed into stereotypes and expectations based on American media representations. American media seems to struggle in allowing for diverse representations of racial and ethnic minority folx. While the stereotypes may be the stories and experiences of some South Asians, they are frequently poorly portrayed and do not leave room for the richness and diversity present among South Asian Americans who have different journeys and experiences. The connection to South Asian American identity, therein, lies in how much South Asian Americans can relate to these representations and how they are forced to navigate U.S. society based on others' assumptions, influenced by one-sided media portrayals. However, there have been positive shifts in representing the lives of South Asian Americans as portrayed in recent shows such as "Never Have I Ever" and "Sex Life of College Girls", produced by Mindy Kaling, in presenting possible lives of second and third-generation stories.

Family and Community

When considering generational differences, it is imperative that we understand the tension between individualism, defined as "having an independent self-construal and striving for one's own best interests" (Lou et al., 2012, p. 664; Phinney et al., 2000), and collectivism, which emphasizes the importance of family and community in the development and understanding of the individual and the decisions they make (Lou et al., 2012). The valuing of family and community is also reflected within Ibrahim et al.'s (1997) model.

Allocentrism, which is often confused with collectivism, is another useful perspective to consider especially for South Asian American communities. Allocentric groups, similar to collectivistic groups, value family and community, but dictate that the individual is interdependent on the community or family (the idea of a "we-self" rather than a "myself"; Farver et al., 2007; Roland, 1996), and that individuals should be more concerned with the needs of the others in the group (family) instead of or at the expense of their own needs (Lay et al., 1998; Maiter & George, 2003). Within an allocentric context, the solo journey that individuals may undertake in an attempt to forge their own identities may be seen as rebellion and interpreted negatively by the individual's family (Somerville & Robinson, 2016). The resulting conflict can lead to stress and tension, given the individual's access to multiple cultural frameworks related to what autonomy and identity look like (Giguère et al., 2010; Lou et al., 2012; Masood et al., 2009). The needs and desires of family and community may overshadow the needs and desires of the individual to explore their interests and develop their various identities. However, balance is difficult to achieve when an individual cannot explore their interests, may want to please their family, and is also being told they are rejecting their culture and values (Alexander et al., 2021). Experiences of racism and pressures that South Asian Americans experience from the outside world may only further complicate this journey.

We see the emergence of various forms of acculturative stress as it relates to family and community for South Asian Americans. Acculturative stress refers to the emotional conflict and pressure that results from negotiating multiple cultural identities (Berry, 1997) and has been associated with diverse mental health outcomes including depression, anxiety, and substance abuse across numerous racial and ethnic minority groups, including South Asian Americans (Hwang & Ting, 2008; Inman et al., 2014; Tummala-Narra et al., 2012). A study by Tummala-Narra et al. (2016), for example, found that acculturative stress experienced by a sample of 16 South Asian American adolescents was negatively associated with psychological well-being and negatively impacted participants' bicultural identity development. Research has also found that family support can help mitigate the mental health impacts of acculturative stress (Tummala-Narra et al., 2012), which is ironic as family can also be a contributor to acculturative stress, depression, and lowered coping ability (Samuel, 2009). Another study by Bhattacharya and Schoppelrey (2004) highlighted a unique acculturative stress experience where many children of first-generation South Asian American immigrant parents are subject to a cultural expectation to perform well in school. This expectation to perform highly creates stress, which can result in youth and adolescents rejecting and subsequently becoming isolated from their family and culture. As such, while family can be an important source of support in the face of stressors, it can also be heavily implicated in acculturative stress.

Individuals feeling the negative impacts of acculturative stress may also try to mitigate its effects by attempting to assimilate into mainstream U.S. culture or separate and immerse themselves into their native culture. However, individuals who are more assimilated into the mainstream U.S. culture or separated from it tend to experience higher levels of mental health issues (Mehta, 1998; Park et al., 2013). More specifically, a study by Needham et al. (2018), using Berry's bicultural model (Berry, 1997), found that South Asian individuals who were more separated from mainstream U.S. culture displayed higher levels of depressive symptoms than individuals who identified as integrated, even after accounting for social support. These results underscore the importance of understanding the different factors that may lead to acculturative stress. Numerous generations can experience acculturative stress (Karasz et al., 2019), which is directly tied to experiences of perceived racial discrimination (Kaduvettoor-Davidson & Inman, 2013; Tummala-Narra et al., 2012). Therefore, context is extremely important when trying to understand identity-based experiences of South Asian Americans.

Case Study Discussion

Anjali's parents were married in India and moved to Chicago, Illinois in the late 1980s, where she was born. As her parents came from modest middle-class backgrounds in India, they were hopeful that by immigrating to the U.S. they may be able to better provide for their children and help to financially support their families (i.e., parents and siblings) back home in India. While both of Anjali's parents voluntarily immigrated to the U.S., they often vocalize their longing for their home country and disapproval of "American" social and familial norms. Although they may describe themselves as being integrated into the mainstream U.S. culture, they often exhibit more of a separated presentation (e.g., identifying more with Asian Indian values and collectivistic cultural traits, while rejecting mainstream U.S. culture, such as more individualistic cultural characteristics). Anjali and her younger brother, who is 20 years old, on the other hand, have been trying to develop a more integrated cultural identity, aiming for a balance between their Indian heritage and mainstream U.S. culture.

While growing up, Anjali and her family had access to their South Asian American community, as there were pockets of South Asian immigrant communities within the Greater Chicago area. While Anjali only visited India a few times during her childhood, her paternal grandparents would often come to visit and stay with her family in the U.S., and recently permanently moved to the U.S. to live with her parents. She used to enjoy her grandparents' visits for all the delicious treats her grandmother would make, such as ladoo and kaju ki barfi (e.g., Indian sweets); however, she would also be frustrated by the language barrier, as they only speak Hindi. While Anjali is receptively bilingual (i.e., when someone is able to understand a second language, such as an English speaker understanding Hindi or Spanish, but is unable to or does not feel comfortable speaking it), she would often be made fun of by her grandparents and extended relatives in India when trying to speak Hindi. Additionally, Anjali has recently noticed what she feels as a "regression" in her parents in terms of attempting to place more "restrictions" on her life. She feels that this is a direct influence of her grandparents, who have more conservative and traditional views. For example, Anjali has lived in her own apartment since graduating from college and has recently encountered conflicts with her parents and grandparents due to her grandparents' views that she should live at home until she is married.

While growing up, Anjali experienced name-calling, such as "ABCD" and "Brownie" from South Asian Americans and non-South Asian Americans alike. Many of Anjali's friends did not identify as South Asian, which often made her feel like an outsider, forcing her to code-switch to fit into the various groups to which she belonged. Teachers frequently placed high academic expectations on Anjali due to her status as an Asian, specifically South Asian, American, and the Model Minority myth, while providing minimal support. Despite struggling in her math classes and receiving limited support from teachers, she was still expected to take accelerated math courses by her parents and teachers.

Given her experiences with stereotyping and labels, here are a few things that we recommend be explored in a clinical setting:

1   How has Anjali been impacted by the stereotypes and labels that have been placed on her by the various groups she has been a part of, such as her family, South Asian American community members, extended family, and non-South Asian peers and teachers, etc.?
2   How may have Anjali internalized these stereotypes and labels? How would this internalization influence her personal identity development?

3   How might these stereotypes and labels present themselves in her romantic relationship with Mark? Are they being perpetuated in the relationship? If yes, then how?

Applying perceptions and the impact of media representation to the case study of Anjali, there are a few different facets of her identity the authors recommend clinicians consider when developing their case conceptualization and treatment plan:

1   What are stereotypes that Anjali has seen in the media that may impact the way she sees herself as a South Asian American, and how have those stereotypes impacted her self-identity and her identity in relation to others? Also, what media figures was she exposed to as a child/teen, as this will influence her identity development?
2   How has Anjali been asked to assimilate, accommodate, or modify who she is based on her significant other's perceptions of who South Asians are? With her partner, Mark, how has his knowledge of South Asian Americans, specifically related to Anjali and her family, been influenced by the media?
3   Thinking about topics such as the Model Minority myth and its pervasive representation on the screen, how does that stereotype fit with or clash with Anjali's identity?
4   How do the portrayals of South Asian Americans in Western media force Anjali to work as a cultural broker with her non-South Asian American friends as well as with her parents, who also see specific representations of South Asians with which they may not agree?

Identity Theories and Application to South Asian American Identity

The historical and social context used to frame this chapter aids in adequately understanding the origins and applications of psychological frameworks that researchers and practitioners can use to support the well-being of South Asian Americans. While there are numerous frameworks through which it is possible to understand identity development, the authors will be focusing on ethnic identity development for South Asian Americans from a family and community perspective with care toward sociopolitical and racist experiences.

South Asian American Identity Development Model

Ibrahim et al. (1997) introduced a culturally specific model focused on South Asian American identity development. The model acknowledges that cultural identity is built upon a social-cultural context, which includes both cultural and religious influences, making the development and understanding of cultural identity a complex process. Additionally, the model highlights that identity development may differ among South Asian American immigrants and South Asian Americans born in the U.S. It proposes that although first-generation South Asian American immigrants may relate more to their home culture as opposed to American culture, they still undergo a dynamic process of racial identity formation due to their context related to immigration, their identities, the sociopolitical climate, and other factors, such as the colonial history of South Asia (Kaduvettoor-Davidson & Weatherford, 2018). The model outlines the immigrant generation's cultural identity development will likely encounter the first stage of *acceptance* of the cultural difference between their home and host (U.S.) culture, without experiencing their cultural identity as a burden or barrier. In the *dissonance* stages, the immigrant generation will begin to experience limitations due to cultural differences from mainstream American culture. In the *resistance and immersion,* or third, stage this generation faces a crisis, tries to reconnect with their home culture, and responds to the mainstream dominant culture with rejection. During the *introspection* stage, individuals experience security in their cultural identity while accepting positive traits of the majority culture. Finally, Ibrahim et al. (1997) describe the *synergistic articulation and awareness* stage as a time when the individual develops a subjective blended cultural identity based on accepting and rejecting characteristics from both the dominant and immigrant cultures.

Ibrahim et al. (1997) noted that future generations born within the U.S. will experience cultural identity development differently from the immigrant generation, which may include negotiation of cultural values, denial, and/or the use of other methods to deal with challenges. Additionally, the model suggests that each progressive generation born in the U.S. will become more acculturated to the dominant culture over time in accordance with their respective identities and sociopolitical contexts. Due to these very different socio-cultural experiences, an individual's generational status would be important to consider when working with a South Asian American client in a clinical setting. Additionally, research has found that for some South Asian American communities (i.e., the Asian Indian American community), racial/ethnic identity development may be a lifelong process (Iwamoto et al., 2013). Such findings may generalize to other South Asian American communities and should be considered within a psychotherapeutic context. Furthermore, Ibrahim et al. (1997) identified six broad cultural characteristics that are believed to overlap across a variety of South Asian American communities (i.e., self-respect/dignity/self-control; respect for family; respect for elders; awareness and respect for community, which at times is considered as a form of extended family; fatalism; and humility). Many of these factors impact identity development and the subsequent well-being of South Asian American individuals.

While this model provides a foundational understanding, it is important to take into consideration the complexities that can influence a South Asian American client's identity development that may not be fully captured by a single model or theory. When trying to understand South Asian American identity, one must acknowledge that it is not a "single" identity. Rather, "South Asian American" is a broad term used to describe multiple cultural identities. As mentioned throughout this chapter, South Asian and South Asian American communities are extremely diverse, with a variety of languages, cultures, traditions, beliefs, nationalities, etc. Thus, a theory focused on the "South Asian American identity" may feel reductionist to those within the community. Identity development is further complicated by individuals' immigration generation and journey as well as their other identities (i.e., gender identity, religious identity, educational background, socio-economic status, etc.). Additionally, this model primarily focused on the Asian Indian and Pakistani American communities, which may limit its generalizability to other South Asian American communities.

Racism and Identity Theories

Critical Race Theory (CRT) is a useful perspective to mention here as it analyzes race and ethnicity in the broader social, political, and historical context in which it has developed (Delgado & Stefancic, 2017). Furthermore, it also emphasizes the socially constructed nature of race, in that race was constructed based on skin color or phenotypic characteristics (O'Hearn, 1998; Chavez et al., 2003), as well as the social distance or power dynamics between various groups of people (Delgado & Stefancic, 2017; Smedley & Smedley, 2005). However, racial and ethnic identity should be thought of as dynamic as it changes across time and context. This is especially important considering the South Asian diaspora to the U.S., as well as the increasing diversity (e.g., socioeconomic statuses, classes, castes, religions, etc.) of the individuals within the South Asian American community. Subsequently, the results of the studies explored in the following section speak to the complicated nature of racial identity development for South Asian Americans from family systems lens, a larger societal perspective, and via experiences of racism.

South Asian American individuals' families play a large role in identity-development related stress, which may stem from the family's fear of their child losing their parents' culture (Inman et al., 2014). However, family can also serve as a protective factor against experiences of discrimination and racism, which, too, can impact mental health and identity development (Iwamoto et al., 2013). Experiences of racism on their own, however, are also ample enough to influence how comfortable South Asian Americans feel in expressing or repressing different parts of their identities. As such, these are two factors that must be considered when understanding the identity-related struggles of South Asian Americans.

Previous racial identity theories, such as those created by Cross (1995), proposed that various races and ethnicities enter life without awareness of race. While this may be true at birth, research has shown that infants as young as three months old can distinguish between their race and other races, demonstrating that racial differences are evident at a physical level (Kelly et al., 2005). Accordingly, the idea of racial identity evolved to reflect the dynamic nature of its evolution from unconscious to conscious (Parham, 1989). Parham (1989), in particular, stated the need for a racially triggering event to foster this progression from unconscious to conscious (e.g., "storm and stress"), an idea that has been endorsed by subsequent authors, such as Quiñones-Rosado (2020). For example, in a phenomenological study that explored the experiences of Asian Indian American participants, researchers found that participants' racial/ethnic identity was developed within their social context, which included their experiences with discrimination, racism, and stereotypes (Iwamoto et al., 2013). Therefore, social context and race-based experiences become salient to the racial identity developmental process. It should be noted, however, that other identity theorists have struck down the idea of a "storm and stress" racial event that triggers racial identity exploration and development (Quintana, 2007).

Quiñones-Rosado (2020) proposed that racial identity can be seen as a developmental process that consists of five stages (i.e., *naive, acceptance, resistance, redefinition,* and *internalization*). In each stage, the child develops their relationship with their identity, which is influenced by their sociopolitical environment, which includes experiences of racism and discrimination. The model describes that during the first stage, *naive* stage, the child is unaware of race and the implications of their own race. Over time and through experience, a child from a minoritized background is exposed to the dominant race and will begin to accept the social portrayal of racial superiority and inferiority. As they enter the *resistance* stage, which may occur in adolescence or adulthood, the individual will begin to experience psychological and emotional distress due to sociopolitical surroundings. This stage is described as a time of questioning, challenging, and/or confronting narratives and others who may comply with a White supremacist culture. Within the *redefinition* stage, the individual begins to reframe and redevelop their narratives of White supremacy, develop a newfound appreciation for their racial community, and create a more self-affirming racial identity, which is guided by individual experience and critical thought. Finally, in the *internalization* stage the individual internalizes their racial identity, which is impacted by sociopolitical-cultural experience as well as their other social identities, such as gender identity, socioeconomic, religious, sexual orientation, etc. (Quiñones-Rosado, 2020).

Numerous studies have found that racism and discrimination impact the physical and mental health of all groups, especially Asian Americans (Cheng, 2020; Ahrens, 2020). Studies specifically focusing on South Asian Americans (first and second generation) also confirm this relationship between perceived discrimination and higher rates of mental health struggles (e.g., increased stress, depression, and lower self-esteem; Kaduvettoor-Davidson & Inman, 2013; Needham et al., 2018; Tummala-Narra et al., 2012). When talking about experiences related to racism and discrimination, South Asian American Muslims, in particular, also must be visualized in an attempt to address the rampant Islamophobia that has existed within the U.S. since the 9/11 terrorist attacks. Much research focusing on individuals who identify as Muslim as well as South Asian American individuals who appear to be Muslim to others confirms the fact that racism exists and impacts their mental health in this particular racialized context (Samari et al., 2018; Verma, 2006).

The results of these studies and others focused on experiences of racism for South Asian Americans also support the theories centered on the complex relationship between social context and ethnic identity. Some studies have shown that higher ethnic identity identification appeared to exacerbate the impact of racial discrimination; yet, the same studies also found the opposite, in which higher ethnic identity can be protective against the negative effects of racial discrimination (French & Chavez, 2010; Greene et al., 2006). The heightened effects are particularly pronounced for individuals who have high ethnic affirmation or pride in their ethnicity (Phinney, 2000), as compared to individuals who have low ethnic affirmation (Greene et al., 2006). Furthermore, we know that experiences of discrimination can impact and sometimes hinder identity development (Okamoto et al., 2009). Therefore, understanding a South Asian American client's experiences of racism and discrimination is imperative when attempting to understand ethnic identity, as they are intrinsically linked.

In the case of Anjali, as a child, she was unaware of her racial differences until she went to school and would get comments from her non-South Asian peers about the color of her skin or her food being "smelly" and "gross." Anjali went through a phase of outwardly resisting her Asian Indian heritage, which put her into conflict with her parents and other South Asian peers. However, over time, she transitioned to the resistance and redefinition stages of questioning and opposing the racist comments from her peers and redefining her relationship with her culture and her non-South Asian peers. As such, it would be helpful to explore with Anjali her experiences with her family, community, and with racism and discrimination to better understand if and how cultural identity is important to Anjali, how to support her cultural identity development, as well as if and how experiences of racism have impacted her identity. Below are some questions the authors recommend exploring with Anjali, particularly, how these events in her life might relate back to her mental health:

1   What does Anjali like or dislike about her South Asian American culture? What elements of her culture and ethnic identity have helped or harmed her in her life? How much does she relate to her ethnic identity?
2   What does Anjali's ethnic culture, religion, caste, etc. look like in her expression of them and in her personal and professional relationships?
3   What has Anjali's personal history/childhood been like with regards to embracing, shunning, or being in conflict with her various cultural identities?
4   What expectations around her gender identity, physical appearance, and culture has she experienced from her non-South Asian American community?
5   What are some salient positive or negative events related to Anjali's ethnic/racial identity that have been formative in her development such as racism or discrimination, as well as family/community events?

Ibrahim et al.'s (1997) model mentions the acceptance phase, which may not apply to Anjali, given that she was born in the U.S. As such, she may not have experienced an acceptance of cultural differences in the way that her parents, who immigrated to the U.S., might have. Similarly, her experience with around acculturation will differ from that of her parents'. Given Anjali's questions and struggles around her multicultural identity, it can be conceptualized that Anjali is currently in the *resistance and immersion* stage within the Ibrahim et al. (1997) identity development model. Furthermore, it can be interpreted that her struggles in this stage are a form of acculturative stress. She has experienced trouble negotiating her Asian Indian and American identities, a struggle that is complicated by her parents' expectations of her. Questions that the clinician may consider include:

1   What is the role that Anjali's family plays in her personal decision -making process?
2   What are Anjali's expectations of her family? What does she feel are her family's expectations of her?
3   Where does she fall along the identity development spectrum? What are some of the challenges Anjali has faced as she tries to reconnect with her home culture?
4   How have these challenges and experiences impacted her relationship with individuals from the dominant culture (American)?
5   What are some of the key struggles and tensions she faces with integrating her multiple identities and how are those struggles influenced by her familial needs and expectations?

Clinical Recommendations

Given the heterogeneity within the South Asian American community, it is important to invite South Asian American clients to share their personal narratives and how they relate to their identities. Thus, approaching the client with cultural humility and developing one's (the clinician's) cultural knowledge can aid in the development of the therapeutic relationship, an essential part of psychotherapeutic healing (Hook et al., 2013; Lo & Fung, 2003; Tervalon & Murray-García, 1998; Vera & Speight, 2003). It can be beneficial to incorporate a multicultural approach (American Psychological Association, 2017; Bernal et al., 2009; Fouad & Arredondo, 2006; Owen et al., 2015; Sue et al., 1992; Sue, 2002) along with other evidence-based interventions (Ibrahim et al., 1997) in therapy with clients from historically minoritized backgrounds, such as South Asian Americans. It is important to note that many South Asian Americans may not consider themselves to be Asian American, making it important for clinicians to be cautious of generalizing recommendations that have been provided for other Asian groups.

Cultural psychotherapy (LaRoche, 2013) is one such approach. The method outlines three phases of therapy. During phase one, therapists may initially take on the role of the "expert," learn the client's language and form of expression, understand their distress, and are encouraged to focus on clients' needs (including setting culturally and spiritually salient therapeutic goals; Ibrahim et al., 1997), safety, as well as harm and symptom reduction with cultural humility and thoughtfulness. By doing so, the therapist can avoid pathologizing behaviors, thoughts, beliefs, and values that are rooted in cultural norms and, instead, incorporate indigenous/culturally salient healing practices along with evidence-based psychotherapies. The second phase in the cultural psychotherapy model centers around the therapist trying to gain a holistic understanding of the client's lived experiences (i.e., individual, relational, and contextual), which parallels Ibrahim et al.'s (1997) clinical recommendations. The second phase is appropriate to begin once it has been confirmed that the client has not had any recent psychological crises, has developed skills for emotional regulation, a trusting therapeutic relationship has been developed, and the client is comfortable challenging the therapist. The final phase is focused on promoting client empowerment. It must be noted that many clients drop out of therapy prior to phase three. This stage of therapy is largely influenced by the client exploring and acting on their desire to bring change to unjust social situations. Cultural psychotherapy provides a variety of recommendations for clinicians to utilize in supporting their clients in this phase (Refer to LaRoche, 2013 for the detailed approach). More recent psychotherapeutic approaches parallel LaRoche's (2013) phase three, encouraging mental health professionals to promote (radical) healing in minoritized clients by taking a strengths-based approach and supporting clients in acting toward social change and against oppressive situations (French et al., 2020).

Another approach that the authors recommend incorporating is liberation psychotherapy, which aims to decolonize mental health. Decolonization in this context refers to increasing awareness of and moving away from a Euro-American, White, colonial-centric foundation of psychology and psychological healing and toward honoring and including diverse cultural perspectives that have often been ignored in psychology such as those of Black, Indigenous, and People of Color cultures/communities, as well as reclaiming psychological healing (Bhatia, 2020). Liberation psychotherapy acknowledges that minoritized communities carry with them intergenerational and oppression-related trauma, such as postcolonial stress disorder (Comas-Díaz, 2020). In order to promote healing in a culturally humble way, it is vital for clinicians to incorporate indigenous and culturally salient healing practices into psychotherapy with cultural minorities, such as South Asian Americans (Ibrahim et al., 1997). This could include psycho-spiritual healing, the incorporation of cultural arts in therapy, and the development of a mutually impactful relationship with the client (Comas-Díaz, 2020). For example, a clinician supporting an elderly Pakistani Sikh immigrant woman presenting with depressive symptoms may explore how incorporating the client's spiritual practices of going to the local gurdwara (e.g., Sikh temple) could promote social connection, behavioral activation, and increase positive emotions. From the authors' (Sharma & Swami) collective clinical experiences and research, Table 4.2 provides a summary of broad clinical recommendations for supporting South Asian Americans.

In the case of Anjali, the therapist assigned to work with Anjali identified as a cisgender second-generation Asian Indian American woman in her 40s. Her therapeutic work was guided by a Relational Cultural approach as well as a cultural psychotherapy model, as outlined in the chapter. The clinician met with Anjali for a total of 60 sessions over the course of a year and a half. During the initial sessions with Anjali, the therapist focused on addressing any crises or urgent symptoms, building culturally sensitive rapport, making space to discuss differences and similarities between the two of them, and exploring Anjali's narrative as a South Asian American woman. While the client and therapist shared a lot of cultural similarities, the therapist was thoughtful to not make assumptions about Anjali's experiences.

Through the process of careful exploration, the therapist and Anjali together decided to focus on helping Anjali explore and build a relationship with her cultural identity, while also addressing her feelings of guilt and shame for being neither American nor Asian Indian enough. To begin the journey, the therapist went through the Cultural Identity Checklist-Revised (CICL-R; Ibrahim, 2016) with Anjali to invite a space of reflection. She also provided the client with psychoeducation about therapy and cultural identity development through discussions throughout the sessions. As therapy progressed, Anjali was guided to reflect on her experiences with racism, sexism, cultural expectations from family and friends, and her current interracial and multicultural romantic relationship. She was encouraged to explore how these experiences may relate back to her blended cultural identity development. The therapist used a cost-benefit analysis intervention to support Anjali in exploring the

Table 4.2 Clinical Recommendations for Psychotherapy with South Asian Americans in Exploring Identity

The Role of questions in therapy	It is helpful to keep the following factors in mind when presenting questions to a South Asian American client: the client's age, gender identity, current class, and class background, educational level, profession, role in family, immigration status, and level of acculturation. This list is not exhaustive but provides a starting point for clinicians. Additionally, it may be helpful for the clinician to explore the client's comfort in questioning authority and people in power (i.e., parents, elders, teachers, doctors, and religious leaders) when they disagree. These factors may also influence the client's comfort in asking questions in therapy.
Family involvement	It is important for the clinician to be aware and thoughtful of if and when it may be appropriate to involve other family members in the client's healing journey. Accessing formal mental health treatment is highly stigmatized in South Asian communities, and so clients may steer away from family involvement. The authors suggest that clinicians maintain a culturally humble approach and avoid potential assumptions and stereotypes of South Asian American families. Contrastingly, the insistence on boundaries between the client and family may lead to conflict for the client (Durvasula & Mylvaganam, 1994). Thus, it is important to work with the client without making assumptions about their relationship with family and community, as well as desired external involvement.
Psychoeducation	A client may be unfamiliar with therapy and its expectations, making psychoeducation, or education on the therapeutic process, the presenting concerns, and subsequent treatment (Dahl et al., 2020) a powerful tool and intervention to incorporate into the healing journey, especially in the beginning treatment. Such an approach can help facilitate the client's understanding of therapy (Segal, 1991). Furthermore, it can also help combat cultural stigma that might be associated with formal mental health services. In the cultural psychotherapy model, LaRoche (2013) states that during the beginning of therapy, it may be necessary for the clinician to take the stance of the expert when developing a culturally sensitive therapeutic alliance. For example, a therapist could validate the client's hesitation to talk about their emotions (i.e., you may not feel comfortable talking about your feelings as it is not often encouraged in society).
Identity exploration	Therapy can be a place for the client to explore their personal cultural identity, views, and values (Shariff, 2009). It may be helpful for the psychotherapist to guide the client in conducting a cost-benefit analysis (e.g., outline the advantages and disadvantages) of their various cultural identities, as they explore an authentic way of blending these identities (Shariff, 2009, p. 39), while being aware that identities are fluid and ever-changing.
Role play	While western base therapists may encourage clients to potentially confront individuals in their lives who may be contributing to the client's distress, that may not feel safe, respectful, or culturally salient to an individual from the South Asian American community. For this reason and others, it may be helpful to include role play in therapy, such as the Gestalt two-chair technique. This approach can also help individuals who are struggling with identity-related issues (Shariff, 2009, p. 39). Such methods can provide the client a safe space to practice difficult conversations, increase confidence in verbalizing their thoughts, and confront potential undesired relational dynamics. Additionally, the role playing can be beneficial to the client regardless of them acting it out in reality, as it can provide an emotional release in a contained and safe environment

cultural values and characteristics that feel more salient to her personal cultural identity. As she became more confident with her cultural identity, Anjali expressed interest in wanting to respectfully share her relationship with Mark with her parents. Over multiple sessions, the therapist incorporated various role-playing exercises, including the Gestalt two-chair technique. This provided Anjali with a safe space to experience emotional release, process her fears around talking to her parents, and practice her conversations to feel prepared to talk to her parents. After about one and half years in therapy, Anjali made significant progress in feeling more confident and comfortable with her Asian Indian American cultural identity and began to have conversations to help bridge the gap between herself and her parents to empathetically understand each other's cultural identity experiences. The therapist and Anjali continued working together on different therapeutic goals.

Challenges and Complicating Factors in the Clinical Treatment

There were several challenges that were encountered throughout the course of therapy. Initially, Anjali expressed concerns with privacy, given that the therapist and client were a part of the same cultural community, despite the clinician's assurance of professionalism and rules around confidentiality and privacy. Additionally, the client worried that the clinician may judge her emotional struggles, relationship with her parents, and opinions/grievance with her elders. Anjali was hesitant to disclose personal details, reactions, and opinions. The clinician noticed the client's hesitation and addressed it by using a process comment (i.e., stating the observation of what was happening in the therapeutic space; Tasca et al., 2014) and provided reassurance to the client. She also normalized Anjali's fears and worries about therapy. The therapist also used appropriate self-disclosure to strengthen the therapeutic relationship as well as to create a safe and trusting space (LaRoche, 2013). Within the initial ten sessions, the client expressed frustration with not seeing improvement at a faster speed. The clinician normalized and validated Anjali's frustration as well as provided her with education about the process of therapy to help her develop realistic therapeutic expectations. Other challenges included Anjali feeling empowered following role-playing scenarios in the clinical setting, but then feeling defeated and resistant to therapy after her real-life conversations with her parents did not go as intended. The therapist normalized these occurrences, validated Anjali's difficulty in broaching issues with her parents, and acknowledged her courage in taking the steps to do something she had not previously done.

Reflection Questions

1   What type of experiences have you had in working with South Asian Americans in counseling?
2   Regarding South Asian American identity, what areas do you feel you need to learn more about?
3   What difficulties do you anticipate in working with Anjali as a client?

Summary

The current chapter provided a general overview of the history of South Asian American immigration in the U.S., stereotypes and labels, and popular media depictions in relation to South Asian American identities. It also explored various identity development theories, including Ibrahim et al.'s (1997) South Asian American identity development model, acculturative stress, and the effects of racism and discrimination on racial and ethnic identity development. Finally, the authors provided clinical recommendations for mental health professionals to consider when working with South Asian American clients. We followed Anjali's experiences throughout the chapter to explore the concepts that were discussed. Her experiences are only one of numerous that South Asian Americans may have, given the diversity of race, ethnicity, socioeconomic status, caste, religion, and language, to name a few, present within the community. We emphasize that clinicians working with South Asian Americans maintain a humble and open perspective as well as a willingness to learn about the various intersectional issues impacting South Asian Americans and their identity development, especially within the broader sociopolitical context. The authors (Sharma & Swami) suggest that individuals working with South Asian American clients seek culturally relevant training, supervision, and consultation, such as through the Division on South Asian Americans and/or by connecting with South Asian American clinicians. The experiences of South Asian Americans have been historically invisible and swept into generalizations about Asian Americans. However, we cannot ignore that racial and ethnic identity development will always be largely influenced by social contexts. As such, we hope that this chapter provides an introduction to the increasing complexity of South Asian American identities that are ripe for exploration

Suggested Resources

Books

*   Bhatia, S. (2007). *American karma: Race, culture, and identity in the India diaspora.* New York University Press.
*   Ibrahim. F.A & Heuer, J.R. (2016). *Cultural and social justice counseling: Client-specific interventions.* Springer
*   Iyer, D. (2017). *We too sing America: South Asian, Arab, Muslim, and Sikh immigrants shape our multiracial future.* The New Press.

Organizations

*   SAALT: South Asian Americans Leading Together (https://saalt.org/)

References

Abraham, M. (2002). Addressing domestic violence among South Asians in the United States. *Hofstra Horizons, Fall 2002*, 12–16.

Ahrens, R.P. (2020). Statement before the house ways and means committee on "The Disproportionate Impact of COVID-19 on Communities of Color". *COVID-19 impact on Asian American and Pacific Islander Mental and Physical Health.* Retrieved from https://waysandmeans.house.gov/sites/democrats.waysandmeans.house.gov/files/documents/OCA%20Testimony.pdf

Alexander, A.J., Khera, G.S., & Bedi, R.P. (2021). Bicultural identity and self-construal in-family among Indian American emerging adults: A mixed-methods study. *Journal of Adult Development*, *28*, 1–14. 10.1007/s10804-020-09356-y

American Psychological Association. (2017). Multicultural guidelines: An ecological approach to context, identity, and intersectionality. Retrieved from http://www.apa.org/about/policy/multicultural-guidelines.pdf

Anonymous (2017, October 15). *The problem with Priyanka Chopra and South Asian anti-Blackness.* Wear Your Voice Mag. https://www.wearyourvoicemag.com/the-problem-with-priyanka-chopra-south-asian/

Bablak, L., Raby, R., & Pomerantz, S. (2016). 'I don't want to stereotype ... but it's true': Maintaining whiteness at the centre through the smart Asian stereotype in high school. *Whiteness and Education*, *1*(1), 54–68. 10.1080/13613324.2015.1122661

Balram, D. (2018, December 14). *Anti-blackness in South Asian communities – how do we break the cycle?* Media Diversified. https://mediadiversified.org/2018/12/14/anti-blackness-in-south-asian-communities-how-do-we-break-the-cycle/

Bernal, G., Jiménez-Chafey, M.I., & Domenech Rodríguez, M.M. (2009). Cultural adaptation of treatments: A resource for considering culture in evidence-based practice. *Professional Psychology: Research and Practice*, *40*(4), 361–368. 10.1037/a0016401

Berry, J.W. (1997). Immigration, acculturation, and adaptation. *Applied Psychology: An International Review*, *46*(1), 5–68. 10.1111/j.1464-0597.1997.tb01087.x

Bhatia, S. (2020). Decolonizing psychology: Power, citizenship and identity. *Psychoanalysis, Self and Context*, *15*(3), 257–266. 10.1080/24720038.2020.1772266

Bhatia, S., & Ram, A. (2018). South Asian immigration to United States: A brief history within the context of race, politics, and identity. In M. J. Perera, & E. C. Chang (Eds.), *Cross-cultural research in health, illness and well-being: Vol. 1. Biopsychosocial approaches to understanding health in South Asian Americans* (pp. 15–32). Springer International Publishing. 10.1007/978-3-319-91120-5_2

Bhattacharya, G., & Schoppelrey, S.L. (2004). Preimmigration beliefs of life success, postimmigration experiences, and acculturative stress: South Asian immigrants in the United States. *Journal of Immigrant Health*, *6*(2), 83–92. 10.1023/B:JOIH.0000019168.75062.36

Chae, H.S. (2004). Talking back to the Asian model minority discourse: Korean-origin youth experiences in high school. *Journal of Intercultural Studies*, *25*(1), 59–73. 10.1080/07256860410001687027

Chavez, A.F., Guido-DiBrito, F., & Mallory, S.L. (2003). Learning to value the "other": A framework of individual diversity development. *Journal of College Student Development*, *44*(4), 453–469. 10.1353/csd.2003.0038

Cheah, C.S., Wang, C., Ren, H., Zong, X., Cho, H.S., & Xue, X. (2020). COVID-19 racism and mental health in Chinese American families. *Pediatrics*, *146*(5). 10.1542/peds.2020-021816

Cheng, H.-L. (2020). Xenophobia and racism against Asian Americans during the COVID-19 pandemic: Mental health implications. *Journal of Interdisciplinary Perspectives and Scholarship*, *3*(3). https://repository.usfca.edu/jips/vol3/iss1/3

Cherng, H.-Y. S., & Liu, J.-L. (2017). Academic social support and student expectations: The case of second-generation Asian Americans. *Asian American Journal of Psychology*, *8*(1), 16–30. 10.1037/aap0000072

Comas-Díaz, L. (2020). Liberation psychotherapy. In L. Comas-Díaz & E. Torres Rivera (Eds.), *Cultural, racial, and ethnic psychology book series. Liberation psychology: Theory, method, practice, and social justice* (pp. 53–68). American Psychological Association. 10.1037/0000198-004

Cross, W.E., Jr. (1995). *The psychology of nigrescence: Revising the Cross model.* In J. G. Ponterotto, J. M. Casas, L. A. Suzuki, & C. M. Alexander (Eds.), *Handbook of multicultural counseling* (pp. 93–122). Sage Publications.

Dahl, V., Ramakrishnan, A., Spears, A.P., Jorge, A., Bigio, N.A., & Chacko, A. (2020). Psychoeducation interventions for parents and teachers of children and adolescents with ADHD: a systematic review of the literature. *Journal of Developmental and Physical Disabilities*, *32*(2), 257–292. https://doi-org.hmlproxy.lib.csufresno.edu/10.1007/s10882-019-09691-3

Dasgupta, S.R. (1998). Gender roles and cultural continuity in the Asian Indian immigrant community the U.S. *Sex Roles: A Journal of Research*, *38*(11–12), 953–974. 10.1023/A:1018822525427

Delgado, R. & Stefancic, J. (2017). *Critical race theory (Third Edition).* New York: New York University Press. 10.18574/9781479851393

Durvasula, R.S. & Mylvaganam, G.A. (1994). Mental health of asian Indians: Relevant issues and community implications. *Journal of Community Psychology*, *22*, 97–108.

Farver, J.M., Xu, Y., Bhadha, B., Narang, S., & Lieber, E. (2007). Ethnic identity, acculturation, parenting beliefs, and adolescent adjustment: A comparison of Asian Indian and European American families. *Merrill-Palmer Quarterly*, *53*(2), 184–215. 10.1353/mpq.2007.0010

Fouad, N.A. & Arredondo, P. (2006). *Becoming culturally oriented: Practice advice for psychologists and educators.* American Psychological Association.

French, S.E., & Chavez, N.R. (2010). The relationship of ethnicity-related stressors and Latino ethnic identity to well-being. *Hispanic Journal of Behavioral Sciences, 32*(3), 410–428. 10.1177/073 9986310374716

French, B.H., Lewis, J.A., Mosley, D.V., Adames, H.Y., Chavez-Dueñas, N.Y., Chen, G.A., & Neville, H.A. (2020). Toward a psychological framework of radical healing in communities of color. *The Counseling Psychologist, 48*(1), 14–46. 10.1177/0011000019843506

Giguère, B., Lalonde, R., & Lou, E. (2010). Living at the crossroads of cultural worlds: The experience of normative conflicts by second generation immigrant youth. *Social and Personality Psychology Compass, 4*(1), 14–29. 10.1111/j.1751-9004.2009.00228.x

Greene, M.L., Way, N., & Pahl, K. (2006). Trajectories of perceived adult and peer discrimination among Black, Latino, and Asian American adolescents: Patterns and psychological correlates. *Developmental Psychology, 42*(2), 218–236. 10.1037/0012-1649.42.2.218

Gupta, A., Szymanski, D.M., & Leong, F.T.L. (2011). The "model minority myth": Internalized racialism of positive stereotypes as correlates of psychological distress, and attitudes toward help-seeking. *Asian American Journal of Psychology, 2*(2), 101–114. 10.1037/a0024183

Hahm, H.C., Ozonoff, A., Gaumond, J., & Sue, S. (2010). Perceived discrimination and health outcomes: A gender comparison among Asian-Americans nationwide. *Women's Health, 20*(5), 350–358. 10.1016/j.whi.2010.05.002

Hook, J.N., David, D.E., Owen, J. Worthington, E.L., & Utsey, S.O. (2013). Cultural humility: Measuring openness to culturally diverse clients. *Journal of Counseling Psychology, 60*(3), 353–366. 10.1037/a0032595

Huang, S. (2005). The new white flight. *The Wall Street Journal.* Retrieved from https://www.wsj.com/articles/SB113236377590902105

Hwang, W.C., & Ting, J.Y. (2008). Disaggregating the effects of acculturation and acculturative stress on the mental health of Asian Americans. *Cultural Diversity and Ethnic Minority Psychology, 14*(2), 147–154. 10.1037/1099-9809.14.2.147

Ibrahim, F.A. (2016). Appendix A: Cultural identity check-list-revised. F. A. Ibrahim & J. R. Heuer (Eds.), *Cultural and social justice counseling: Client-specific interventions* (pp. 239–240). Springer International Publishing.

Ibrahim, F.A., Ohnishi, H., & Sandhu D.S. (1997). Asian American Identity development: A culture specific model for South Asian Americans. *Journal of Multicultural Counseling and Development, 25*, 34–50. 10.1002/j.2161-1912.1997.tb00314.x

Inman, A.G., Devdas, L., Spektor, V., & Pendse, A. (2014). Psychological research on South Asian Americans: A three-decade content analysis. *Asian American Journal of Psychology, 5*, 364–372. 10.1037/a0035633

Iwamoto, D.K., Negi, N.J., Partiali, R.N., & Creswell J.W. (2013). The racial and ethnic identity formation process of second-generation Asian Indian Americans: A phenomenological study. *Journal of Multicultural Counseling and Development, 41*(4), 224–239. 10.1002/j.2161-1912.2013.00038.x

Karasz, A., Gany, F., Escobar, J., Flores, C., Prasad, L., Inman, A., Kalasapudi, V., Kosi, R., Murthy, M., Leng, J. & Diwan, S., (2019). Mental health and stress among South Asians. *Journal of Immigrant and Minority Health, 21*(1), 7–14. 10.1007/s10903-016-0501-4

Kaduvettoor-Davidson, A., & Inman, A.G. (2013). South Asian Americans: Perceived discrimination, stress, and well-being. *Asian American Journal of Psychology, 4*(3), 155–165. 10.1037/a003 0634

Kaduvettoor-Davidson, A., & Weatherford, R.D. (2018). South Asian identity in the United States. In M. J. Perera & E. C. Chang (Eds.), *Cross-cultural research in health, illness and well-being: Vol. 1. Biopsychosocial approaches to understanding health in South Asian Americans* (p. 33–49). Springer International Publishing. 10.1007/978-3-319-91120-5_3

Kelly, D.J., Quinn, P.C., Slater, A.M., Lee, K., Gibson, A., Smith, M., Ge, L., & Pascalis, O. (2005). Three-month-olds, but not newborns, prefer own-race faces. *Developmental Science, 8*(6), F31–F36. 10.1111/j.1467-7687.2005.0434a.x

Kim, P.Y., Kendall, D.L., & Cheon, H.S. (2017). Racial microaggressions, cultural mistrust, and mental health outcomes among asian american college students. *American Journal of Orthopsychiatry*, *87*(6), 663–670. 10.1037/ort0000203

LaRoche, M.J. (2013). *Cultural psychotherapy. Theory, methods and practice*. Sage.

Lay, C., Fairlie, P., Jackson, S., Ricci, T., Eisenberg, J., Sato, T., Teeaar, A., & Melamud, A. (1998). Domain-specific allocentrism-idiocentrism: A measure of family connectedness. *Journal of Cross-Cultural Psychology*, *29*(3), 434–460. 10.1177/0022022198293004

Lee, S.J. (2015). *Unraveling the "model minority" stereotype: Listening to Asian American youth*. Teachers College Press.

Lo, H.-T., & Fung, K.P. (2003). Culturally competent psychotherapy. *The Canadian Journal of Psychiatry*, *48*(3), 161–170. 10.1177/070674370304800304

Lou, E., Lalonde, R.N., & Giguère B. (2012). Making the decision to move out: Bicultural young adults and the negotiation of cultural demands and family relationships. *Journal of Cross-Cultural Psychology*, *43*(5), 663–670. 10.1177/0022022112443414

Maiter, S., & George, U. (2003). Understanding context and culture in the parenting approaches of immigrant South Asian mothers. *Affilia*, *18*(4), 411–428. 10.1177/0886109903257589

Masood, N., Okazaki, S., & Takeuchi, D.T. (2009). Gender, family, and community correlates of mental health in South Asian Americans. *Cultural Diversity and Ethnic Minority Psychology*, *15*, 265–274. 10.1037/a0014301

Mehta, S. (1998). Relationship between acculturation and mental health for Asian Indian immigrants in the United States. *Social & General Psychology Monographs*, *24*(1), 61–78.

Muffuletto, S.L. (2018). Effects of American media representation of South Asian Americans. *Digital Access to Scholarship at Harvard*. Retrieved from http://nrs.harvard.edu/urn-3:HUL. InstRepos:37799749

Museus, S.D. & Kiang, P.N. (2009). Deconstructing the model minority myth and how it contributes to the invisible minority reality in higher education research. *New Directions for Institutional Research*, *142*, 5–15. 10.1002/ir.292

Needham, B.L., Mukherjee, B., Bagchi, P., Kim, C., Mukherjea, A., Kandula, N.R., & Kanaya, A.M. (2018). Acculturation strategies and symptoms of depression: The Mediators of Atherosclerosis in South Asians Living in America (MASALA) Study. *Journal of Immigrant and Minority Health*, *20*(4), 792–798. 10.1007/s10903-017-0635-z

O'Hearn, C.C. (1998). *Half and half: Writers on growing up biracial and bicultural*. Pantheon.

Okamoto, J., Ritt-Olson, A., Soto, D., Baezconde-Garbanati, L., & Unger, J.B. (2009). Perceived discrimination and substance use among Latino adolescents. *American Journal of Health Behavior*, *33*(6), 718–727. 10.5993/ajhb.33.6.9

Owen, J., Tao, K.W., Drinane, J.M., Hook, J., Davis, D.E., & Kune, N.F. (2015). Client perceptions of therapists' multicultural orientation: Cultural (missed) opportunities and cultural humility. *Professional Psychology: Research and Practice*, *47*(1), 30–37. 10.1037/pro0000046

Parham, T.A. (1989). Cycles of psychological Nigrescence. *The Counseling Psychologist*, *17*(2), 187–226. 10.1177/0011000089172001

Park, I.J.K., Schwartz, S.J., Lee, R.M., Kim, M., & Rodriguez, L. (2013). Perceived racial/ethnic discrimination and antisocial behaviors among Asian American college students: Testing the moderating roles of ethnic and American identity. *Cultural Diversity and Ethnic Minority Psychology*, *19*(2), 166–176. 10.1037/a0028640

Phinney, J.S., Ong, A., & Madden, T. (2000). Cultural values and intergenerational value discrepancies in immigrant and non-immigrant families. *Child Development*, *71*(2), 528–539. 10.1111/1467-8624. 00162

Quiñones-Rosado, R. (2020). Liberation psychology and racism. In L. Comas-Díaz & E. Torres Rivera (Eds.), *Cultural, racial, and ethnic psychology book series. Liberation psychology: Theory, method, practice, and social justice* (pp. 53–68). American Psychological Association. 10.1037/ 0000198-004

Quintana, S.M. (2007). Racial and ethnic identity: Developmental perspectives and research. *Journal of Counseling Psychology*, *54*(3), 259–270. 10.1037/0022-0167.54.3.259

Roland, A. (1996). *Cultural pluralism and psychoanalysis: The Asian and North American experience*. Routledge.

Samari, G., Alcalá, H.E., & Sharif, M.Z. (2018). Islamophobia, health, and public health: A systematic literature review. *American Journal of Public Health, 108*(6), e1–e9. 10.2105/AJPH.2018. 304402

Samuel, E. (2009). Acculturative stress: South Asian immigrant women's experiences in Canada's Atlantic provinces. *Journal of Immigrant & Refugee Studies, 7*(1), 16–34. 10.1080/15562940802 687207

Segal, U.A. (1991). Cultural variables in Asian Indian families. *Families in Society, 72*(4), 233–241. 10.1177/104438949107200406

Shariff, A. (2009). Ethnic identity and parenting stress in South Asian families: Implications for culturally sensitive counselling. *Canadian Journal of Counselling, 43*(1), 35–46. https://cjc-rcc. ucalgary.ca/article/view/58908

Smedley, A., & Smedley, B.D. (2005). Race as biology is fiction, racism as a social problem is real: Anthropological and historical perspectives on the social construction of race. *American Psychologist, 60*(1), 16–26. 10.1037/0003-066X.60.1.16

Somerville, K., & Robinson, O. (2016). Keeping up appearances within the ethnic community: A disconnect between first and second generation South Asians' educational aspirations. *Canadian Ethnic Studies, 48*(2), 99–117. 10.1353/ces.2016.0015

Sue, D. (2002). *Multicultural therapy: Encyclopedia of Psychotherapy*. Elsevier Science.

Sue, D.W., Arredondo, R., & McDavis, R.J. (1992). Multicultural counseling competencies and standards: A call to the profession. *Journal of Multicultural Counseling and Development, 20*, 64–88. 10.1002/j.2161-1912.1992.tb00563.x

Tasca, G.A., Francis, K., & Balfour, L. (2014). Group psychotherapy levels of interventions: A clinical process commentary. *Psychotherapy, 51*(1), 25–29. 10.1037/a0032520

Tervalon, M. & Murray-García, J. (1998). Cultural humility verses cultural competence: A critical distinction in defining physician training outcomes in multicultural education. *Journal of Health Care for the Poor and Underserved, 9*(2), 117–125. https://muse.jhu.edu/article/268076

Thakore, B.K. (2016). *South Asians on the U.S. Screen: Just Like Everyone Else?* Lexington Books.

Tummala-Narra, P., Alegria, M., & Chen, C.-N. (2012). Perceived discrimination, acculturative stress, and depression among South Asians: Mixed findings. *Asian American Journal of Psychology, 3*(1), 3–16. 10.1037/a0024661

Tummala-Narra, P., Deshpande, A., & Kaur, J. (2016). South Asian adolescents' experiences of acculturative stress and coping. *American Journal of Orthopsychiatry, 86*(2), 194–211. 10.1037/ ort0000147

Vera, E.M., & Speight, S.L. (2003). Multicultural competence, social justice, and counseling psychology: Expanding our roles. *The Counseling Psychologist, 31*(3), 253–272. 10.1177/0011000003 031003001

Verma, R. (2006). Trauma, cultural survival and identity politics in a post-9/11 era: Reflections by Sikh youth. *Sikh Formations: Religion, Culture, Theory, 2*(1), 89–101. 10.1080/17448720600779877

Wu, C., Qian, Y., & Wilkes, R. (2020). Anti-Asian discrimination and the Asian-white mental health gap during COVID-19. *Ethnic and Racial Studies, 44*(5), 819–835. 10.1080/01419870.2020.1851739

Yoo, H.C., & Castro, K.S. (2011). Does nativity status matter in the relationship between perceived racism and academic performance of Asian American college students? *Journal of College Student Development, 52*, 234–245. 10.1353/csd.2011.0031

5 South Asian American Multiracial, Multi-Heritage, and Diaspora Identities

Jude Bergkamp, Sarika Persaud, Aishwarya Lonikar, and Anastasia Khan

Case Overview

Lakshmi is a 41-year-old Indo-Trinidadian woman residing in an urban area of the Northeastern U.S. She has a husband, Rajiv, 35, and a son, Vijay, 13, who was born in the U.S. Lakshmi and Rajiv both identify as Hindu, and are both first-generation immigrants, from Trinidad & Tobago and Guyana, respectively. They are both of South Asian ancestry. Lakshmi sought psychotherapy to help to deal with the stress and anxiety of ongoing court proceedings, which she managed without assistance from family, friends, or legal counsel. Lakshmi recently had a case filed against her anonymously with Child Protective Services (CPS), where she was under risk of being deemed psychologically unfit to care for her son.

Introduction

The growth of the South Asian population in the U.S. (SAALT, 2019) points to the likelihood that the demand for mental health services will increase, and clinicians will be called upon to provide culturally sensitive treatment. While the cultural differences between South Asian American individuals is already vast, this chapter takes up the challenge to explore an even deeper level of distinction, that of multi-racial, multi-heritage, and diaspora identities. It is important to consider the historical thrust of colonization across the globe, the formation of diaspora communities, and the inevitability of multi-racial heritages (Oonk, 2007). Questions of identity development and the psychological impact of movement from a cultural homeland in the midst of these migrant waves are central to the field of psychology (Chandra, 2011). It is important for clinicians to have an appreciation of the impact of colonization, the multitude of migrant journeys, and the multiracial and diaspora identities of the South Asian and South Asian American clients they serve.

While many chapters have addressed the South Asian American community as a whole, this chapter explores the variations of South Asian identity that have been shaped by multicultural, multi-heritage, and diaspora communities. The case study Lakshmi will explore and focus on Indo-Caribbean South Asian American identities and experiences. Through the case study, clinical themes and interventions will be explored. This chapter will explore the impact of coloniality for South Asian multicultural, multi-heritage, and diaspora individuals currently living in the U.S.

Terms and Definitions

The interactive levels of cultural and ethnic difference within and between the South Asian American population can be astonishing. As mentioned, the focus of this chapter is on the

DOI: 10.4324/9781003081548-5

aspects of South Asian and South Asian American individuals that identify as multi-heritage, multi-racial, and part of the diaspora journey influenced by historic colonial forces. Terms and definitions can be helpful in understanding the influences upon the individual, providing a conceptual mapping that is essential for culturally sensitive assessment and treatment. Yet, there is also a risk in applying terms to an individual in a manner that is not congruent with their own identification. As such, the authors encourage a balance of conceptual understanding and cultural humility when working with this population.

Multi-Racial and Multi-Heritage

For purposes of this chapter, race is considered the external phenotypic perception used for categorization and resultant social privilege allocation. This occurs at all levels of categorization including interpersonal, family, community, institutional, and systemic.

Multi-Racial

Multi-racial means that an individual's parents represent two or more distinct races that have come together. Traditionally, multi-racial relationships have been restricted under the guise of eugenic principles of racial purity. Historically, social shame has been leveraged to socially engineer bloodline continuity. Thus, multi-racial individuals have historically lived on the margins and have experienced a distinct form of racism, ostracized by both parts of their racial communities (Poston, 1990; Rockquemore et al., 2009; Root, 1998; Stonequist, 1937). First, second, or third generation immigrants can have both multi-heritage and multi-racial aspects to their identities. In addition, the diaspora dynamic inherently involves multi-heritage nature that adds the complexity of identity development, personal experience, relationship issues, and psychological functioning.

Multi-Heritage

Multi-heritage refers to the blending and clashing of two or more distinct cultural influences that impact the formulation of an individual's identity development and inform their values and morals (Yampolsky et al., 2013). This can include the geographic influence of living in two different regions of the world in a single lifetime, or two individuals from very different cultures joining together establishing an intimate and familial relationship, and the child of such a union receiving culturally different messages from their parents.

DIASPORA

The term diaspora refers to the reconstruction of communities of migrant individuals, attempting to hold true to their cultural heritage while inhabiting a new country and culture and Toloyan (1996) makes an important distinction in that people living outside their ancestral land are not necessarily diasporic in nature, as they may pursue the full acculturation into their current lived country. In contrast, diaspora communities fled the despoliation of indigenous resources and assets of their homeland in an attempt to retain and re-establish parts of their traditions, customs, and structures once settled in a new place. It is imperative that clinicians attempt to understand an individual's migration journey and the diaspora drive and dynamics to provide effective clinical care.

IMMIGRANT EXPERIENCES

First Generation Immigrant Experience   As the term connotes, a first generation immigrant is an individual who was born and naturalized in their country of origin prior to immigration (Choules, 2006; Golash-Boza, 2016; Tummala-Narra, 2021). In some cases, South Asians may come to the U.S. in early adulthood in search of promising employment. Others who may be fleeing a natural disaster or political turmoil may arrive later in life, causing increasing personal upheaval. And children may find themselves in this confusing transition, without a clear understanding of the circumstances and loss (Daftary, 2020). Considering the developmental stage at the time of immigration can be useful in informing the individual's experience and impact of this major life transition (Tummala-Narra, 2021).

Second Generation Immigrant Experience   The children of immigrants to the U.S. have naturalized citizenship by birth. The families of these individuals have various degrees of acculturation and may or may not hold true to the customs and traditions of their homeland. Inevitably, these individuals straddle two cultures and hold numerous contradictions that elude those with homogeneous cultural identities. Second generation people have the unmapped task of constructing an identity under the dual gaze of their Western counterparts and their expectant family.

Third Generation Immigrant Experience   In addition, as authors we understand it is also important to consider third generation South Asian American experiences where the individual is U.S.-born with two U.S.-born parents with at least one foreign-born grandparent. The chapter will focus on first and second generation South Asian immigrant experiences.

In some cases, South Asians may come to the U.S. in early adulthood in search of promising employment or better educational opportunities for their children, as in the case of Lakshmi described above. While Indo-Caribbean immigrants such as Lakshmi did not have to contend with a language barrier to acculturation (however some may have dealt with language barriers), as Indo-Caribbean people primarily speak English, accent (e.g., British Creole accent) still provides an othering linguistic marker. Lakshmi spoke of feeling Indian, but never finding community with first-generation immigrants from South Asia, despite living in an area heavily populated with Bengali- Punjabi-, Hindi-, and Urdu-speaking immigrants. She recognized the fact of a shared cultural heritage with South Asian people, and yet, felt foreclosed on exploring aspects of her identity related to South Asia. Similarly, while she had been able to find employment and start her family in the U.S., she never felt quite "American" enough, even calling the U.S., "a white people's country." It became difficult to disentangle her burgeoning paranoia and mistrust of others caused by her mental illness from normal challenges in acculturation and building community, especially as it came to her ability to connect even with other Indo-Caribbean people.

The families of these individuals have various degrees of acculturation and may or may not hold true to the customs and traditions of their parent's homeland. Inevitably, these individuals straddle two cultures and hold numerous contradictions that elude those with homogeneous cultural identities. Second generation people have the unmapped task of constructing an identity under the dual gaze of their Western counterparts and their ex-pectant family. Diverging from their first generation immigrant parents, the challenge of second-generation adolescents may include forging a congruent Western identity while simultaneously preserving the family culture that the previous generations fought so hard to export and keep alive.

COLONIZATION AND COLONIALITY

Colonization refers to the historical large-scale expansion of nation-states by taking control of foreign land and the indigenous populous utilizing supremist philosophy. Colonization refers to the process of establishing outpost colonies that centralize these efforts. Thus, colonization is the act, while colonialization is the intention and rationale motivating the behavior. The most profound example of mass colonialization is that of the Colonial Era in which Western European countries, such as England, France, Spain, Prussia (Germany), and the Netherlands, traveled to lands that were considered "discovered" or "new," including Africa, Latin America, Australia, North America, and Asia. These European countries' expansionist efforts were supported by an ideology of supremacy instrumentalized through the institutions of religion, science, economics, and the military. This ideology was driven by the European Enlightenment and the coming of modernity, including capitalism, urbanization, the decentralization of the home as center of industry, and militarization. Both the U.S. and South Asia have been influenced and formed by colonial forces, primarily the British, yet in dramatically different ways.

Distinct from historical acts of colonialization are the powerful remnant forces of coloniality. Coloniality refers to the often-unspoken, hierarchical system of influence and power that has governed interactions between countries since the beginning of the colonial era. This hierarchy places formal colonies at the bottom of the global power structure and the most vigorously colonizing states at the top. Although specific countries have formed, changed, and disintegrated throughout history, thereby altering the ordering of states within the hierarchy of coloniality, the hierarchical framework itself persists. In today's globalized society it can be seen across the realms of politics, economics, and cultural influence, where many of the most influential countries are also former colonizing powers (Quijano & Wallerstein, 1992). This dynamic results in the active reenactment and reification of colonial worldview and practice that permeates our education, relationships, economics, and psychology. Coloniality is a powerful influence on western psychology's definition of what is functional, normal, and healthy.

To reiterate, while colonialization is not a metaphor, and instead refers to historical atrocities, while coloniality is the current manifestation that permeates our daily lives (Bhatia, 2018). The chapter on Casteism, Colonization, and Colorism will explore colonialism in more detail, and has been explored here to help understand Lakshmi, an Indo-Tranidadian client in the case study discussion.

Multi-Racial Identity Development Models

Poston (1990) Biracial Identity Development Model incorporates more insights from monoracial identity development. This model begins with *personal identity* in which the young person is unaware of their multi-racial identity. The *choice of group orientation* where the person is pressured by family, peers, and social groups to choose a singular identity. The *enmeshment/denial* stage involves a loyalty-pull where they choose one parent culture over another, resulting in guilt and grief. The next stage of *appreciation* is required to progress. The final stage of *integration* is where the individual establishes a secure, valued, and coherent racial identity.

In the same year, Root (1990) offers a typography to illustrate the unique dilemma of multi-racial individuals with four possibilities; acceptance of the identity society assigns, identification of both racial groups, identification of a single racial group, or identification of a new racial group. The mix of external pressures and personal choice results in an idiosyncratic journey in identity. The author emphasizes that pressures from family, geographic location, and the intensity of oppression all influence development.

Rockquemore (1999) resembles the four options above to highlight the fluid and dynamic nature of multi-racial individuals. In the *singular identity* the individual sides with one of their monoracial parents. A *border identity* person holds their multi-racial aspect as central. With a *protean identity* they freely move between racial groups, identifying differently according to context. The *transcendent identity* person claims no racial categorization and emphasizes their own individuality.

The application of these models can aid the clinician in the consideration of the unique psychological weight and work that identity development and modification demands for the South Asian and South Asian American multi-heritage, multi-racial, and diaspora population. Primarily, clinicians are encouraged to use these models to assist in raising awareness of their own identity formation, particularly the ease and societal support provided them in this important psychological process. This, to cultivate diligence in that for this population, there is nothing established and there are no specific models. Both the clinician and client will be inventing and imagining this important work together.

Case Study Discussion

Lakshmi is a 41-year-old Indo-Trinidadian woman who has been married to her husband, Rajiv, 35, for 15 years. Lakshmi and Rajiv are both first-generation immigrants, from Trinidad & Tobago and Guyana, respectively. They are both of South Asian ancestry. They have a school-aged son, Vijay, 13, who was born in the U.S. Lakshmi sought psychotherapy to help to deal with the stress and anxiety of ongoing court proceedings, which she managed without assistance from family, friends, or legal counsel. Lakshmi recently had a case filed against her anonymously with Child Protective Services (CPS), where she was under risk of being deemed psychologically unfit to care for her son. While the CPS call was made anonymously, Lakshmi had reportedly been bringing her son to school late quite often, and that teachers had complained that she had behaved in a concerning and aggressive manner with them (details of her behavior were not reported), which could have been grounds for a CPS call from the school. Similarly, Lakshmi reported that once, Vijay had a school friend come over to play. Lakshmi was paranoid about entering the home, and allegedly made the boys stay outside in the cold weather with her, and disallowed them from entering the home even to use the bathroom, forcing them to urinate in the backyard. Lakshmi reported that this school friend's parent, or perhaps a neighbor, could also have been responsible for the CPS call for these reasons. Therefore, weekly psychotherapy for Lakshmi and Vijay was also mandated as a part of her CPS case.

However, a variety of other symptomology soon revealed itself. Lakshmi believed that men from a secret, international organization were behind the CPS case. She believed that these men were surveilling, stalking, and intimidating her. Lakshmi believed that their intention was to make her look crazy, and to make others lose respect for her and other women in society. She believed that the past US President, Donald Trump, was a part of this group as well, and that the men currently intimidating her could be traced up to him. Therefore, Lakshmi found it difficult to trust others, especially men, who could offer her help, including physicians, lawyers, and government workers. (Her therapist, the writer, is an Indo-Caribbean woman.) Lakshmi even revealed that she believed her husband, Rajiv, was being influenced by this group. Lakshmi also began to report a number of somatic symptoms that she believed came about due to discrete poisoning of the air around her home by the secret male group.

Rajiv did not participate in individual or family therapy, and was not involved with Vijay's school life. Lakshmi reported that Rajiv believed it was her job as Vijay's mother to take care of these things by herself. Lakshmi reported that Rajiv had been occasionally physically and emotionally abusive toward Vijay, including insulting him for not being masculine enough, and using physical threats (such as slapping) to make Vijay comply with his behavioral demands. Otherwise, Lakshmi reported that Rajiv was uninvolved in parenting, and seemed to mostly ignore Vijay's presence in the home. Unfortunately, the therapist was unable to make contact with Rajiv to confirm any of Lakshmi's accounts of events in the home.

In the case study, Lakshmi and Rajiv are first generation immigrants whose national and personal identities were formed in their home countries. Their marriage further constitutes a multi-heritage dynamic as Lakshmi and Rajiv were from different geographic and culturally distinct areas, and began a multi-heritage family.

Vijay is a second-generation immigrant who was born in the U.S., and thus a naturalized citizen, unlike his parents. While there is innate privilege and security in citizenship, the instability and risk of his parent's national allegiance (e.g., between home country and site of migration) can dramatically impact Vijay's sense of place. In addition, he has the unprecedented task of forging his own identity, both as a person and a citizen, from a frame of reference far from that of his parents. He too can be considered multi-heritage, as he inherits the distinct cultural influences of his parents, the diaspora legacy of his family, and his new home of the U.S.

With regard to the case study presented, a number of factors were observed which may be of interest in considering how differences in language, culture, and social status may affect diagnosis and treatment. Firstly, one may note cultural factors which influence perceptions of trust and safety in the clinical encounter.

- As consistent with research on barriers to mental health help-seeking with Indo-Caribbean clients, shame and stigma about mental illness, fear of negative to mental health help-seeking, and negative beliefs about mental health services (Arora & Persaud, 2019) tended to contribute to Lakshmi's defenses around acknowledging her alleged maltreatment of her son, as well as her psychotic symptoms. Lakshmi was guided to first speak about her mental health in terms that were comfortable for her, such as referring to it as "stress," to make her more comfortable with the therapy relationship.
- While there is high respect for doctors and other professionals in Indo-Caribbean culture (as well as other South Asian cultures), in the case presented, these politics of respect made Lakshmi more cautious at first about opening up to her therapist about topics that required more vulnerability. Initially, she remained symptoms-focused, and was less likely to delve into details of interpersonal dynamics in her family, or to speak about emotions that came up when others may have mistreated her. The therapist gently reminded Lakshmi whenever appropriate about the differences in interacting with a therapist (versus other types of doctors), and that speaking about her feelings would mitigate feelings of stress. Greater time and space was given to Lakshmi to become comfortable with a client-centered approach.
- Once Lakshmi became more comfortable with the nature of the therapeutic relationship, her conversational style began to resemble more of the casual, informal style of speaking common in the Caribbean, known in some regions as "gyaffing" (Simone, 2014). Gyaffing involves a long, meandering conversation, usually without an imposition of time limit. It is a common way for Caribbean people to bond and seek informal counseling from their peers. In Caribbean culture, a person may show

up to a friend's house to gyaff for hours, and it is understood that the conversation remains confidential. For this reason, Lakshmi may have had a similar approach to therapy sessions. This allowed for a level of informality to interactions that is unique to the cultural context. The therapist had to navigate issues of therapeutic frame, such as retaining the time and length of sessions, while understanding that too much "Western" professionalism could cause damage to the development of the working alliance. The therapist would introduce certain transitional gestures to indicate that the session was coming to a close, so as to continue to allow the flow of conversation, but to also retain the structure of the therapeutic frame. For example, while the therapist would usually end a session with a client and have them leave her office on their own, the therapist found it beneficial and more culturally appropriate to continue chatting with the client about non-clinical issues (e.g., what the client was planning on cooking for dinner, their method of preparing it) on the way to the waiting room to see her out.

- Because of shame and stigma present in Indo-Caribbean culture around topics of mental health, it is common for clients to speak in third person terms ("When people have depression ...") rather than in the first person ("When I am depressed ..."). The clinician is advised to gently lead the client back to speaking about personal experience as a way to make contact with repressed affect, or to reintroduce the rationale behind a client-centered approach as necessary.

Treatment Considerations

Lakshmi's major conflict seems to stem from a core sense of helplessness. While she consistently proves to seek she can do things on her own and attempts to assert her independence, she has disavowed her own anger at being abandoned and hurt, especially by men in her life. Dependence may remind her of her own disavowed helplessness, and so, she avoids attempts at connection and support from others. Lakshmi rejects her own desire for dependence, suppressing it into the unconscious. This combination of complex trauma history (i.e., abuse, neglect, generational trauma) and dysfunction in emotional regulation, especially her overreliance on suppression, may have led to the presence of positive psychotic symptoms, including delusions (i.e., the secret group of men out to control her) and hallucinations (i.e., certain somatic symptoms, sounds she reported hearing which indicated that she was being surveilled). During the clinical sessions, Lakshmi had difficulty identifying and sharing her deeper experiences, and tended to express emotions somatically—feeling heavy, sore, and low energy. Even when professing to weepiness, she was resistant to connecting these symptoms to feelings of grief or sadness. Understandably, vulnerability can feel risky to Lakshmi, as she has faced real danger in the past with people she may have been vulnerable with (e.g., her husband).

Lakshmi's conflictual relationship with control seems to stem from her early life relationships. Lakshmi had experienced abandonment, emotional neglect, and abuse from both parents. While she likely sought affection and care from caregivers early in life, her attempts at seeking nurturance were often met with rejection or violence. Lakshmi has remained in a marriage where she was treated as powerless, and her reality testing abilities deteriorated to a point where she displayed limited judgment in her treatment of herself and others. Overall, Lakshmi seems to have developed a conception of herself as not worthy of love.

By suppressing her fear of being out of control, especially repeatedly at the hands of men in her life, Lakshmi's anxieties eventually manifested as a persecutory delusion of an all-powerful group of males whose purpose was to malign and hurt her. Her initial anxieties may have been compounded by cultural and generational experiences of women being treated as powerless. The therapist clinical framework in this case takes into account the impact of colonization on the client. A colonial history of indentured women being treated as sexual objects may have further compounded her rationalization of the treatment she received from her husband in their marriage. There was a poignant truth to her delusions—in many ways, her fear of control by a powerful, male-controlled institution likely reflected endemic patriarchal control in Indo-Caribbean culture, a generational legacy, fomented in times when Indo-Caribbean men themselves felt emasculated by European colonial powers.

Lakshmi projects her own disavowed helplessness onto her son, Vijay. He is both the recipient of her control when she fears he may individuate from her by having his own desires and interests, and is the recipient of her disgust when he seeks physical and emotional closeness. Emotional intimacy was rarely found in her family, and in her relationships, was often tied to mistreatment or abuse. In times where she did seek closeness, it was often inappropriate or unboundaried. Lakshmi seemed to trust the therapist, who is also an Indo-Caribbean woman, despite her paranoia of almost everyone else she encountered. However, with the therapist, she frequently asked inappropriately personal questions about the therapist's life, and often engaged the therapist in conversation well past the end of their session time, even after multiple attempts to end every session.

Repeated abandonment and abuse in her relationships led to internalized beliefs of herself as bad and worthy of blame. This was compounded by a cultural atmosphere that stigmatizes mental health help-seeking. Lakshmi often showed up late to her sessions, which she explained was due to trying to lead the men who she believed were following her off of her trail. However, while Lakshmi always had a lot of content to fill the entire session time with, she often repeated that she knew she had no anxiety (or other mental illness), and that she was only attending therapy because it would help her court case. In reality, it seemed likely that Lakshmi was ashamed to admit that she did need help, as this would mirror cultural beliefs that people who seek mental health treatment are weak, crazy, or unintelligent.

While the clinician treating Lakshmi identifies as Indo-Caribbean as well, a rarity in itself, her education, and upbringing happened in primarily Western settings. As connected as the clinician herself could be to her cultural identity, it is inescapable that Eurocentric, white supremacist ideals would permeate her training experiences in psychology. Whatever the racial or cultural identities of the clinician, one must remain aware of how coloniality affects not only their theoretical approach to therapy, but the therapeutic relationship itself. (This could be understood as a type of transference and countertransference in the psychodynamic model).

The therapeutic relationship can be a site where the language of the personal narrative is returned to its original intention—a tool by which the individual learns, just as in infancy, to negotiate the needs of self and other, outside of the self-other divide as inherited from colonial society (Spivak, 1988). The therapeutic alliance can be an opportunity for an individual, even within the context of coloniality, to make their language, their story, feel to be intimately their own again.

For the non-white clinician and client, moments of cultural connection can feel like pockets of comfort to which they both may feel, consciously or unconsciously, alien to. At other times, the association may not have a comforting effect—reminders of specific oppressions faced within one's own cultural context can be unearthed in clinician-client relationships where there is a shared cultural background. The clinician often indulged Lakshmi in culturally relevant modes of connection, a style of talking known as "gyaffing" in the Caribbean, which was casual, non-goal directed, and often humorous or teasing. This method of therapeutic intervention highlights the ways in which culturally defined power and respect create safety, helping the client feel heard and supported in the therapeutic setting.

Applying Concepts of Colonization and Coloniality to Case Study

Both Lakshmi and Rajiv are inherently impacted by the legacy of colonial diaspora that forcibly transferred their parents and grandparents from various parts of India to Trinidad and Guyana respectively. The aspect of involuntary servitude on the psychology of their families is evident in the many levels of exploitation experienced. Of note, Guyana's independence from the British was as recent as 1966 (Britannica, 2021). Further, the diaspora dynamic can inform the motivation of Lakshmi and Rajiv's decision to immigrate to the U.S., especially due to the political and economic impacts of colonialism.

Regarding the aforementioned definition of multi-heritage, they both share the general Indian identity and similar family backgrounds. This may not always be the case considering the vast cultural differences within India itself. Also, their marriage introduced the difference in the cultures of Trinidad and Guyana. Thus, Vijay will inherit the influences of his family's diaspora journey, the multi-heritage influences of India, Trinidad, and Guyana, and his own unique identity as a U.S. citizen without generational validation.

Furthermore, Vijay is exposed to parenting practices which may originate from his parents' racial or colonial trauma. This could contribute to challenges in emotional reconciliation with his cultural identity. For example, Rajiv's use of corporeal punishment with Vijay represents a history of slaves and indentured servants learning how to use violence to shape the behavior of children from white slave masters (Patton, 2017); however, Rajiv allegedly considers corporeal punishment as a part of his cultural duty as a father, as he was likely disciplined in the same ways.

Lakshmi's attachment relationship with her son, Vijay, could best be described as anxious-ambivalent. Lakshmi described Vijay as clingy, annoying, weak, and described feeling physically disgusted when he would come close to her body for a hug. On the other hand, Lakshmi was quite protective of her son. She did not allow him to have friends, as she was afraid that others would bully him for being "a weak child," though he physically presents as slightly larger than other children his age. Lakshmi described various attempts at sabotaging her son's friendships, including mistreatment of friends that he invited over to her home to play with him. She expressed frustration at her son as being "too American," which she often used to refer to his attempts at asserting age-appropriate self-efficacy (e.g., how he set aside time to do his homework). She reflected fondly on times that she had brought him to Trinidad and had seen him fitting in well with children there. However, she rarely allowed him to engage in such friendships with children at their home in America. In other words, his Americanness became associated with his individuation, and thus, was viewed as a threat to their relationship.

Conceptualizing Lakshmi's current situation within a historical context that combines the impacts of diaspora and multi-heritage forces can assist the clinician in relevant assessment and treatment. The insidious colonial ghosts of the past begin to reveal themselves in the case study. The multi-heritage issues between the families of Lakshmi and Rajiv should not be underestimated, as the result is abuse and isolation that has roots in cultural taboos and stereotypes regarding their marriage. While Rajiv is clearly responsible for his abusive behavior, it is also possible that a colonial mindset and gender socialization reinforced his sexist beliefs regarding his marriage and treatment of Lakshmi. Further, the parent-child relationship is characterized by muli-heritage conflict in which Vijay's efforts to acculturate to American norm and find a place among his peers is sabotaged by his mother's protective impulses.

Working in South Asian Diaspora Settings

Psychological Stressors, Vulnerabilities, and Resilience

In South Asian diaspora populations which are twice or more-removed from their original diasporic site (e.g., Indo-Fijians settled in the United Kingdom), it is difficult to disaggregate data on South Asian diaspora and multiracial groups, as they tend to be subsumed into other racial or ethnic categories (e.g., Asian, South Asian) (Islam et al., 2010). Therefore, more research is needed to understand particular risk factors for mental illness for multiracial South Asian groups, as well as for South Asian diaspora groups which have further immigrated out of their original diasporic site.

Even within once-removed South Asian diaspora settings, such as the Caribbean, Fiji, and countries in Eastern Africa, there is a paucity of research on psychological risk factors for these populations. Many sites of the South Asian diaspora are currently classified as developing nations. Risk factors of mental illness and suicidality particular to developing countries in Asia, South America, and Africa have been identified. While poor education, social isolation, limited access to healthcare services, a history of mental illness, and poverty are also associated with suicide in developing countries, just as in industrialized nations, additional factors specific to developing nations include rapid industrialization, feelings of powerlessness in family conflict, parental disagreement with romantic relationships or romantic relationship failure, intergenerational conflict, exam failure, and domestic violence (Gerbasi et al., 2014; Milner & De Leo, 2010; Vijayakumar, 2004).

Other risk factors for mental illness in countries with a significant South Asian diaspora population are culture-specific. In one study that included data from fifteen Caribbean territories, Indo-Caribbean people were more likely to glorify suicide as a courageous act, or as a means to avoid shame and disgrace (Brown et al., 2017). In Guyana and Trinidad, the highest rates of suicide across the population were found in people of East Indian (i.e., South Asian) descent, with risk factors including pressure and expectations (e.g., high academic expectations, family pressure about marriage or romantic relationships), perceived lack warmth when seeking emotional support, limited coping skills, ease of access to means of dying by suicide (e.g., pesticides), and exposure to means of dying by suicide (Arora et al., 2020; Hutchinson et al., 1999). Similarly, in the Fiji islands, suicidality in people of Indian descent was linked to romantic relationship failure, financial problems, academic problems, and intergenerational conflict (Aghanwa, 2000).

Furthermore, in nations where agriculture is a major industry, a common feature of many formerly colonized nations, farmers who suffer from impoverishment due to competition from larger agricultural corporations have suffered higher rates of suicide, reportedly as a route to escape their financial and job-related stressors (Scutti, 2014; Shiva et al., 2000; Simms, 1999). However, there appear to be specific links between colonialism, indentured servitude, and mental illness in South Asian diaspora communities, which reveal stressors outside of the norm for agricultural laborers. In the era of European indentured servitude, suicides of workers on sugar plantations in the Caribbean and Fiji greatly outpaced the rates of suicide for agricultural workers in India (Nath, 1970). During an era of colonization, a disruption in aspects of cultural power hierarchies may occur, which caused sudden changes to family systems, kinship, societal roles, and individual responsibilities toward the collective (Kral, 2012). This disruption to cultural and institutional systems may cause significant stress to the individual, which could increase the

risk of mental illness and suicide (Chandler & Lalonde, 2008). During the European colonial period, suicide was often seen as one of the only escapes from slavery or indentured
servitude (Warren, 2016). By the early 19th century in the Caribbean, suicide had already
become a common act of insubordination by laborers against European plantation owners
as a sort of "inward protest" against the sociocultural disconnection and violence of their
indenture, along with other deliberate acts of self-harm (Mangru, 2005; Mangru, 2017;
Snyder, 2015).

Further, as the power hierarchies of colonial society contributed to feelings of emas-
culation and disempowerment in men, colonial reports detail accounts of men displacing
their rage through increased violence toward women (Bahadur, 2016). Severe mental illness, homicidal behavior, and suicidality were widely observed as a means for indentured
women to escape widespread sexual violence, as gender ratios on plantations tended to
greatly skew toward a male majority (Bahadur, 2016). There is evidence in formerly colonized societies for the effects of intergenerational transmission of trauma on mental
illness, especially regarding trauma related to political injustice (Cairns & Lewis, 1999;
Kinzie et al., 1998; Weingarten, 2004). Therefore, as formerly colonized nations continue
to struggle with the social, political, and economic impacts of colonialism, so too do they
grapple with the generational impacts of colonial-era trauma on community institutions,
power hierarchies, and gender dynamics. A limited amount of research is available on
protective factors for mental illness in South Asian diaspora settings. In a study conducted
with Indo-Guyanese youth and adults, positive social support and community involvement were identified as perceived protective factors against mental illness (Arora et al.,
2020). Specifically, positive social support was described as the presence of trusted others
in the community who could inquire about an individual's changes in behavior, or who
could be relied on for emotional support, coupled with a non-judgmental and validating
nature. Affiliation with various cultural and religious institutions was identified as a
protective factor, in that participants found that these activities provided viable methods
for coping with distress, coupled with opportunities for individuals to form bonds and
explore talents that brought meaning to their lives. Affiliation with religious institutions
was also identified as a protective factor for Indo-Trinidadian people (Ali & Maharajh,
2005). However, when religion was used to shame or blame an individual for their mental
illness (e.g., being told that not praying enough is a cause of depression), it was perceived
as a threat to mental health (Arora & Persaud, 2019).

Clinician Awareness and Humility

When learning about culturally different groups, there is always the risk of over-
generalizing acquired group knowledge to the individual. Further, when the clinician is
unaware of their own social privilege and positionality, stereotyping becomes an increased
threat to treatment effectiveness. Thus, it is important for the reader to learn about the
different shades of the South Asian community with humility and self-awareness. The
authors posit that to understand the contemporary psychological issues of South Asian
American individuals, it is imperative to understand their historical journey coupled with
an awareness of our social privilege as a citizen and clinician.

Psychology has been a trailblazer of cultural consideration in the realm of human services. The field has produced revolutionary theories from the historic Clark study to
contemporary implicit bias (Clark & Clark, 1939; Banaji & Greenwald, 2013). These
theories have also had real societal implications. The Clark studies provided insight into
the power of racial socialization that was pivotal in the desegregation of schools (Clark &
Clark, 1939). And the current understanding regarding the inevitability of implicit bias has

been integrated into legal and corporate policies and even found its way into political discourse (Merica, 2016). Understanding the role that culture plays in clinical issues has been an important principle in psychology, making the specialty of multicultural psychology a major consideration in education, research, and practice. This, again, points to the importance for the clinician in the case study to remain vigilant of the inescapable influence of bias and socialization as they work with Lakshmi and her family.

For all the strong emphasis on culture in psychology, there are still some limitations, both in concept and implementation. The field has long emphasized the importance of our fund of cultural knowledge of those different from the norm, thus being focused on the other. Yet, it has seldom acknowledged the culture of the societal norm, or the colonial influences that continues to keep this norm intact. Specifically, there has been limited attention to the fact that graduate psychology education is laden with WEIRD (Western, Educated, Industrialized, Rich, and Democratic) values (Christopher, 2014). Multicultural curriculum usually has segments of books and lectures dedicated to African Americans, Latin Americans, Asian Americans, and American Indians but nothing on European Americans let alone the acknowledgment of whiteness (Ridley, 2021). This points to the risk that traditionally trained clinicians, despite good intention, could do harm simply due to the lack of privilege awareness. The engrained external clinical focus could mask the values of whiteness that influence decisions regarding case conceptualization, diagnosis, and assessment.

The field has also put a focus on the interpersonal relationship and the cultural influences within the individual client (Shah & Tewari, 2019; Sharma et al., 2020). Yet, psychology has traditionally not explored the relationship between a client's culture and the systems of institutionalized oppression that uses cultural identification to allot resources and benefits to some and not others. This conflation of culture with societal issues of privilege and power can be used as a convenient proxy to avoid acknowledging difficult issues of oppression in the domains of race, sex, gender, class, etc. Further, the field of psychology has yet to come to terms with its own colonial past of white supremacy. A past formulated within a capitalist, imperialist, and hegemonically Western mindset that can be conceptualized as a distinctly European value system of health, normality, and pathology.

Recently, the field has begun an important move from increasing the fund of cultural knowledge of others to a refocusing on understanding ourselves, as clinicians, as cultural beings with our own hegemonic identity formation. The foundational work of scholars such as McIntosh (1988), Tatum (1994), Helms (1984; 2017), Spanierman & Smith (2017), Goodman (2015), and Case & Cole, (2013) suggest it is critical for psychologists to begin reflecting on their social privilege awareness to provide ethical and multiculturally competent treatment and services. As the 2017 revision of the American Psychological Association Multicultural Guidelines states, "Psychologists aspire to recognize and understand historical and contemporary experiences with power, privilege, and oppression" (American Psychological Association, 2017). Social positioning, or the mapping of our own socially conferred privilege and disadvantage, has a burgeoning emphasis as well.

What happens when a well-intentioned clinician has an acquired knowledge of the culturally different client, but does not have a clear awareness of their own social position, areas of privilege, and unexplored cultural identity? Specifically, what could be the impact and consequence for Lakshmi and her family when the clinician carries acknowledged, socially conferred power (Bergkamp et al., 2022)?

Even our drive to be helpful and advocate for others less fortunate than us can serve to sabotage our efforts. Without an awareness of our own social location, which shapes our worldview and provides our sense of agency, we can naively make uninformed suggestions that can impact assessment, treatment planning, interventions, and outcomes. More importantly, it can impact the therapeutic alliance, one of the primary common factors of psychotherapy (Nierkens et al., 2019). This relates to concepts such as our savior or missionary complex, performative allyship, and empty advocacy. At the deepest of levels, it could result in a type of forced assimilation that encourages the erasure of native cultures, shames ethnic identity, and imposes values of whiteness.

Thus, for clinicians working with the populations addressed in this chapter, the ideal is a combination of knowledge of the other coupled with an awareness of their own social positioning and a continuous reflective process of inherent hegemonic influences on their perception. We suggest that clinicians begin with understanding their own social privilege, exploring intersecting identities and attending to the embodiment of their own status power as professional clinicians. Black and Stone (2005) provides a comprehensive definition of social privilege:

> First, privilege is a special advantage; it is neither common nor universal. Second, it is granted, not earned or brought into being by one's individual effort or talent. Third, privilege is a right or entitlement that is related to a preferred status or rank. Fourth, privilege is exercised for the benefit of the recipient and to the exclusion or detriment of others. Finally, a privileged status is often outside of the awareness of the person possessing it (p. 244).

The proposed antidote for inadvertently enacting a savior complex or engaging in performative allyship is to ensure that clinician decisions are scaffolded by an awareness of social position. Spanierman and Smith (2017) outline six steps toward this goal. The following six steps are modified to speak beyond White allyship and consider allyship in all social identity domains. These six steps involve 1) gaining a nuanced understanding of institutional oppression and social privilege; 2) enacting a continual process of self-reflection about one's own racism, biases, and positionality; 3) commitment to promoting equity from a position of privilege; 4) taking responsibility for actions against racism, discrimination, and the status quo on multiple levels; 5) participate in solidarity work with people of marginalized groups; 6) encounter resistance from other socially privileged individuals (p. 609).

In addition, Melton (2018) provided guidelines to address clinical role complexities regarding allies, activists, and advocates in ethical and competent ways. They suggest that psychologists should take part in self-reflection that is intentional to diminish biases and expand cultural humility and critical consciousness, that psychologists are considerate and deliberate in choosing activities of allyship, activism, and advocacy, that psychologists hold themselves and their colleagues accountable, and finally, that psychologists have a plan in place to maintain their competence and wellness.

The reader is encouraged to take time to cultivate a mindful practice of identifying their social position and explore how their privilege informs and shapes thoughts, emotions, perceptions, and behavior. Further, considering how these aspects of identity impact their clinical work and how they integrate knowledge of the culturally different other. This is an important concept throughout this chapter and book.

Community-Based Interventions and Outreach

In collectivistic cultures, individuals can often identify informal groups and institutions which are trusted caretakers of emotional health, especially when access to professional mental healthcare is scant. In diaspora groups, existing structures of community counseling and conflict resolution were often transported along on the journey from South Asia to the site of migration. For example, there are detailed accounts of the panchayat system being used as a community decision-making body in Indo-Fijian indenture (Lal, 2012). A panchayat is a group of several community-selected decision makers, usually men, who help to resolve marriage issues, land disputes, and whose values are ideally representative of the village(s) which they belong to. While members of the panchayat were often selected due to their social status (e.g., caste, religious authority, wealth), they could also be selected based on their ability to faithfully counsel and guide issues of group tension. While a panchayat may not be an appropriate replacement for professional mental health services, and can even reinforce social values which cause various social oppressions, clinicians, and researchers can collaborate with existing recognized social institutions to train them in counseling skills, mental health outreach, and mental health referral procedures—in other words, what are referred to as gatekeeper trainings.

Gatekeeper trainings often serve to reinforce existing social support systems in the community, which ensures that they provide more permanent institutional change (Isaac et al., 2009). In many diaspora settings, schools are already a trusted site for mental health help-seeking for both students and parents (Arora & Persaud, 2019). Although many diaspora settings have limited access to professional healthcare facilities (e.g. hospitals, counseling clinics), schools are often much more plentiful. If schools are used as a site for mental health treatment, this could greatly increase youth access to mental health services. Similarly, cultural and faith-based institutions can be utilized as a site for adult mental health outreach. For example, South Queens Women's March, a non-profit which conducts outreach to the Indo-Caribbean community in New York City, created a guide for combatting gender-based violence as a training tool for faith leaders (South Queens Women's March, 2021). Clinicians and researchers are encouraged to explore the possibility of collaborating with existing arts, advocacy, and recreational groups where emotional wellness may already be related to the purpose of the group's work, though may not be identified explicitly as a mental health organization.

Community Interventions and Case Study Discussion

Lakshmi reported having few friends in the Indo-Caribbean community in the U.S., and limited engagement with local cultural organizations that she may have had contact with when she lived in Trinidad (e.g., temples). Her isolation from her social circle is likely due to paranoia or social anxieties related to her burgeoning struggles with mental illness. However, when she was more involved in community activities, such as when she first immigrated to the U.S. or early in her marriage to Rajiv, may have presented some opportunities for preventative intervention. Had trusted figures in her social circles been trained in mental health gatekeeper skills, or had she been presented with psychoeducation on identifying gender-based violence, it is possible that the signs of her mental illness could have been caught earlier, and referrals could have been provided for the aid she required.

Nevertheless, in her current state of limited social contact, Lakshmi still does her grocery shopping in Indo-Caribbean neighborhoods, and Vijay does attend school in a neighborhood with a large South Asian diaspora population. More community-level mental health outreach by local advocacy organizations could still reach Lakshmi as she goes about her daily routines. For example, a community organization could provide free and accessible mental health screenings on main thoroughfares of the Indo-Caribbean ethnic enclaves where she does her shopping, and could provide resources on seeking referrals and navigating the U.S. healthcare system. Similarly, teachers and administrators at Vijay's school could be trained in mental health interventions adapted for the immigrant groups present in his neighborhood.

Summary

As the U.S. population reaches a demographic turning point and the South Asian American community within the country continues to grow, the demand for mental health services from this group will likewise become greater. The minority and multi-racial identity development models can be useful in exploring the immense variety of experiences of South Asian American multiracial, multi-heritage, and diaspora clients, and can help clinicians develop a more nuanced understanding, we must move from increasing the store of cultural knowledge of others toward a focus on clinician humility and self-awareness. Moreover, to understand the present-day psychological issues that South Asian Americans individuals experience, it is necessary for clinicians to investigate and recognize both their own social privilege as citizens and mental health practitioners, as well as their clients' unique experiences within the context of their own identity formation, their family's journey, and the consequences of past and present colonial influences.

Self-reflection is the first step toward gaining a better understanding of one's own thoughts and feelings about one's own culture and one's understanding of other cultures. Part of cultural humility involves an understanding that the clinician must continually revisit their ideas of social privilege, oppression, biases, discrimination, and prejudice. It is easy to stagnate and assume that the work is done after momentary self-reflection. However, just like a client's healing is a long-term and continual process, a clinician's understanding, allyship, activism, and advocacy should also be a long-term and continual process. A clinician must also remain aware of their own well-being, and it is also very important that the clinician practice mindful-based interventions to avoid burn-out, self-blame, and shame during this process of self-reflection and exploration.

Reflection Questions

Before working with clients from Multiracial, Multi-Heritage, and Diaspora South Asian American communities, clinicians could consider the following questions to help guide their treatment and interventions:

1 What are the psychological impacts on individuals' identity development as a result of being multi-heritage, multi-racial, and belonging to a diaspora community?
2 What assumptions are you making as a clinician sitting across from a South Asian American client?
3 How can clinicians support South Asian American clients and communities, individuals who identify as multi-heritage, multi-racial, or belonging to a diaspora?

Suggested Resources

- South Asian American Digital Archives (SAADA) https://www.saada.org
- Caribbean Hindustani (Indo-Caribbean history archives) http://www.caribbeanhindustani. org
- Girmit (Indo-Fijian history) http://girmit.org
- Sana Aiyar, "Indians in Kenya: The Politics of Diaspora" (Podcast, *South Asian Studies*) https://podcasts.apple.com/us/podcast/sana-aiyar-indians-in-kenya-politics-diaspora-harvard/id427197319?i=1000490766818
- Dilemmas of the Diaspora podcast series with Shana Narula https://podcasts.apple. com/us/podcast/dilemmas-of-the-diaspora/id1529917876

- "Claim us if you're famous" on the complications of Kamala Harris' multiracial Black & South Asian identity (Podcast, *NPR Code Switch*)

References

American Psychological Association. (2017). Psycextra dataset. In *Multicultural guidelines: An ecological approach to context, identity, and intersectionality*, 2017: (501962018-001). essay.

Aghanwa, H.S. (2000). The characteristics of suicide attempters admitted to the main general hospital in Fiji islands. *Journal of Psychosomatic Research*, *49*(6), 439–445. 10.1016/S0022-3999(00)00193-8

Ali, A., & Maharajh, H.D. (2005). Social predictors of suicidal behaviour in adolescents in Trinidad and Tobago. *Social Psychiatry and Psychiatric Epidemiology*, *40*(3), 186–191. 10.1007/s00127-005-0846-9

Arora, P.G., & Persaud, S. (2019). Suicide among Guyanese youth: Barriers to mental health help-seeking and recommendations for suicide prevention. *International Journal of School & Educational Psychology*, *0*(0), 1–13. 10.1080/21683603.2019.1578313

Arora, P.G., Persaud, S., & Parr, K. (2020). Risk and protective factors for suicide among Guyanese youth: Youth and stakeholder perspectives. *International Journal of Psychology*, *55*(4), 618–628.

Bahadur, G. (2016). *Coolie woman: The Odyssey of indenture*. Oxford University Press.

Banaji, M., & Greenwald, A. (2013). *Blind spot: Hidden biases of good people*. Delacorte Press.

Bergkamp, J. , Martin, A. , & Olson, L. (2022). Social privilege: Flipping the coin of inequity. In J. L. Chin, Y. E. Garcia, & Blume A. (Eds.), *The Psychology of Inequity, Volume 1: Motivations and Beliefs*. Praeger Press.

Bhatia, S., & Priya, K. R. (2018). Decolonizing culture: Euro-American psychology and the shaping of neoliberal selves in India. *Theory & Psychology*, *28*(5), 645–668. 10.1177/0959354318791315

Black, L.L., & Stone, D. (2005). Expanding the definition of privilege: The concept of social privilege. *Journal of Multicultural Counseling and Development*, *33*, 243–255. 10.1002/j.2161-1912. 2005.tb00020.x.

Britannica. (2021). Independence of Guyana. In *Encyclopædia Britannica*. https://www.britannica. com/place/Guyana/Independence

Brown, C.R., Hambleton, I.R., Sobers-Grannum, N., Hercules, S.M., Unwin, N., Harris, E.N., Wilks, R., MacLeish, M., Sullivan, L., & Murphy, M.M. (2017). *Social determinants of depression and suicidal behaviour in the Caribbean: A systematic review*. BMC Public Health, 17. http://dx.doi. org.ezproxy.cul.columbia.edu/10.1186/s12889-017-4371-z

Cairns, E., & Lewis, C.A. (1999). Collective memories, political violence and mental health in Northern Ireland. *British Journal of Psychology; Leicester*, *90*, 25–33.

Case, K.A. & Cole, E.R. (2013). Deconstructing privilege when students resist. In K. A. Case (Eds.), *Deconstructing privilege: Teaching and learning as allies in the classroom* (pp. 34–48). Routledge.

Chandler, M.J., & Lalonde, C.E. (2008). Cultural continuity as a moderator of suicide risk among Canada's first nations. In L. Kirmayer, & G. Valaskakis (Eds.). *Healing Traditions: The Mental Health of Aboriginal Peoples in Canada*, (pp. 221–248). University of British Columbia Press.

Chandra, S. (2011). Global indian diasporas: Exploring trajectories of migration and theory. *Journal of World History*, *22*(1), 177–181. n https://doi-org.antioch.idm.oclc.org/10.1353/jwh.2011.0010

Choules, K. (2006). Globally privileged citizenship. *Race, Ethnicity & Education*, *9*(3), 275–293.

Christopher, J.C., Wendt, D.C., Marecek, J., & Goodman, D.M. (2014). Critical cultural awareness: Contributions to a Globalizing psychology. *American Psychologist*, *69*. 645–655.

Clark, K.B., & Clark, M.P. (1939). Segregation as a factor in the racial identification of Negro preschool children. *Journal of Experimental Education*, *8*, 161–163.

Daftary, A.-M. H. (2020). Living with uncertainty: Perceptions of well-being among latinx young adults in immigrant family systems. *Family Relations*, *69*(1), 51–62.

Gerbasi, M.E., Richards, L.K., Thomas, J.J., Agnew-Blais, J.C., Thompson-Brenner, H., Gilman, S.E., & Becker, A.E. (2014). Globalization and Eating disorder risk: Peer influence, perceived social norms, and adolescent disordered eating in Fiji. *International Journal of Eating Disorders*, *47*(7), 727–737. 10. 1002/eat.22349

Golash-Boza, T. (2016). Feeling like a citizen, living as a Denizen. *American Behavioral Scientist*, *60*(13).

Goodman, D.J. (2015). Oppression and privilege: Two sides of the same coin. *Journal of Intercultural Communication*, *18*, 1–14.

Helms, J.E. (1984). Toward a theoretical explanation of the effects of race on Counseling: A black and white model. *The Counseling Psychologist*, *12*(4), 153–165.

Helms, J.E. (2017). The challenge of making whiteness visible: Reactions to four whiteness articles. *The Counseling Psychologist*, *45*(5), 717–726. doi:10.1177/0011000017718943

Hutchinson, G., Daisley, H., Simeon, D., Simmonds, V., Shetty, M., & Lynn, D. (1999). High rates of paraquat-Induced suicide in Southern Trinidad. *Suicide and Life-Threatening Behavior*, *29*(2), 186–191. 10.1111/j.1943-278X.1999.tb01055.x

Isaac, M., Elias, B., Katz, L.Y., Belik, S.-L., Deane, F.P., Enns, M.W., & Sareen, J. (2009). Gatekeeper training as a preventative intervention for suicide: A systematic review. *Canadian Journal of Psychiatry*, *54*(4), 260–268.

Islam, N.S., Khan, S., Kwon, S., Jang, D., Ro, M., & Trinh-Shevrin, C. (2010). Methodological issues in the collection, analysis, and reporting of granular data in Asian American populations: Historical challenges and potential solutions. *Journal of Health Care for the Poor and Underserved*, *21*(4), 1354–1381. 10.1353/hpu.2010.0939

Kinzie, J.D., Boehnlein, J., & Sack, W.H. (1998). The effects of massive trauma on cambodian parents and children. In *International handbook of multigenerational legacies of trauma* (pp. 211–221). Springer. 10.1007/978-1-4757-5567-1_14

Kral, M.J. (2012). Postcolonial suicide among inuit in arctic canada. *Culture, Medicine, and Psychiatry*, *36*(2), 306–325. 10.1007/s11013-012-9253-3

Lal, V.B. (2012). *Chalo Jahaji: On a journey through indenture in Fiji*. ANU Press.

Mahmud, T. (2013). Cheaper than a slave: Indentured labor, colonialism and capitalism. *Whittier L. Rev.*, *34*, 215.

Mangru, B. (2005). *The elusive El Dorado: Essays on the Indian experience in Guyana*. University Press of America.

Mangru, B. (2017). *Champions of Indo-Guyanese welfare 1838-1938*. Adams Press.

McIntosh, P. (1988). White privilege: Unpacking the invisible knapsack. Excerpt from White Privilege and Male Privilege: A Personal Account of coming to see Correspondences through Work in Women's Studies. *Wellesley College Center for Research on Women*.

Melton, M.L. (2018). Ally, activist, advocate: Addressing role complexities for the multiculturally competent Psychologist. *Professional Psychology: Research and Practice*, *49*(1), 83–89.

Merica, D. (2016, April 21). *Protesters interrupt Clinton rally*. CNN. https://www.cnn.com/2016/04/20/politics/hillary-clinton-race-implicit-biases

Milner, A., & De Leo, D. (2010). Suicide research and Prevention in developing countries in Asia and the Pacific. *Bulletin of the World Health Organization (WHO)*, 795–796. https://doi.org//entity/bulletin/volumes/88/10/09-070821/en/index.html

Nath, D. (1970). *A history of Indians in Guyana*. London, D. Nath.

Nierkens, V., Hartman, M.A., Nicolaou, M., Vissenberg, C., Beune, E.J.A.J., Hosper, K., van Valkengoed, I.G., Norcross, J.C., & Lambert, M.J. (Eds.). (2019). *Psychotherapy relationships that work (Third, Vol. Volume 1, evidence-based therapist contributions /, Ser. Oxford clinical psychology)*. Oxford University Press. http://dx.doi.org.ezproxy.cul.columbia.edu/10.1186/s12888-016-1059-3

Oonk, G. (2007). *Global indian diasporas: exploring trajectories of migration and theory (Ser. Iias publications series. edited volumes, 1)*. Amsterdam University Press. 10.5117/9789060535358

Patton, S. (2017). *Spare the Kids: Why Whupping Children Won't Save Black America*. Beacon Press.

Poston, W.S.C. (1990). The biracial identity development model: A needed addition. *Journal of Counseling & Development*, *69*(2), 152–155.

Quijano, A. (2007). Coloniality and modernity/Rationality. *Cultural Studies*, *21*(2/3), 168–178.

Quijano, A., & Wallerstein, I. (1992). Americanity as a concept, or the Americas in the modern world-system. *International Social Science Journal*, *44*(134), 549.

Ridley, C.R., Mollen, D., Console, K., & Yin, C. (2021). Multicultural Counseling competence: A construct in search of operationalization. *The Counseling Psychologist*, *49*(4), 504–533. 10.1177/0011000020988110

Rockquemore, K.A. (1999). Between black and white: Exploring the biracial experience. *Race and Society*, *1*, 197–212.

Rockquemore, K.A., Brunsma, D.L., & Delgado, D.J. (2009). Racing to theory or retheorizing race? understanding the struggle to build a multiracial identity theory. *Journal of Social Issues*, *65*, 13–34.

Root, M.P.P. (1990). Resolving "other" status: Identity development of biracial individuals. *Women & Therapy*, *9*, 185–205.

Root, M.P.P. (1998). Experiences and processes affecting racial identity development: Preliminary results from the biracial sibling project. *Cultural Diversity and Mental Health*, *4*(3), 237–247.

SAALT. (2019, May 15). South Asians by the numbers: Population in the U.S. has grown by 40% since 2010 | Saalt. *Saalt.org*. https://saalt.org/south-asians-by-the-numbers-population-in-the-u-s-has-grown-by-40-since-2010

Scutti, S. (2014, October 14). Suicide rates highest in Guyana, may be explained by clustering effect. *Medical Daily*. http://www.medicaldaily.com/suicide-rates-highest-guyana-may-be-explained-clustering-effect-306982

Shah, S., & Tewari, N. (2019). Cognitive behavior therapy with South Asian Americans. In G. Y. Iwamasa & P. A. Hays (Eds.), *Culturally responsive cognitive behavior therapy: Practice and supervision*, 2nd ed. (pp. 161–182). American Psychological Association.

Sharma, N., Shaligram, D., & Yoon, G.H. (2020). Engaging South Asian youth and families: A clinical review. *The International Journal of Social Psychiatry*, *66*(6), 584–592.

Shiva, V., Jafri, A.H., Emani, A., & Pande, M. (2000). Seeds of suicide: The ecological and human costs of Globalisation of agriculture. *Seeds of Suicide: The Ecological and Human Costs of Globalisation of Agriculture*. https://www-cabdirect-org.ezproxy.cul.columbia.edu/cabdirect/abstract/20026792341

Simms, A. (1999). Selling suicide: Farming, false promises and genetic engineering in developing countries. http://agris.fao.org/agris-search/search.do?recordID=GB2013202425

Simone, A. (2014, September 15). West indian word of the week: GYAFF. Retrieved March 16, 2021, from http://rewindandcomeagain.com/west-indian-word-of-the-week-gyaff/

Snyder, T.L. (2015). *The power to die: Slavery and suicide in British North America*. University of Chicago Press.

South Queens Women's March. (2021). Interfaith toolkit to combat gender-based violence. https://www.southqueenswomensmarch.org/resources

Spanierman, L.B., & Smith, L. (2017). Roles and responsibilities of white allies: Implications for research, teaching, and practice. *Counseling Psychologist*, *45*(5), 606–617.

Spivak, G.C. (1988). Can the subaltern speak? In C. Nelson & L. Grossberg (Eds.), *Marxism and the interpretation of culture* (pp. 271–313). University of Illinois Press.

Stonequist, E.V. (1937). The problem of the marginal man. *The American Journal of Sociology*, *41*, 1–12.

Tatum, B. (1994). Teaching white students about racism: The search for white allies and the restoration of hope. *Teachers College Record 94*(4), 462–476.

Toloyan, K. (1996). Rethinking diaspora(s): Stateless power in the transnational moment. *Diaspora*, *5*, 3–35.

Tummala-Narra, P. (2021). *Trauma and racial minority immigrants: Turmoil, uncertainty, and resistance*. APA.

Vijayakumar, L. (2004). Suicide Prevention: The urgent need in developing countries. *World Psychiatry*, *3*(3), 158–159.

Warren, W. (2016). *New England bound: Slavery and colonization in early America*. W. W. Norton & Company.

Weingarten, K. (2004). Witnessing the effects of political violence in families: Mechanisms of intergenerational transmission and clinical interventions. *Journal of Marital and Family Therapy; Hoboken*, *30*(1), 45–59.

Yampolsky, M.A., Amiot, C.E., & de la Sablonnière, R. (2013). Multicultural identity integration and well-being: A qualitative exploration of variations in narrative coherence and multicultural identification. *Frontiers in Psychology*, *4*, 126. 10.3389/fpsyg.2013.00126

6 Impact of Gender Socialization and Cultural Norms on South Asian Americans

Shanta Kanukollu and Rahul Sharma

Case Overview

The case of Binal, a 20-year-old cisgender second-generation Muslim Bangladeshi-American female who identifies as queer, will be used to illustrate key issues and concepts discussed in this chapter. While this client enters therapy due to "problems with relationships," it becomes evident to the clinician that she also struggles with a deep-rooted fear of being abandoned by her family and a core belief of not being "enough," which Binal explained as always feeling inadequate and imperfect. Binal grew up just outside of Philadelphia with her older brother (age 23), her two parents, and her paternal grandmother. She describes her family as "somewhat traditional Bengali but trying really hard to be American," which she further explained as trying to fit into American culture. Her issues and struggles are also tied to gendered expectations implicitly placed on her by her family, their immigrant community, and her own understanding of herself as a second-generation American confronting gender norms both within her community and in the society at large. She says she has "a complicated relationship with Islam." She is currently in a relationship with a Bengali-American man, which has surprised her since she thought she would "never ever date anyone Bengali." After providing a review and discussion of the literature on gender socialization within the South Asian American (SAA) cultural context, the authors use Binal's case as a way to illustrate how these gendered themes may come to life in clinical settings.

Introduction

This chapter will begin with a focus on the context of gender socialization and gender role expectations for men and women in South Asian American (SAA) cultures. This context will be followed by discussion of the evolving gender socialization process within SAA communities today. The influence of family, community, generation, immigration & acculturation, and religion will be discussed, as each of these elements inform the blueprint of how SAA beginning in childhood are expected to behave or perform their gender. (It should be noted that gender socialization with many cultures is predicated on conforming to a gender binary.) The consequences of conforming or not conforming to gendered norms will be addressed, including how gendered expectations may affect the mental health of SAA communities in the United States. A case study will help illustrate significant themes pertinent to SAA clients and individuals. Finally, therapeutic considerations and discussion questions will be provided, along with a listing of relevant resources.

Gender socialization has been defined as the process through which children learn about the social expectations, attitudes, and behaviors associated with one's gender (Barker, 2006). Possible ways that parents might influence children's gender development include role modeling and encouraging different behaviors and activities in sons and daughters.

DOI: 10.4324/9781003081548-6

(Bussey & Bandura, 1999). For the purposes of this discussion, gender socialization refers to the process by which SAA populations receive gendered expectations and make meaning of how they experience the world given their gender identity. As will be discussed, there are a multitude of factors that affect the gender socialization process for SAA communities. This chapter aims to highlight some of those factors, anchoring the discussion with consideration of essential information for clinicians working with SAA clients in therapy.

The authors of this chapter recognize that our own lived experiences, the intersections of our own identities and concordant layers of privilege and oppression undoubtedly impact our understanding of gender and gender socialization in the SAA context. While we have conducted e work related to managing how these identities impact our work with clients, as authors we acknowledge that our life experiences will inevitably "show up" in this chapter. Therefore, we find it important to share a bit about who we are, for readers to appreciate our perspective, potential biases, and lenses through which we make sense of SAA gender socialization.

Author 1 (SNK) identifies as a second-generation, cisgender, heterosexual Indian-American female from a Hindu Brahmin background. She was born and raised on the East Coast (New Jersey) of the United States with exposure to a tight-knit SA community prior to moving to the Midwest (Michigan) for her doctoral education. From an early age, Author 1 was given access to religion and spirituality through a non-denominational organization, based in India, and eventually completed a portion of her primary education in a small village in South India. It was this experience that lay the seeds for her future self-reflection on identity, privilege and the meaning of culture. In 2010 she completed a dual-PhD in Clinical Psychology and Women's Studies, with a dissertation exploring myths about child sexual abuse and attitudes toward help-seeking among SAA young adults. She spent some formative school years in India, which provided her with an appreciation for the religious, socioeconomic, and cultural diversity of her family's country of origin. She currently resides in the Midwest (Chicago), where she lives with her partner and two daughters, who compel her to think about how she is raising two young girls in America today. This author and her partner often comment on how they were raised differently from one another, despite their shared identities (both second-generation, of the same caste, and from families from similar parts of India), due to the varying ways in which their parents adapted to life in the U.S. This has led them to have different narratives about what it means to be Indian-American, which has contributed to many rich conversations about gender socialization, culture and parenting. Author 1 currently works in a private practice setting where her patients are predominantly SAA. These experiences have contributed to her understanding of gender, immigration and the SAA community.

Author 2 (RS) identifies as a second-generation, cisgender, heterosexual Indian-American male from a Hindu (Arya Samaji sect) Brahmin background. He was born and raised in Michigan, the youngest of four, the child of parents born and raised in Kenya. He had the opportunity to travel many times to Kenya, forming an initial interest in issues of identity and difference. As an undergraduate at The University of Michigan, he began to facilitate workshops on gender and gendered violence as a trained peer educator. At this time, he began thinking about gender socialization specifically within a South Asian context, and in particular, South Asian men's roles in addressing their own privilege and addressing sexism within the community. In 1998, he completed his doctorate in Clinical Psychology, completing a dissertation that examined a group treatment program specifically for South Asian men in Canada who were court ordered for domestic violence offenses. He led many workshops and trainings, specifically on South Asian American gender socialization. He currently resides in Evanston, IL with his partner and two teenage children. As the parent of a SAA son and daughter, he often thinks about the implications of the dynamic interplay of race and gender and how his children navigate these complexities.

In conferring with each other about the subject of this chapter, we noted that many SAAs are keenly aware of many gendered expectations placed upon them. While there are variations, in our clinical, as well as personal experiences, the overarching expectations and pressures seem quite uniform, and any divergence that manifests is in the *degree of pressure* by family, peers, and community to adhere, and in the *strategies* SAAs employ to contend with these expectations. Clinicians working with SAA clients in therapy have the opportunity to provide an important space to "unpack" how they make meaning of their gender identity. They can also assist clients in actively navigating the complex messages they receive regarding what is expected of them based on how others perceive their gender and gender roles, and explore strategies utilized in response to these complexities.

Gender Socialization in the South Asian American Context: An Overview

Primary socialization, occurring in infancy and childhood, is the initial process of learning the ways of a society or group. The four most studied agents of socialization are family, peers, education, and media (Fulton, 2017). From the present authors' personal and clinical experiences, it seems these agents of socialization need to be contextualized within an intersectional framework to fully appreciate the process of gender socialization within the SAA community. Additionally, factors specific to the immigrant experience should be taken into consideration including a client's (and their family's):

- Relationship to their country of origin
- Experiences they were afforded or not afforded based on their gender
- Identification with or exposure to a religious or spiritual path
- Desire to conform/not conform to their community's values
- Level of acculturation to their host country

While we will highlight some of these issues further in the case study of Binal, included later in this chapter, we argue that these two women cannot be presumed to have similar issues based on gender and race classification alone. They will each have varying contextual factors and experiences that will impact how they parent and socialize their children, which could easily be glossed over by an untrained or unaware clinician. Exploring how each contextual factor plays a role in their lives will be crucial for a clinician working with them to have a more complete picture of their presenting concerns.

A common stereotype of the SAA family is one with a clear patriarchal structure and adherence to rigid, traditional gender roles. The 'gender story' in the SAA home can be complex. While there is evidence of an egalitarian mindset with regards to some aspects of gender role expectations in SAA communities, as well as evidence of resistance against rigidity, there is a concurrent, pervasive transmission of traditional gender ideology.

Many SAA females are encouraged by their families to pursue academic and career goals. This is consistent with changes in the Indian subcontinent as well; Fuller and Narasimhan (2008) explain that due to the emancipation through professional careers and individual income, young women's hierarchical position changes in relation to their in-law families. Bhandari and Titzmann (2017) argue that while the South Asian family can be oppressive and dominant in structure on the one hand, especially with regard to gender roles and duties, the family system also has transformative abilities—becoming a space to externalize resistances, especially for women in the domains of love and work. In this process, the family system itself undergoes transformation.

These instances of resistance and transformation directly battle the stereotype of South Asian and SAA women as submissive or subservient. Examples of prominent SAA women who have taken on positions of power and leadership include: Dr. Sadaf Jaffer, the Mayor of Montgomery Township, New Jersey, the first South Asian American woman to serve as the mayor of a municipality in New Jersey, and the first Muslim woman mayor of any municipality in the United States; Meena Harris, the Head of Strategy and Leadership at Uber and Founder & CEO of Phenomenal Woman Action Campaign, which supports women's organizations and of course; Nikki Haley, former two-term Governor of South Carolina and Ambassador to the United Nations; and Kamala Harris, the first South Asian and Black woman to become Vice President- Elect in the United States. Indeed, "South Asian women lag behind men in literacy, workforce participation, reproductive rights and most other areas. Yet the region's array of female leaders put the rest of the world to shame" (Akl, 2011). Bhandari and Titzmann (2017) summarize it well:

> Being largely dominated by a patriarchal lineage and a family system, South Asian societies are witnessing changes as evident in the increasing participation of women in the workforce, the rise of youth culture that shapes the experience of new intimacies, and a public discourse of love and companionship, as well as amendments to existing laws and the enactment of new laws. The [South Asian] family therefore, finds itself propagating continuity of certain normative behavior as it is also compelled to adjust its norms and values.

These contradictions within SAA culture can make it challenging for clinicians to have a comprehensive understanding of their SAA clients and their families. This challenge might be met by providers ensuring they ask a variety of questions about their client's up-bringing, including their family's gendered expectations and pressures. Sample questions for clinicians to consider asking their SAA clients specifically focused on counseling considerations and interventions are listed in the subsequent section of this chapter.

Acculturation

Acculturation adds a layer to the gendered story for the SAA family as it plays a major role in the immigrant family's adaptation and is influenced by gender-based cultural norms and expectations (Sharma et al., 2020). Acculturation has traditionally been defined as the process by which individuals grasp and absorb values, beliefs and behaviors of the host culture into their natal perspective (Berry, 1980). It has also been viewed as the "the cultural change which results from the continued firsthand contact between two distinct cultures" (Nwadiora & McAdoo, 1996). Berry (1997) describes acculturation as a bidimensional process where one may identify highly or temperately with both their culture of origin, and with the host culture, resulting in four modes: assimilation, separation, integration, and marginalization. In acculturation discourse, bicultural integration (i.e., high identification with both culture of origin as well as host culture) is often posited as the ideal.

For families where members are in different acculturation modes (as is often the case), there may be psychological stress and interpersonal conflict with regards to expectations about relationships, achievements and behaviors. Indeed, it can be argued that acculturation is related to endorsement of traditional gender ideology. Research has shown that this can be a source of contention specifically between SAA girls and their families, and affects the levels of assimilation and integration possible for these youth (Masood et al., 2009). This may be exemplified in the differing demands placed on male and female children in the SAA home. SA culture, while traditionally favoring the male gender, idolizes femininity as a symbol of chastity, modesty, and motherhood. Girls more than boys, bear the burden of being demure in dress, submissive in deportment, limiting/abstaining from premarital sex and sexual experimentation (Ekanayake et al., 2012). Additionally, the burden of preserving cultural and religious customs and traditions in a new land often falls on girls (Dasgupta, 1998; Mahalingam & Haritatos, 2006).

As described in the case of Binal, her family adapted in many ways to Western culture, but also did their best to maintain ties to Bangladeshi culture. Berry (2006) refers to the high identification with both host culture as well as culture of origin as bicultural integration. Despite the benefits of being able to adapt to two cultures and find a sense of belonging in each,, the process of acculturation often involves acculturative stress (Berry, 2006). Due to this stress, Binal may struggle with whether to resist or conform to cultural expectations of femininity and with her ethnic identity. Immigrant communities often use binaries, such as "American" and "South Asian" (or Indian, Pakistani etc.), to frame behavioral expectations (Bacchus, 2017). In Binal's case, these rigid constructs may do her a disservice in regards to her ethnic and sexual identities because she often feels torn in deciding what set of expectations to adhere to. Given the importance of acculturation level on an immigrant family's sense of belonging and identity, it would be important for a clinician working with Binal to appreciate where she lies on the spectrum of both gender and ethnicity, and to explore where she (and her family) see themselves in regards to Berry's model of acculturation.

The Importance of Marriage

The pressure placed on females in the SAA home often manifests in the domain of marriage and sexuality, including the presence of premarital sex, expectations for partner choice, type of marriage and beliefs about dating. Evidence suggests that SAA males often experience more conflict on academic-related items (i.e., being compared to others academically and time allocation for study and recreation) while their female counterparts experienced greater conflict on sociocultural items (i.e., issues of dating and collective decision-making processes) (Rahman & Witenstein, 2013). Women's sexuality has often served as a battleground for contesting or conforming to ethnic boundaries (Bacchus, 2017); and the average SAA female is acutely aware of this phenomenon. The following are quotes from SAA clients in therapy sessions with the authors over the years:

> *If I don't get married before my brother does, it's going to be so embarrassing for my family.*

> *If people find out about who my sister is dating, my parents would die of a broken heart. She clearly doesn't care enough about them and is more focused on herself.*

> *I was sexually harassed by someone the other day and I know I can't tell my parents. They would ask me what I was wearing and why I was out by myself. They would blame me and be embarrassed that it happened as opposed to being angry on my behalf. That's the first thing that entered my mind after it happened.*

> *There's no way I can tell my parents that I don't even want to get married. Because then they'll start asking why, and I would need to tell them more about who I am than I am ready to. I'd rather just play along for now.*

Indeed, marriage is often seen as the cornerstone of the U.S. South Asian family and community (Ternikar, 2008; Kniss & Numrich, 2007). Additionally, ethnic community and religious expectations reinforce adherence to accepted standards of behavior for women and girls. These sociocultural expectations in addition to intensified parental concern that children will become "Americanized," lead to separation (from one's own culture of origin) rather than assimilation in many U.S. South Asian families.

Feminist scholarship has critiqued the institution of the South Asian American family as hetero-normative, patriarchal, exclusionary, and hierarchical. As Chayanika Shah (2005) writes, "[q]ueer, feminist, Dalit [the name for people belonging to the lowest caste in India, characterized as 'untouchable'] and left politics have all engaged theoretically and practically in an attempt to critique and transgress the familiar boundaries of marriage and family." Furthermore, there is critique on the entanglement of family and caste as factors of oppression on the South Asian subcontinent (John, 2005; Rao, 2005). John, furthering the Dalit critique of caste-based marriage alliances, states that the anti-caste movements, beginning during the early 19th century, were alternate ways of politicizing the institutions of marriage and family "by addressing sexuality, gender, caste and religion altogether" (2005). Clinicians working with SAA clients in therapy will better their understanding of the robust history of critique and resistance to gendered oppression in SA cultures. For example, it would be empowering for Binal to know the history of South Asian American women that have stood against gendered oppression, as much of what she was taught about feminism has often highlighted European and European American women.

Although there is variation regarding the practice of intimate relationships, courtship and arranged marriages, dating and premarital sexual behaviors, it is usually viewed as unacceptable. The lack of acceptance applies more so for girls and women as not adhering to prescribed behaviors may compromise a family's ability to secure a "good" husband for their daughters (DasGupta, 1998). Indeed, traditional arranged marriage practices persist among some U.S. South Asian families, particularly those living in suburban and small town locales. Many adolescents and young adults of this cultural background also reportedly accept ethnic and/or parental limitations on their socialization, and trust elders to make sound decisions regarding mate selection (Hickey, 2011). Similar to the mindset of many other ethnic minority communities, chastity and "purity" for females is considered valuable within the South Asian context as it relates to whether an individual comes from a "good" family and reflects a woman's sense of modesty, allegiance to cultural norms and commitment to family harmony. In the case of Binal, she definitely experiences pressure to remain chaste and pure in the eyes of her family, knowing that any deviation from that will bring shame to the entire family. Interestingly, while scholarship has delineated the specific ways in which the family promotes inequality and asymmetrical gender roles, another set of literature has highlighted women's agency in dealing with the structures and norms of various forms of oppression. (Bhandari & Titzmann, 2017).

It should be noted that searches on clinical and sociocultural literature on South Asian American male gender socialization of men has yielded few results. While there is more written about the impact of gender socialization of SAA females, there is very little focus on the process of negotiating masculinity across cultural contexts for SAA men. In a study exploring attitudes toward seeking psychological help, authors have suggested that the pressures men experience "to appear strong and in control" may exacerbate the already prevalent issue of stigma and shame regarding mental health, and prevent them from seeking psychological services (Arora et al., 2016). Clinicians will do well to be alert to this possible phenomenon. The impact of patriarchy and male gender privilege on so many aspects of SAA men's lives can also not be underestimated (Sharma, 2000).

Growing research points to a diversity inherent in the U.S. South Asian population with regards to marriage practices and gendered expectations. Evidence from a qualitative study of young women of South Asian descent in the U.S., for example, suggests that there are variations in the extent to which mothers enforce traditions surrounding premarital sex as some allow dating to prepare for marriage (Deepak, 2004) while others do not. Furthermore, semi-arranged marriages are growing in popularity among South Asian Americans (Hickey, 2017) with men and women having choice over who they marry with just some input or friendly "introductions" by the family/community. Ethnographic works have demonstrated that, far from being passive recipients, SA women have their own strategies to negotiate with familial suppression (Jeffery & Jeffery, 1996; Raheja & Gold, 1994; Thapan, 2009). In a study of South Asian Canadian young adults, Gravel et al. (2016) reveal how premarital sexuality in emerging adults of South Asian descent is not uniform and bound to the traditional sexual values of their heritage culture that encourage abstinence before marriage.

These nuances should caution clinicians to avoid generalizations about SAA clients and urges diligence in exploring each individual's narrative about their gender and their family or community's gendered expectations with regard to intimacy and relationships. What is important is to provide space in conceptualization, and when appropriate, in therapy to deftly contend with these nuances.

Gender and Impact of Family

As mentioned earlier in this chapter, the SAA family plays a crucial role in the gender socialization of subsequent generations. The way in which gender expectations manifest in a family are likely impacted by the specific dynamics of that family unit. Below are a few examples of how family may impact the ways in which males and females are treated, parented, and understood in the home by their family. The themes below are not exhaustive given the heterogeneity of the South Asian diaspora in regards to religion, geographic region of origin, caste, socioeconomic level, educational attainment, acculturation level and immigration history, but the authors offer a few family related dynamics that may be important to consider when working with a SAA client.

Male vs. Female Preference

A preference for male children in the South Asian context may play a role in how female children are treated in the home. As Das Gupta et al. (2003) state, "as long as daughters continue to be totally absorbed into their husband's home and cannot contribute to their parents' welfare, son preference will continue to persist even though adult women are integrated into education and formal employment." In the case of Binal, she is aware that it was perfectly acceptable for her father's parents to be cared for by her mother, while it would have not been acceptable to have her maternal grandparents live with the family. Though she loves her paternal grandparents, she has always felt this was an unfair system. This may manifest in how close daughters feel to their parents, how they monitor their bodies and behaviors, in the opportunities afforded to them and in their views of traditional gender ideology. It should be noted, however, that this dynamic may or may not play a role within a South Asian-American family and does not uniformly manifest across families in the South Asian subcontinent either.

Research shows that son preference is especially strong only in the Northern part of India (Das Gupta et al., 2003). This may be related to a kinship system in the Southern parts of India where there is a mutual reliance between married women and their families—the parents receive some physical and other types of supports from their daughter while the daughters continue to receive support from parents, as needed (Das Gupta et al., 2003). The persistence of male preference will likely manifest (or not play a role at all) based on where a family is from in India, their value for traditional gender roles, and the level of their adaptation to Western values and level of urbanization. The authors have found little research in the SAA context regarding how the preference for males plays out in the SAA home; but it would be remiss to ignore data from countries of origin as we also consider this dynamic in the host countries.

In parts of Canada, for instance, son preference was found to persist among second-generation mothers of South Asian ethnicity (Wanigaratne et al., 2018). South Asian immigrant women in another Canadian study were also found to have an abnormally high share of boys after a first-born girl, suggesting sex-selective mechanisms to achieve this outcome. (Adsera & Ferrer, 2020). In the United Kingdom, The Pink Ladoo Project—"a global gender equality campaign dismantling patriarchy by encouraging South Asian families to abandon sexist customs and celebrate girls' births"—was founded by lawyer and social activist, Raj Khaira, after the negative reactions she witnessed to her sister's birth (www.pinkladoo.org).

Anecdotal and clinical evidence, however, suggests an equal preference for sons and daughters in many SAA homes but differences in how they are expected to behave and in what responsibilities they are given. Both face different pressures and seem to be expected to play specific roles in the home, sometimes due to their gender and at other times, due to their family's broader expectations. Again, here are some quotes from SAA clients we have worked with:

> *My father never made me and my sister feel like we were second-class citizens growing up [as females]. But when it came time to participate in a specific puja [religious ceremony], we were surprised by how we weren't allowed to participate.*

> *No one ever said this to me explicitly but it was always clear that I should stay closer to home for college [as the female], while my brother was allowed to go anywhere he wanted. If I ask my parents about this now, they would probably think I was crazy and deny that they wanted this … but it was in the air.*

> *I feel so much shame that I live far away from home and am marrying someone who is not Indian. As the older child and as the son, I just feel like I'm supposed to do better.*

Again, how these roles and expectations come alive within a family are likely related to a family's level of acculturation, how connected they feel to their country/culture of origin, how gender is understood in their family, and other factors such as loss or trauma, that complicate the expectations placed on both sons and daughters in a home.

Family Structure

Recent research indicates that the role played by daughters is intensified when there is no other female present in a family. In a study that explored how maternal loss impacted father-daughter relationships in the South Asian American home, analyses revealed that all daughters seemed to take on additional responsibilities in their families (Sharma & Natrajan, 2018). It was evident that fathers consciously or unconsciously encouraged stereotypical gender roles in their daughters and did not see this as problematic. This expectation of women to place others' needs ahead of their own, respect their elders, and be caregivers is consistent with patriarchal ideals in and out of the South Asian cultural context, but may be emphasized when there are limited social supports upon immigration (Sharma & Natrajan-Tyagi, 2018). In the case of Binal, a clinician could consider the potential for this gender role expectation due to the fact that she is the only female child in her family system.

Indeed, the caregiving burden has been found to be placed on women in many South Asian families. Gupta and Pillai (2012) point out that Asian Indian female (child/in-law) caregivers experience more burden in providing care for the elderly than their male counterparts. Other research highlights how more wives are seen providing care to their older husbands in India, though adult sons are culturally expected to shoulder caregiving responsibilities. The emigration of men further increases the care burden on women, especially on spouses and daughters-in-law (Ajay et al., 2017; Bongaarts & Zimmer, 2002). For Indian daughters, traditional norms emphasize that once a daughter is married, she is no longer obligated to care for her own parents as her obligations for caregiving are now transferred to her parents-in-law (Gupta et al., 2009; Lamb, 2005). However, research and anecdotal evidence indicates that daughters do assume responsibility for parent care when a son is not available due to emigration or when a parent is widowed (Pillai et al., 2012). These findings are consistent with broader caregiving research work that has shown that women are more likely to experience a great amount of role conflict as they attempt to juggle occupational demands and the demands of caregiving (Hooyman & Kiyak, 2011). Oftentimes, this is due to the ways in which women have been socialized to be "nurturers" and caregivers in a home or because of the inadvertent expectation that they are better equipped emotionally to manage the grief and complex emotions that come with aging parents.

Emphasis on Family Honor

A noteworthy family dynamic that may also govern the behaviors of both sons and daughters in a SAA home is the concept of upholding family honor, preserving and maintaining a positive reputation. These values lead to a salient paradigm that ensures children behave within certain gendered boundaries. The common Hindi and Urdu phrase "Log Kya Kehenge," meaning "What will people say?," captures the essence of this dynamic, as it evokes the fear of public opinion on one's personal life, as well as one's family's standing in society. A number of high-profile South Asian Americans, including comedians Hasan Minaj and Lilly Singh, have brought this phrase into mainstream culture, showcasing the deep impact it has on their generation's psyche. In the case study of Binal discussed later in the chapter, the role of this dynamic becomes clear: though this client feels conflicted about this, a part of her strives to make her parents and extended family proud, which she interprets as needing to meet their expectations and therefore hide her sexual identity. There is an understanding between her and her partner that discussing the nuances of their relationship and the history of her sexual partners would create a panic and fear in her family, evoking a worry about how others in their community will regard them.

It should be noted that, to date, there is limited literature on family issues and mental health considerations for gay, lesbian, bisexual and transgender communities within SAA populations. To the authors' knowledge, most of the SAA research and ethnographies surrounding family life and other relevant dynamics have developed their hypotheses and analyses around heterosexual interactions. This is unfortunate as it positions SAA males and females as stereotypically heterosexual, cisgender and in contrast to counterparts of the "opposite" sex alone. With such an unfortunate gap within the literature, it is imperative for the clinician working with SAA individuals to explore how their client sees and understands themselves in regards to sexuality and gender identity. Binal's case is an example of how assumptions cannot be made about a client's sexuality, regardless of current partner choice. Clinicians should be mindful not to presume heterosexuality. Indeed, while the literature is sparse, one journal article has noted: "queer South Asian diaspora has become more visible and vocal about asserting their unique identity" (Adur & Purkayastha, 2017). These authors point out that the very nature of these identities transgress traditional notions of gender role conformity (Adur & Purkayastha, 2017). Thus, clinicians will do well to familiarize themselves with language and discourse that does not presume a binary of gender. Further, familiarity with culturally specific South Asian LGBTQ resources, locally and nationally will be of great benefit to some clients.

Stigma and Other Consequences for Not Conforming to Gender Norms

Many South Asian American cultures govern social behavior and expectations with shame, which is not only reflected individually, but in many cases brings shame on an entire family (Karasz et al., 2019). Gender socialization, to a large degree, is strongly reinforced, with tremendous social, physical, economic, and existential consequences for non-adherence. Gender-based violence can be seen as mechanisms to maintain control and reminders that there are severe consequences for not fulfilling the expectations of one's ascribed gender. And much of this tremendous pressure is unduly placed on women. This pressure is important to consider in terms of clinical presentation and issues. Some of the traditional tenets in South Asian cultures, which extend to pressure on South Asian American women from our clinical experiences, include:

- It being considered "dishonorable" if cultural norms not adhered to (e.g., becoming pregnant out of wedlock, dating for too many years before getting engaged, living with partner before marriage)
- Females being pressured to get married younger than their male counterparts due to "getting too old" for attractiveness or child bearing.
- Single men and women identifying as anything other than heterosexual or cisgender
  - In terms of second-generation SAA lesbian women, Islam (1998) notes "the fact that there is no word for lesbians in Bengali, Hindi or Urdu is a linguistic clue to cultural and structural organization of sexuality in the respective societies."

While it is true that much of the pressure of gender role conformity in South Asian cultures are placed on women, and that men typically are afforded many more privileges, and are socialized with concordant sense of entitlement, South Asian men experience pressure to conform as well, which may manifest in such ways as feeling more keenly shame or stigma in seeking help (Arora, Metz, & Carlson, 2016). Additionally, non-traditional South Asian men may feel the pressures of pursuing lucrative professional careers, being breadwinners for the family, and may be criticized for taking a hands-on approach to raising children or performing shared domestic duties with their partners as viewed by other traditional family members. Such expectations have brought upon criticism of males as a consequence to evolving toward greater gender equality.

Case Study Discussion

The case of Binal, a 20-year-old cisgender, Bangladeshi-American female, who identifies as queer, will be used to illustrate key issues and concepts discussed in this chapter. While this client enters therapy due to "problems with relationships," it becomes evident to the clinician that she also struggles with a deep-rooted fear of being abandoned by her family and a core belief of not being "enough." Binal feels this way regardless of how hard she works or how well she performs at work or school. She is also aware that because of her achievement and drive, she may appear to be a "stereotypical Asian American" because she is a member of a community labeled as "the model minority." Binal grew up just outside of Philadelphia with her older brother (age 23), her two parents, and her paternal grandmother. (Her paternal grandfather died when she was five.)

Her issues and struggles are also tied to gendered expectations implicitly placed on her by her family, their immigrant community, and her own understanding of herself as a second-generation American. She noted that she always found it unfair that her brother didn't seem to experience nearly the amount of pressure she did to conform to gender roles. She reflected: "It was easier for him to break the rules, and Amma and Baba rarely got as angry with him." She added

> But it's not like we're SUPER conservative—I think we are pretty relaxed compared to other Bangladeshi families, but when it came to me, WOW—my parents, and sometimes even my brother, seemed to all of a sudden get psycho traditional on me.

When asked about her grandmother's role in these expectations, "well, it's mixed. I definitely knew that she wanted me to be 'a good Muslim girl' and even though she doesn't get me completely, she makes me want to make her proud."

When asked about her religious identity, she says she has "a complicated relationship with Islam." She adds, however, that her family's identification as Muslim "has been a problem" given the stigma of this religious background in the sociopolitical context of the United States today. She feels like her parents "overcompensate" for this stigma by prominently displaying the American flag in their front yard after 9/11, and becoming "diehard" Philadelphia Eagles and 76ers fans.

> It's a little over the top, but I guess it's cute seeing them all dressed up in team jerseys in the sports arenas while packing halal meals for themselves as they tailgate with neighbors and friends. A speck of brown in a sea of white and black.

She adds that her father often would say, "we can't be as American as our neighbors, but we must try to fit in."

When asked what brought her in for therapy, she replied "problems with relationships." When asked about previous romantic relationships, Binal replied: "Well ... I've had sex with men and with women ... AND I hate the term bisexual, so if you use that word with me, you and I are going to have a problem." The intake counselor asks her if there is a term she prefers, and she says "I guess I'm ok with queer—though I'm not that into labels in general." As therapy continues, you come to find out that Binal is estranged from her family because, per her report, "they just don't get me and accept the way I am." She also refers to not being "the good Muslim Bengali girl they expect me to be." You use this opportunity to say "tell me more about what makes for a "good Muslim Bengali girl." Binal opens up to you at this point, telling you what her family expects of her, and how she has always rebelled against what she sees as "backwards thinking." She shares that her family was often anxious about "what others will say" in regards to who she spent time with, what she wore and how often she attended community events. Upon inquiry by the clinician, she also shared: "I guess a part of me also does fall into that trap of worrying about bringing shame to the family." This made her want to disengage from the family since she is "such a problem" for them and was tired of struggling with her and her family's experience of shame regarding so many of her life decisions. Now that she is dating a Bangladeshi-American male, she sometimes wonders if she's "falling into the trap" of doing what is expected of her as opposed to "finding the right person for me."

There are many factors—namely, culture, sociopolitical context, family, and the intersection of identities—that appear to be impacting Binal's sense of self and overall mental health. In terms of culture, Binal appears to be caught between cultural expectations of her culture of origin (Bangladeshi) while contending with expectations from her host culture (U.S.). The sociopolitical impact of racism, sexism, and Islamophobia cannot be ignored. Understanding family dynamics from a nuanced cultural perspective is also important, recognizing that influences beyond the nuclear family must be considered. Since Binal's sense of self is informed in part by her identity development, including race, gender, religion, sexual orientation, and more dimensions of identity, all of these must be considered in addressing Binal's case.

In terms of presenting problems, it may be important to consider any biological predispositions for anxiety and depression. When asking about Binal's family history of these diagnoses, a clinician may find that someone of her background may not have knowledge of this since mental health diagnoses were not talked about in the family. There may have been no language for psychological disorders and even if there was, there is often shame and stigma in talking about it them, due to pressures to "keep up appearances" related to the family value or preserving the family reputation. Anecdotally, a number of SAA clients often do not know about their family's psychiatric, psychological, or medical histories due to a silence surrounding traumatic events or highly emotional content.

This gap in intergenerational knowledge is consistent with intergenerational trauma research, which describes one of the central clinical features to be the silence that occurs in families surrounding traumatic experiences (Evans-Campbell, 2008; Fossion et al., 2003; Herman, 1992; Mussell et al., 2004; Nagata & Cheng, 2003). The trauma remains a "secret" trauma not verbally expressed; unacknowledged but with the potential to be passed on nonetheless (Byers & Gere, 2007). The first generation has difficulty in communicating the trauma, and with silence as the only means of expression, discontinuity occurs in the historical legacy of the family (Fossion et al., 2003). In the case of Binal, it may be worth exploring her knowledge of her family's history, including potential traumatic experiences that may have never been fully acknowledged, yet may have an impact on Binal's well-being.

The conflict Binal feels in terms of being in a romantic relationship with someone that would potentially meet her family's expectations in fulfilling her gender role (by being of the same ethnicity and religion) must be addressed. She appears to identify with a sense of resisting gender disparity and gender-based oppression, and may feel she is conforming to what her culture expects of her. An appreciation of this conflict with all its nuances related to gender, sexuality, and identity, must be considered.

In the authors' experiences of working with SAA's, we wish to highlight a few considerations with this case study. Clinicians working with SAA clients should:

- Pay close attention to client's language, especially around self-identification—note the therapist above reflecting back and enquiring about 'good Muslim Bengali girl'. Even if a clinician may feel they understand what these terms, identities, or expectations placed on them mean to the client, it can be a powerful method of empathic joining to ask clients to "say more" about what the particular phrases mean to them.
- Use any opportunity to create spaces for clients to share (and perhaps deepen the client's own reflection on) their own gender socialization from both their family of origin and from social influences. Listen for moments where such a line of exploration seems warranted.

- Throughout the therapeutic process, place the client at the vanguard of these issues and "get behind the curtain with them" as they attempt to navigate these complexities. For example, a clinician could ask "what's it like for you to get these conflicting messages of how you are supposed to conform to gendered expectations (from your family and/or community)?" Or, in this case, there is an opportunity to assess the family's acculturation by asking "you mentioned your parents being 'a speck of brown in a sea of black and white'—tell me more about what that was like for you growing up."
- Explore how gender was performed or how gender roles were modeled in the client's home. A clinician could ask, for example, "What did you observe around specific gender roles with your parents or the adults in your community?" and "How has this influenced how you identify and how you engage in the world?"

Clinical Stories

In addition to anecdotes shared thus far, the authors wish to convey important breakthroughs in therapy with SAA in therapy and gender issues. Author 2 (RS) is often reminded of working with an Indian-American male in therapy who was struggling with his sense of manhood as a physical injury compromised not only his physical strength, but also made him prone to crying spells. It was the clinician's assessment that the client's religious beliefs as a Hindu were important to him. The clinician was able to integrate aspects of Hindu mythology (in this case, The Mahabharata & Bhagavad Gita) to position a clinical "reframing" of the concept of strength. The client was comforted by this culturally meaningful point of reference and its' integrating with psychotherapy techniques. Therefore, it is important to explore the varied factors that play a role in mental health; knowledge may prove useful in providing effective clinical services to SAAs.

Author 1 (SNK) relates that there are multiple cases where the issue of anxiety, often to the point of panic disorder and related issues, can be largely traced to the amount of pressure placed on SAA women in therapy. The provision of a space to "unpack" the magnanimity of that pressure, and the potential for relief that can occur when the therapist deftly navigates these complexities with the client, is vital. It cannot be stressed how powerful therapy can be in providing a much needed space to address issues typically not validated, explored or named in the SAA community with regard to stress and mental health.

Thinking Outside the Box (or Outside the Therapy Room): The Role of Outreach & Psychoeducation

Author 2 (RS) wishes to share experiences in addressing SAA gender socialization through innovative outreach programming. For the past 30 years, he has been designing culturally specific dialogues on gender for SAA communities. His experience has taught him that there is a yearning to collectively "unpack" expectations and pressures placed upon individuals and groups. The judicious use of humor, innovative techniques, and an ability to validate experiences have been powerful. Because of the stigma associated with mental health, clinicians might want to think about partnering with cultural organizations or student groups. For example, screening a movie like Monsoon Wedding and holding a well-facilitated discussion gender, stigma, shame, sexual assault, and more may be needed. Hosting a workshop that encourages community members to discuss intimate partner violence in the community, accountability, and more may also be quite beneficial. These outreach events could be followed by a provision of resources, and through evaluation forms, a sense of what other forums community members may wish to attend, or even co-create.

Therapy and Identity Issues

Working with South Asian patients may require us to consider our own biases and assumptions, regardless of our ethnic background and heritage. For the South Asian therapist, overidentification with a patient is one possible dynamic that may emerge in the treatment room. While commonalities between therapist and patient can create rapport, a sense of safety, and a strong sense of empathy from the clinician's end, it can certainly contribute to some challenges too. The concept of countertransference, defined "as a therapist's emotional entanglement with a client" (Stefana, 2017), has been researched and discussed at length within the field of Psychology, but we discuss here the ways in which it might play out between a SAA therapist and patient.

Considerations for the SAA Therapist

There may be assumptions on the part of SAA clinicians, for example, that their client's experiences mirror ones they experienced themselves. This may gloss over important differences between the experiences of the therapist and client, impacting the ways in which a presenting issue may be processed or discussed. Over-identification with a client may also lead to an empathic rift from the therapist's end when a client does not interpret or respond to a cultural experience in the way the therapist may have in their own personal life. Using the case study discussed above, Binal says to her South Asian American therapist: "Well, you know how South Asian parents can be." You have an opportunity to keep "one foot in, one foot out"—the foot in me maintenance of a perhaps much-needed sense of connection and identification with the therapist, and the foot out being maintenance of some level of clinical neutrality. An effective response would be: "I think I DO know what you mean—but I'd still like to hear from you what that means to *you*."

Considerations for the Non-SAA Therapist

The non-SAA therapist may bring a different set of assumptions into the therapeutic setting with a SAA client, based on their familiarity and exposure to the SAA community. One dynamic that frequently comes into play, for example, is the confusion on the part of the non-SAA therapist at how a seemingly "successful," adult SA client is afraid to share certain aspects of their life with their families. It is commonplace for SAA adults to hide who they are dating or what they do in their recreational time from their families, based on how traditional their families might be in regards to dating, premarital sex, and beliefs regarding gender ideology. As highlighted in a recent exploratory study of South Asian Muslims (Couture-Carron, 2020), many younger members of this community still engage in dating despite cultural norms prompting fear of parenting and community reactions. Indeed, second-generation Americans are at the crossroads between meeting their parents' cultural expectations and selecting new ethnic options that may conflict with ancestral traditions (Bacchus, 2017). This might be a decision a non-SAA therapist may struggle to understand, based on their own identities and lived experiences. It would be remiss to label this secrecy within the family as pathological when in fact, it may be a natural process by which children of immigrants construct ethnic boundaries.

Similarly, it is not uncommon for SA clients in therapy to hide that they are in therapy at all from their family members. This is related to the social stigma surrounding seeking professional mental health services and talking about one's mental health in the SAA community. This, in turn, is related to courtesy stigma, 'the contagion effect of social stigma from the "marked" individual to family members' (Moses, 2014), which has been seen to be a significant barrier to help-seeking among SA (Bradby et al., 2007). The fear is that family members may be discriminated against or valued differently if someone in their family unit is "marked" by mental illness. Elias (2015) summarizes it well—"In a community that valorizes endurance, stoicism is the lionized mode of existence—especially when the community in question, is in America and subjected to the social pressure of conforming to a model minority stereotype."

The non-SAA therapist would benefit from exploring how salient the Model Minority identity is for their SAA client, and how open they might be with their family about such topics. Regardless of ethnic background, it is imperative for a therapist working with SAA clients to challenge their biases, to provide a non-judgmental stance and ensure they are not pathologizing decisions made by the first or second-generation SAA client, that may be more culturally normative.

Summary

In this chapter, we have emphasized the enormity of gender role expectations placed upon SAA populations. While it is complicated by the process of acculturation, family structure, religion, migration history and so much more and there are divergent responses and strategies employed to either conform or resist these influences, it is clear that gender socialization remains a pervasive source of meaning as well as pressure for SAA individuals and families.

As Tummala-Narra (2013) posits: "Psychotherapy that integrates feminist, multicultural and psychodynamic perspectives can provide a meaningful opportunity for healing." Indeed, we believe that many lenses are needed in order to capture the complexity of the lived experiences of SAA people, and that gender socialization is among the most pressing of factors. What is clear is that spaces are needed (both in the therapy room, as well as in psychoeducational and in community dialogues) that allow SAA men, women, and gender non-conforming people to talk about how gender socialization has affected them, thereby strengthening their ability to navigate these complex inlfuences.

As individuals impacted by our own cultures, gendered identities and life experiences, we will undoubtedly have our own introspective, reflective work to do as clinicians to best serve our SAA clients. We hope this chapter, with the assistance of our case study of Binal, helps our readers have a more nuanced, and less stereotyped view, of SAA clients entering the therapy space. It is also our hope that SAA clients like Binal are provided culturally competent and culturally responsive spaces to comfortably and safely process their experiences in the U.S., undoubtedly made more complex by being children of immigrants. As clinicians ourselves, we hope that this discussion on gender socialization in SAA families urges future clinicians and researchers to explore ways to work with SAA couples, parents, caregivers and families to enhance the psychological well-being of this community overall.

Reflection Questions

Reflection Questions for the Clinician

1   What are the limits of my knowledge about the client's:

- Cultural heritage?
- Gender socialization?
- Migration history?
- Self-identification?
- Culturally relevant support resources?

2   What methods can I utilize to bridge this gap? Judiciously asking the client to share? Research? Consultation?
3   What assumptions do I have about this client? In what ways may I be vulnerable to not identifying with my client? In what ways may I be overidentifying with my client?
4   How much work have I done to examine how my own identities of privilege as well as of oppression affect my therapeutic relationship?
5   What questions are you afraid/nervous to ask?

Questions to ask the client (about themselves):

•   How do you identify?
•   What does your identity mean to you? (Use client's language).
•   What are concerns you may have about someone like me working with you?
•   What about your identity/culture/background would be important for me to know?
•   (Balance doing your homework on your client's background with respectfully requesting more information)—I realize as you're talking that I don't know as much as I should about X aspect of your cultural experience (e.g., religion, ethic identification, etc.). So while that's on me, I do want to know more about it as it will help me understand you more. Would you mind telling me more about X as you have experienced it?

Questions to ask client (about their family):

•   What do you know about your family's immigration story to the U.S.?
•   What do you know of your family's experience with adjusting to life in the U.S.?
•   How much do you think your family's _____ affects their story/life here in the U.S.:

    •   Social class?
    •   Caste?
    •   Educational background?
    •   Religion?
    •   Acculturation experience/process?

•   How connected does your family feel to their South Asian heritage/ancestry?

Suggested Resources

South Asian community organizations with focus on gender-based violence, women's advocacy, and/or community responsivity to gender inequality:
    https://www.sakhi.org/south-asian-womens-organizations-in-the-us-new/

Educational Resources

•   South Asian American Digital Archive (saada.org)
•   The Pink Ladoo Project (www.pinkladoo.org)

References

Adsera, A., & Ferrer, A.M. (2020). Speeding up for a son: Sex ratio imbalances by birth interval among South Asian migrants to canada. *Canadian Studies in Population*, *47*(3), 133–149. 10.1007/s42650-020-00025-9

Adur, S.M., & Purkayastha, B. (2017) (Re)telling traditions: The language of social identity among queer South Asians in the United states. *South Asian Diaspora*, *9*(1), 1–16. 10.1080/19438192.2016. 1199456

Ajay, S., Kasthuri, A., Kiran, P., & Malhotra, R. (2017). Association of impairments of older persons with caregiver burden among family caregivers: Findings from rural South India. *Archives of Gerontology and Geriatrics*, *68*, 143–148.

Akl, A. (2011). South Asian women caught between tradition and modernity. *Voice of America*. https://www.voanews.com/east-asia-pacific/south-asian-women-caught-between-tradition-and-modernity.

Arora, P.G., Metz, K., & Carlson, C.I. (2016). Attitudes toward professional psychological help seeking in South Asian students: Role of stigma and gender. *Journal of Multicultural Counseling and Development*, *44*(4), 263–284. 10.1002/jmcd.12053

Bacchus, N.S. (2017). Shifting sexual boundaries: Ethnicity and pre-marital sex in the lives of South Asian American women. *Sexuality & Culture*, *21*(3), 776–794. 10.1007/s12119-017-9421-2

Barker G. 2006. Presented at United nations division for the advancement of women (DAW). In *Collaboration with UNICEF, Expert Group Meeting: Elimination of all forms of discrimination and violence against the girl child*, September 25–28. Florence, Italy: UNICEF Innocenti Research Centre (EGM/DVGC/2006/EP.3). Retrieved from http://www.un.org/womenwatch/daw/egm/elim-disc-violgirlchild/ExpertPapers/EP.3%20%20%20Barker.pdf.

Berry (1980). *Acculturation as varieties of adaptation*. Westview Press.

Berry, J.W. (1997). Immigration, acculturation and adaptation. *Applied Psychology*, *46*(17), 5–34.

Berry J.W. (2006) Acculturative stress. In P. T. P. Wong & L. C. J. Wong (Eds.), *Handbook of multicultural perspectives on stress and coping. International and cultural psychology*. Boston, MA: Springer.

Bhandari, P., & Titzmann, F.-M. (2017). Family realities in South Asia: Adaptations and Resilience. *South Asia Multidisciplinary Academic Journal*, (16). 10.4000/samaj.4365

Bradby, H., Varyani, M., Oglethorpe, R., Raine, W., White, I., & Helen, M. (2007). British Asian families and the use of child and adolescent mental health services: A qualitative study of a hard to reach group. *Social Science & Medicine*, *65*(12), 2413–2424. 10.1016/j.socscimed.2007.07.025

Bongaarts, J., & Zimmer, Z. (2002). Living arrangements of older adults in the developing world: An analysis of demographic and health survey household surveys. *The Journals of Gerontology Series B: Psychological Sciences and Social Sciences*, *57*(3), S145–S157.

Bussey K., & Bandura A. (1999) Social cognitive theory of gender development and differentiation. *Psychological Review*, *106*, 676–713.

Byers, J.G., & Gere, S.H. (2007). Expression in the service of humanity: Trauma and temporality. *Journal of Humanistic Psychology*, *47*(3), 384–391.

Couture-Carron, A. (2020). Shame, family honor, and dating abuse: Lessons from an exploratory study of South Asian muslims. *Violence Against Women*, *26*(15–16), 2004–2023. 10.1177/1077801219895115

Dasgupta, S.D. (1998). Gender roles and cultural continuity in the Asian Indian immigrant community in the U.S. *Sex Roles*, *38*, 953–974.

Deepak, A.C. (2004). *Identity formation and the negotiation of desire: Women of the South Asian Diaspora in the U.S. (Dissertation)* Retrieved from http://search.proquest.com/docview/61533228?accountid=15115

Ekanayake, S., Ahmad, F., & McKenzie, K. (2012). Qualitative cross-sectional study of the perceived causes of depression in South Asian origin women in Toronto. *BMJ Open*, *2*(1). 10.1136/bmjopen-2011-000641

Elias, P.-A. (2015, September 23). The silence about mental health in south Asian Culture is dangerous. https://newrepublic.com/article/122892/silence-mental-health-south-asian-culture-dangerous.

Evans-Campbell, T. (2008). Historical trauma in American Indian/native Alaska communities. *Journal of Interpersonal Violence*, *23*(3), 316–338.

Fossion, P., Rejas, M.C., Servais, L., Pelc, I., & Hirsch, S. (2003). Family approach with grandchildren of holocaust survivors. *American Journal of Psychotherapy*, *57*(4), 519–527.

Fuller, C.J., & Narasimhan, H. (2008). Empowerment and constraint: Women, work and the family in Chennai's software industry. In C. Upadhya & A. R. Vasavi (Eds.), *In an outpost of the global economy: Work and workers in India's information technology industry* (pp. 190–210). New Delhi: Routledge.

Fulton, C.L. (2017). Gender socialization. In *Counseling women across the lifespan: Empowerment, advocacy, and intervention* (pp. 21–38). Springer Publishing.

Gravel, E.E., Young, M.Y., Darzi, C.M., Olavarria-Turner, M., & Lee, A. M.-S. (2016). Premarital sexual debut in emerging adults of South Asian descent: The role of parental sexual socialization and sexual attitudes. *Sexuality & Culture, 20*(4), 862–878. 10.1007/s12119-016-9362-1

Gupta, D.M., Zhenghua, J., Bohua, L., Zhenming, X., Chung, W., & Hwa-Ok, B. (2003). Why is son preference so persistent in East and South Asia? A cross-country study of China, India, and the Republic of Korea. *Policy Research Working Papers*. 10.1596/1813-9450-2942

Gupta, R., & Pillai, V.K. (2012). Elder caregiving in South-Asian families in the United States and India. *Social Work & Society, 10*(2), 1–16.

Gupta, V. K., Turban, D. B., Wasti, S. A., & Sikdar, A. (2009). The role of gender stereotypes in perceptions of entrepreneurs and intentions to become an entrepreneur. *Entrepreneurship Theory and Practice, 33*, 397–417. 10.1111/j.1540-6520.2009.00296.x

Herman, J. (1992). *Trauma and recovery*. New York: Basic Books.

Hickey, M.G. (2011). American friends are for school ... Indian friends are for everything else': Developmental Characteristics of Asian Indian Children in the United States Words and Silences, 6(1), pp. 58–72. International Oral History Association. https://www.ioha.org/wp-content/uploads/2016/06/23-224-3-PB.pdf

Hooyman, N.R., & Kiyak, A.H. (2011). *Social gerontology: A multi-disciplinary perspective* (9th Ed.). Boston, MA: Allyn & Bacon.

Islam, N. (1998). Naming desire, shaping identity: Tracing the experiences of Indian lesbians in the United States. In S.D. Dasgupta (Ed.). *A Patchwork Shawl: Chronicles of South Asian Women in America*. (pp. 72–96). New Brunswick, NJ: Rutgers University Press.

Jeffery, P., & Jeffery, R. (1996). *Don't Marry Me to a Plowman!: Women's everyday lives in rural North India*. Routledge.

John, M.E. (2005). Feminist perspectives on family and marriage: A historical view. *Economic and Political Weekly, 40*(8), 712–715.

Karasz, A., Gany, F., Escobar, J., Flores, C., Prasad, L., Inman, A., Kalasapudi, V., Kosi, R., Murthy, M., Leng, J., & Diwan, S. (2019). Mental health and stress among South Asians. *Journal of Immigrant and Minority Health Supplement; New York, 21*(1), 7–14.

Kniss, F.L., & Numrich, P.D. (2007). *Sacred assemblies and civic engagement*. Rutgers University Press.

Lamb, S. (2005). Cultural and moral values surrounding care and (in)dependence in late life: Reflections from India in an era of global modernity. *Care Management Journals, 6*(2), 80–89.

Mahalingam, R., & Haritatos, J. (2006). *Cultural psychology of gender and immigration*. Lawrence Erlbaum Associates Publishers.

Masood, N., Okazaki, S., & Takeuchi, D.T. (2009). Gender, family, and community correlates of mental health in South Asian Americans. *Cultural Diversity and Ethnic Minority Psychology, 15*(3), 265–274. 10.1037/a0014301

Moses, T. (2014). Stigma and family. In P. W. Corrigan (Ed.), *The stigma of disease and disability: Understanding causes and overcoming injustices* (pp. 247–268). American Psychological Association. 10.1037/14297-013

Mussell, B., Cardiff, K., & White, J. (2004). *The mental health and well-being of Aboriginal children and youth: Guidance for new approaches and services*. Chilliwack: Sal'i'shan Institute.

Nagata, D., & Cheng, W.J.Y. (2003). Intergenerational communication of race related trauma by Japanese-American former internees. *American Journal of Orthopsychiatry, 73*(3), 266–278. 10.1037/0002-9432.73.3.266.

Nwadiora, E., & McAdoo, H. (1996). Acculturative stress among Amerasian refugees: Gender and racial differences. *Adolescence, 31*(122), 477–487.

Pillai, V.K., Levy, E., & Gupta, R. (2012). Relationship quality and elder caregiver burden in India. *Journal of Social Intervention: Theory and Practice, 21*(2), 39–62.

Raheja, G.G., & Gold, A.G. (1994). *Listen to the Heron's words: Reimagining gender and kinship in North India.* Oxford University Press.

Rahman, Z., & Witenstein, M.A. (2013). A quantitative study of cultural conflict and gender differences in South Asian American college students. *Ethnic and Racial Studies, 37*(6), 1121–1137. 10.1080/01419870.2012.753152

Rao, M.G. (2005). *Should Indians pay more in taxes?* Business Standard. https://wap.business-standard.com/article-amp/opinion/m-govinda-rao-should-indians-pay-more-in-taxes-105021201064_1.html.

Shah, C. (2005). The roads that (E)merged: Feminist activism and queer understanding. In *Because I Have a Voice: Queer Politics in India. Essay.* New Delhi: Yoda Press.

Sharma, N., Shaligram, D., & Yoon, G.H. (2020). Engaging South Asian youth and families: A clinical review. *International Journal of Social Psychiatry, 66*(6), 584–592. 10.1177/0020764020922881

Sharma, P.K., & Natrajan-Tyagi, R. (2018). South Asian American daughter–father relationships in the aftermath of maternal loss. *Women & Therapy, 41*(3-4), 356–379. 10.1080/02703149.2018.1430395

Sharma, R. (2000) (Book chapter). Ending violence against women: The role of South Asian men. In S. Nankani (Ed.), *Breaking the Silence: Domestic Violence in the South Asian-American Community.* Xlibris.

Stefana, A. (2017). *History of countertransference: From Freud to the British object relations school.* Routledge/Taylor & Francis Group.

Ternikar, F. (2008). To arrange or not: Marriage trends in the South Asian American community. *Ethnic Studies Review, 31*(2), 153–181. 10.1525/esr.2008.31.2.153

Thapan, M. (2009). *Living the Body: Embodiment, Womanhood and Identity in Contemporary India.* India: Sage Publications.

Tummala-Narra, P. (2013). Psychotherapy with South Asian women: Dilemmas of the immigrant and first generations. *Women & Therapy, 36*(3-4), 176–197. 10.1080/02703149.2013.797853

Wanigaratne, S., Uppal, P., Bhangoo, M., Januwalla, A., Singal, D., & Urquia, M.L. (2018). Sex ratios at birth among second-generation mothers of South Asian ethnicity in Ontario, Canada: A retrospective population-based cohort study. *Journal of Epidemiology and Community Health, 72*(11), 1044–1051. 10.1136/jech-2018-210622

7 South Asian American LGBTQIA+ People and Communities: Developing Spaces of Empowerment and Liberation in Mental Health Settings

Anneliese Singh (she/they) and Saumya Arora (she/they)

Case Overview

Zoha (they/them) is a queer South Asian American individual who experienced anxiety and dealt with frequent microaggressions. Furthermore, as a nonbinary college student, Zoha presented with feelings of hopeless and isolation—despite being close with their family. As they had begun to embrace their identity, Zoha expressed feelings of gender euphoria. The conflict between Zoha's liberation from the gender binary and their family's perspectives creates distress that stems from colonial rule in South Asia.

Introduction

In this chapter, we provide the case example of Zoha, a queer and trans identified South Asian American, to highlight possible difficulties faced by LGBTQIA+ South Asian individuals in the U.S. We describe LGBTQIA+ communities, including specific definitions and unique South Asian American LGBTQIA+ communities. We then present the history and impact of British, white, and western on South Asian American communities, followed by a reclaiming of South Asian culture on the path to LGBTQIA+ liberation. As we explore South Asian American LGBTQIA+ identity throughout this chapter, we do so by utilizing an intersectional lens (Crenshaw, 1991), which highlights interlocking systems of oppression that create multiple societal inequities impacting the mental and physical health and well-being of South Asian American LGBTQIA+ communities. We end the chapter with clinical interventions focusing on the South Asian American LGBTQIA+ community and conclude by providing discussion questions and additional resources.

This chapter will cover relevant literature about cultural context, including South Asian history and family structures, that is necessary to understand Zoha's narrative. For many South Asians, queerness is viewed as something that stems from "Western" society. Presently, LGBTQIA+ South Asian Americans experience familial disapproval, unacceptance by community and/or in religious circles, and mental distress. In order to better support this community, we will discuss factors that impact identity exploration and therapeutic work with LGBTQIA+ South Asian American clients. The relevant literature will also provide a framework to recognize the transmission of intergenerational trauma that influences Zoha's own experiences.

Throughout this chapter, we explore South Asian American genders and sexualities, as well as ways to support South Asian American LGBTQIA+ communities in mental health settings. Unlike many Asian countries, South Asia has documented early history of the acceptance of LGBTQIA+ identities, but with the impacts of white and western colonization, these views have significantly changed in society with the impacts of colonization imposing rigid gender and sexuality binaries that impact South Asian

DOI: 10.4324/9781003081548-7

American LGBTQIA+ communities—as well as South Asian American cisgender and straight communities—today. For instance, distinct queer and non-conforming populations in South Asia have existed prior to British colonization as culturally distinct groups (e.g., Hijra, Aravani, Thirunangaigal, Khwajasara, Kothi, Thirunambigal, Jogappa, Jogatha, or Shiva ShaktiIt—we describe these communities in later sections in this chapter). Post-colonization, there has been a great shift and political oppression of LGBTQIA+ communities both within South Asian and South Asian American communities.

The first public account of South Asian American LBGTQIA+ communities was in 1918 when Tara Singh and Jamil Singh are separately arrested for "interracial sodomy" in Sacramento, California. There is other history of South Asian American LGBTQIA+ identity from this time forward, however past and current heterosexist stigma has erased much of this history—including the history of resilience to multiple oppressions and the experience of joy and liberation within South Asian American LGBTQIA+ communities. Instead, our South Asian American LGBTQIA+ community history is left with restricted definitions and cultural norms that prioritize straight and cisgender identities, which then gives rise to extensive embedded heterosexism within South Asian American families and institutions within the South Asian American communities (e.g., religious centers, community centers). The influence of British puritanical colonization mixes with U.S.-based heterosexism to give rise to not only a lack of acceptance by South Asian American families of LGBTQIA+ family and community members, but also major mental health impacts for South Asian American LGBTQIA+ communities. In addition, South Asian American LGBTQIA+ communities are often exploring their genders and sexualities outside of their families and in predominantly white spaces, where they can experience the impacts of racism and white supremacy as they are moving through their gender and sexual orientation identity development.

In this chapter, we present a case example to show the mental health challenges and opportunities South Asian American LGBTQIA+ communities face within their families and communities. We describe who LGBTQIA+ communities are, including definitions and unique South Asian American LGBTQIA+ communities. We then describe the history and impact of British, white, and western on South Asian American LGBTQIA+, cisgender, and straight communities, followed by a reclaiming of South Asian culture on the path to LGBTQIA+ liberation. As we explore South Asian American LGBTQIA+ identity throughout this chapter, we do this through an intersectional lens per Crenshaw's (1991) theory that demands exploration of interlocking systems of oppression that create multiple societal inequities impacting the mental and physical health and well-being of South Asian American LGBTQIA+ communities. We end the chapter with clinical interventions focusing on the South Asian American LGBTQIA+ community and share discussion questions and other resources at the end of the chapter. As we begin this chapter, refer to the brief synopsis of Zoha, a South Asian LGBTQIA+ person, mentioned at the beginning of the chapter to highlight the issues our chapter will address. We also include two first-person accounts of South Asian LGBTQ+ people.

LGBTQIA+ South Asian Communities: Terms and Definitions

As we write this chapter, we recognize that the impact of white and western colonization continues even in our use and definition of terms used in LGBTQIA+ South Asian American communities. For instance, we will describe essential terms that mental health practitioners such as "gender," "sex," and "sexual orientation" to ensure we have a strong foundation in LGBTQIA+ mental health. However, we also grieve as we write, as we can also recognize that the dismantling and erasure of LGBTQIA+ identities in South Asia has impacted the way we use language today.

A foundational understanding of South Asian American LGBTQIA+ communities starts with knowing that gender, sex, and sexuality are distinct, but interrelated constructs (APA, 2015). Much has been written about essential terms within LGBTQIA+ communities (Singh & dickey, 2016), and it is important to also note that for each term and definition we share that it is important to seek to understand how South Asian American LGBTQIA+ communities might use and understand these terms for themselves individually. Whereas sex is typically a binary designation assigned at birth (often "female" or "male" and also often erases "intersex" identities), gender is also a binary designation (typically "woman" or "man") assigned to a person based on their sex assignment at birth. The challenge with these binary sex and gender designations is that they are social constructs and are not self-described by the person to whom they are assigned. So, from birth, a person is tagged, labelled, and assumed to have a sex and gender that may not fit them and actually is a "guess" until the person grows into their sex and gender where they can self-identify. This leaves South Asian American communities without more helpful and accurate information about what sex and gender assignment is—and how South Asian American LGBTQIA+ communities can fall well outside of these sex and gender identity labels and boxes. Cisgender people are those who their sex and gender assignments may match how they truly feel their sex and gender are. Trans people are those who sex and gender assignments do not match how they know their sex and gender identities to be. Trans is often used as an umbrella term to include those who identify as transmen, transwomen, transsexual (a more dated term, but used with empowerment by older trans people), and nonbinary. Nonbinary people (or gender-nonconforming, agender, genderqueer, gender-fluid, and more terms) are those who may not ascribe to one gender identity—and/or feel their gender identity shifts and changes over time or is without a gender at all. Nonbinary people often use third person plural pronouns, such as "they/their/them," "ze/hir," or another set of gender-neutral pronouns outside of the "she/her/hers" or "he/him/his" that other cisgender and trans people may use.

Sexuality similarly has had inaccuracies within how this term is used in larger straight communities—but less in terms of a binary (straight and queer for instance) and more in terms of a homogenous assumption that all people are straight. This assumption causes harm to South Asian American LGBTQIA+ communities as there is additional work to self-describe. A famous quiz in the 1970s called the "Heterosexual Questionnaire" (Rochlen, 1977) would often ask, "When did you first realize you were straight" to note how heterosexism (the societal oppression that prioritizes sexuality as being only straight and that LGBQA+ identities are an anomaly). Another hetero-normative assumption is that all people must have sexual attraction, sexual drive, and desire to have sex. With the LGBTQIA+ umbrella, asexual (or "ace") people may or may not ascribe to these definitions of sexual attraction. For instance, some aromantic people may enjoy cuddling and physical touch, but not sexual touch. As we unpack the colonized, white, and western terms within and outside of the LGBTIA+ community, we realize that many of these terms—although essential to know—reflect the embedded assumptions that people do and should have a sex, gender, and sexuality (Dave, 2011). We are not countering these assumptions entirely, but we do raise questions related to adultism (the oppression of young people by older people, manifested by the assumption that older people know younger people's bodies, thoughts, feelings, beliefs better than young people know themselves) that impact this entire discussion and designation of what sex, gender, and sexuality are.

When working with South Asian American LGBTQIA+ communities, it is important to know the specific terms that can describe them within South Asian society. For instance, trans people in South Asian are referred to as the "hijra"—but there may also be no specific terms within South Asian languages that are positive descriptors (Gandhi, 2020). There are references of positivity where hermaphrodites, hijra's are specifically asked to be a part of religious rites despite the stigma. Additionally, for those South Asian American communities immigrating to the U.S., they may use the terms that do not have positive connotations relative to their home language; and, as they learn the terms we have described above, they may think that the English terms make LGBTQIA+ identities a white and western phenomenon. So, there are also many anti-LGBTQIA+ slurs used in South Asian community that are important to become aware of when working with South Asian American LGBTQIA+ communities as they may hear these within their communities and the impact of colonization both within South Asian and the U.S. are important to keep in mind when working with South Asian American LGBTQIA+ communities.

Indigenous Groups in South Asia and LGBTQIA+ Roots

Like indigenous groups in the U.S., indigenous groups that have resided in South Asia since ancient times possess a distinct culture whose existence has been threatened and minoritized since the occupation of non-indigenous peoples in South Asia (Tulanker, 2020). Indigenous knowledge in South Asia has provided essential information for ways of living, such as for healthcare and agriculture (Bandyopadhyay, 2018), medicinal plant usage (Zhasa et al., 2015), and political intervention (Sillitoe, 2000). Ironically, many indigenous tribes are now caste-oppressed within Hinduism and other religions in South Asia, including Sikhism, Buddhism, Islam, and Christianity (Upadhyay, 2020). Despite their contributions to modern day South Asian culture, indigenous tribes face a myriad of inequalities, including poverty, increased mortality, hunger, and illiteracy (Thresia et al., 2022).

Prior to Indo-Aryan migration, indigenous tribes in South Asia embraced gender and sexual fluidity, and these roots must be acknowledged when considering the queerness of pre-colonial South Asia. For example, before the growth of Hinduism and other religions in South Asia, indigenous cultures in South Asia celebrated the gender fluidity of their deities. The various religious beliefs of indigenous groups in South Asia were largely absorbed into what is now known as Hinduism. It is important to pay attention to these dynamics when deconstructing what it means to be LGBTQIA+ and South Asian American. Furthermore, a decolonized approach to counseling South Asian American LGBTQIA+ individuals requires a return to indigenous roots of collective healing and acceptance. See Deepali's first-person account of getting married to her wife in South Asia and navigates both being queer and of two different faiths.

Deepali Gets Married: A First-Person Account

When my wife and I first decided to get married, we definitely knew we would face some big barriers. It wasn't that we were queer that was the problem. Both of our families are pretty progressive and wanted us to be happy and liked the person we chose to be with for life. The problem was that I am Hindu and my wife is Muslim. We ourselves, of course, didn't have trouble with being an interfaith couple, but our families didn't know what to do. Even though India has so many different religions, sects, and ways to practice religion and spirituality, my wife and I had to acknowledge the deep generations of distrust and history between religious groups here. To get through this difficulty, we talked to our parents about what they believed about the other religion—and we were shocked! What they shared had less to do with actual history and more to do with myths that aren't true.

We also talked to them about having an interfaith ceremony. We both value our religions and we wanted to reflect this in our marriage. I am not saying this is a typical story—but for us it worked out. Our families saw a little of their own values in our wedding ceremony and they learned quite a deal about the other religion. For my wife and I, we decided to continue to integrate both of our religions into our lives. We jointly recognize Hindu and Muslim holidays. Moving through our family issues helped us strengthen our own religious faiths.

Naming the Impact of British, White, and Western Colonization on South Asia to Move toward and Reclaim South Asian American LGBTQIA+ Liberation

In Deepali's story, you can see the importance of family ties and religion in South Asian American families. In addition to family and religion, working with South Asian American LGBTQIA+ communities, the impact of colonization is constantly at work underlying the work of mental health practitioners. When we name this impact to ourselves as providers and to our clients in ways that are helpful, we can help reclaim a more positive approach to South Asian American LGBTQIA+ communities and move our communities toward LGBTQIA+ liberation as well. For instance, South Asia has a documented history of accepting same-sex love and gender diversity far before South Asian lands were colonized (Gupta, 2006). During colonization, gender and sexual fluidity were restricted, and shifting views in society fostered homophobic ideologies. As a result, South Asians often deal with homoprejudice and internalized sexual stigma that is rooted in colonial violence (Patel, 2019). Needless to say, colonization had a lasting impact on the wellbeing and safety of LGBTQIA+ people in South Asia.

Prior to colonization, LGBTQIA+ individuals were acknowledged in many ways, including in religious texts, through cultural traditions, and societal acceptance. It's important to first begin with a brief visual of pre-colonization conditions in South Asia. Many historians have found evidence of the existence of LGBQIA+ individuals in ancient South Asia. *The Kama Sutra* has been widely known to depict same-sex love, while Emperor Babur of the Mughal empire documented his infatuation with a boy. Homoerotic poetry emerged in the 1800s, although its traces have been largely removed. Given the erasure of queerness in modern day, it is possible that much of the evidence of LGBTQIA+ societies in pre-colonial South Asia were destroyed, just as other cultural heritage had been stolen or demolished by the British Empire.

During British rule in India, homophobia was institutionalized in South Asia through Section 377 of the British colonial penal code and the anti-sodomy section of Offences against the Person Act 1861 (Novak, 2020). This penal code carried over even after the independence of India, Pakistan, and Bangladesh. Similarly, during the British Ceylon, Article 365A of the Sri Lankan penal code outlawed homosexual male sex in 1885. Even Mahatma Gandhi, who has frequently been seen as a symbol of peace internationally, classified same-sex relations as "unnatural vices." Cissexism was also institutionalized through the labeling of Hijras as a "criminal tribe" under the Criminal Tribes Act of 1871. Due to such sentiments, many South Asians have perceived queerness to be a Western construct. The irony of this challenges the role of the therapist in clinical work with LGBTQIA+ South Asian clients. For these clients, colonial rule plays an impact in the perception of queer identity through a cultural lens, yet often this reflection is not made personally or in clinical work.

During colonization, the queer culture of South Asia had already shifted dramatically, nearly ceasing to exist. Of course, recognition of the third gender has been institutionalized in South Asian countries since then, including in India, Pakistan, and Nepal. In a post-colonial South Asia, the impact and carryover of British rule is still quite prominent, even with India's repeal of Section 377. Religious divides still impact the region of South Asia, and homophobic and sexist attitudes are instilled in South Asian nationalism (Gopinath, 2005; Tulankar, 2020). Queer liberation, then, requires dismantling colonial oppression by returning to and accepting South Asian roots.

Upon migration to the U.S., South Asian immigrants maintained their constructions of gender, specifically the ways in which women represented "home" and family structures embodied South Asian male nationalism (Gopinath, 2005). At the intersection of South Asian identity and sexuality, South Asian sexual minorities may experience a clash between their culture and sexual orientation (Sandil et al., 2015). LGBTQIA+ South Asians face racism and xenophobia within mainstream LGBTQIA+ communities in the U.S. (Gupta, 2006). At the same time, LGBTQIA+ South Asians experience heterosexism and cissexism within their South Asian communities, which view queerness as a byproduct of Western influence. Furthermore, gender diverse LGBQA+ racial minorities report higher psychological distress than their White or cisgender counterparts (Lefevor, 2019).

In general, many researchers have found that stigma and discrimination predict psychological well-being for LGBTQIA+ racial minorities (e.g., Velez et al., 2017). Beyond discriminatory experiences, LGBTQIA+ racial minorities must grapple with cultural histories marked by the trauma and exploitation of colonization, thereby complicating their relationship to sexuality and gender (Scharrón-Del Río, 2018). Thus, the impact of colonization on LGBTQIA+ South Asian Americans has been profound, influencing their narratives of diaspora. LGBTQIA+ South Asians in North America have reported feeling invisible (Patel, 2019), increased psychological distress due to internalized heterosexism (Sandil et al., 2015), and victimization in school settings (Truong et al., 2020). However, it is important to note the differences among South Asians based on country of origin and diasporic narratives. For example, South Asians who migrated to Kenya or Guyana during colonial rule in India, and then generations later migrated to the U.S. have unique cultural experiences and ties to South Asia.

Generally, guidelines to support LGBTQIA+ clients in mental health treatment have focused on the effectiveness of affirmative psychotherapy and incorporating positive psychology into mental healthcare for sexual minority clients. However, these guidelines do not utilize an intersectional approach, failing to address how colonization, White supremacy, heterosexism, cissexism, and other systems of oppression collectively harm LGBTQIA+ racial minorities. Given the history of colonial violence in South Asia, it is necessary to shift to a liberatory framework when working with LGBTQIA+ South Asian Americans. Singh et al. (2020) have called for mental health practitioners to dismantle their reliance on Western and Eurocentric conceptions of counseling, and instead draw from liberation psychology to encourage clients in reclaiming traditional ways of healing. See the first-person account from Jasbir who shares about his gender journey as a Sikh, Punjabi, trans man as he resisted internalized colonization and heterosexism.

Jasbir Affirms His Gender: A First-Person Account

I remember growing up in Delhi with my mom combing my long hair. As Sikhs, we did not cut our hair to honor our religion and our connection with God. Those moments were such bliss. We would be in the courtyard, and mom would comb coconut oil into my hair and then I would let it dry in the sun. For me, my hair length had nothing to do with my gender. All Sikhs have long hair. However, as I grew up, I knew my gender was not "girl-child." I never had the words to talk with my mom about this. I immigrated to the U.S. to begin my college studies, and there I found lots of words to describe my gender: trans, nonbinary, gender-fluid, agender. All of these words felt "right" to me. I was assigned female at birth, but I was not a woman. As I worked with a counselor in the counseling center at my university, I was able to explore my gender and attend a trans support group. I started hormone therapy and all of the anxiety and depression I felt went away. It's been tough for my family in Delhi to understand how to respect my gender, but they try. I have talked to them about the *hijra* and the impact of colonization on our trans South Asian community. I think they are starting to "get" it. I know it will take some time for them to use my correct name and pronouns, but for now I am happy that I can talk with them about what I am going through as a trans person.

South Asian Cultural Heritage and Reclaiming Queerness

Just as Jasbir shared about his gender journey and religion, given the diversity of South Asia as a region, it is important to consider how an LGBTQIA+ South Asian individual defines their own cultural background. The region of South Asia is vast, consisting of several ethnic groups, many with their own distinct languages and cultures. Furthermore, several religions are prominent within South Asia, with religious groups dictating varying views on being LGBTQIA+. Generally, South Asians belong to collectivistic cultures that emphasize group membership. For South Asian Americans, this collectivism, coupled with the pressure of immigrant identity, can create further distress when negotiating being "out" about gender and/or sexual orientation. Weighing the importance of family welfare, differing acculturation strategies may be used to buffer against psychological distress as a result of a clash between one's South Asian culture and their LGBTQIA+ identification (Shariff, 2009; Needham et al., 2017). Again, any lack of acceptance from one's family or South Asian communities should be considered in light of the colonial history of South Asia.

In a post-colonial society, LGBTQIA+ South Asians have made space to represent themselves and have their voices be heard and valued once again. Culturally, there have been many efforts to move toward the acceptance of South Asian queerness. The Hindi movie *Fire* (1996) sparked controversy for its depiction of love between two women, inciting protests by many right-wing parties in India. Nepal's first lesbian movie, *Soongava* (2012), was their entry for the Best Foreign Language Film at the 86th Academy Awards. Although not nominated, the country's decision to submit this movie for consideration indicates a cultural shift toward queer liberation. In the same year, Nepal also held its first gay sports tournament in an effort to promote the view of sexual and gender minorities as equal members of society. In 2015, the Pakistani documentary, *Poshida: Hidden LGBT Pakistan* depicted the lives of a group of LGBT Pakistanis. While efforts continue to be made in South Asian countries to highlight the narratives of LGBTQIA+ individuals, danger also continues to exist in these spaces. LGBTQIA+ individuals frequently are targets of hate crimes, especially in less urban locations, and this is also a reality that must be addressed.

More recently, efforts have continued to amplify LGBTQIA+ voices of South Asians, both in South Asian countries and in the U.S. The representation of *Queer Eye's* Tan France and *The Good Place's* Jameela Jamil on mainstream television has provided role models for many LGBTQIA+ South Asian Americans. Furthermore, LGBTQIA+ South Asian Americans have been able to turn to queer role models in various careers, such as Pakistani-American astrophysicist Nergis Mavalavala and Indian-American politician Gautam Raghavan. Mixed-media artist ALOK founded #DeGenderFashion, a movement to de-gender beauty industries and promote the liberation of all genders through trans-feminism. The existence of such role models alone provides a way for LGBTQIA+ South Asian

Americans to reclaim their queerness with pride. Furthermore, the presence of LGBTQIA+ South Asian Americans in these various spaces can lead to greater familial and community-level acceptance of LGBTQIA+ identity.

Affirming and Liberatory Practice with South Asian LGBTQIA+ Communities

When working with South Asian American LGBTQIA+ communities, mental health practitioners can be aware of both affirmative work and the liberatory practices that can support client wellbeing and empowerment.

Affirmative Practice with South Asian American LGBTQIA+ Communities

Within LGBTQIA+ affirmative practice, there are four major theoretical approaches that are important for mental health clinicians to use: (1) multicultural competence, (2) social justice competence, (2) resilience and trauma, and (3) minority stress model. Multicultural competence refers to the awareness, knowledge and skills that mental health clinicians need to work with South Asian American LGBTQIA+ communities. For instance, with a South Asian American asexual-identified nonbinary person who identifies as disabled, what is the awareness, knowledge, and skills you have as a clinician to work competently with this client affirming their identities? Are there additional readings, consultations, and professional development you need to support them in a way that increases their mental health—and so that you are not relying on your client to educate you about their identities?

A second area of affirming practice with South Asian American LGBTQIA+ communities is social justice counseling competency. In the revision of the 1992 *Multicultural Counseling Competencies (MCCs)* that focused on awareness, knowledge, and skills, the 2015 American Counseling Association *Multicultural and Social Justice Counseling Competencies (MSJCCs; Ratts et al., 2016)* added the role of "action" for counselors to make change on behalf or with their clients with issues of oppression. The authors also shared advocacy interventions that align with counseling interventions across six levels: (1) intrapersonal, (2) interpersonal, (3) institutional, (4) community, (5) public policy, and (global/international). In addition, the MSJCCs ask that counselors examine their own interlocking identities related to privilege and oppression—as well as those of their clients—in their counseling and advocacy practice. For instance, when working with a lesbian cisgender woman Bengali American who is first-generation in the U.S. who is experiencing racial, gender, and lesbian discrimination in her job, you are examining the awareness, knowledge, and skills you have to work with her, but also the action you can take on the six levels to address issues of intersecting oppressions and privileges she has and is experiencing in the workplace.

The third approach to affirming LGTBQIA+ practice is knowing the interaction of resilience and trauma for South Asian American LGBTQIA+ communities. As a mental health clinician, you must strive to identify in the intake session (and beyond) how the traumas of heterosexism, racism, sexism, and other interlocking oppressions have shaped the overall mental and physical health and wellbeing of a South Asian American LGBTQIA+ client. Once these traumas are identified, one can explore the resilience the client has developed in response to oppression (Singh, Hays, & Watson, 2011; Singh & McKleroy, 2011) in order to find ways to enhance this resilience and empowerment for self-advocacy in their lives.

Finally, the fourth area of affirming LGBTQIA+ practice with South Asian American LGBTQIA+ communities is knowing the minority stress model (Meyer, 1995, 2003). In this model, mental health practitioners can be mindful that there may have been ways clients have hidden their identities from people in their families, communities, and even from you as a provider due to anticipated rejection of prejudice events as an LGBTQIA+ person. This minority stress is on top of everyday stress experienced by all people, so it is additive mental health stress that is also socially based and chronic in that it is present in everyday social interactions and interactions with institutions such as school, religious settings, and other community settings. For instance, a Sri Lankan American asexual middle-aged person may have accessed supportive South Asian American LGBTQIA+ community settings—but also may not have disclosed their asexual identity within their community due to fear of being judged as an asexual person within cisgender, straight, *and* LGBTQIA+ environments.

Liberatory Practice with South Asian American LGBTQIA+ Communities

In tandem with affirmative approaches, liberatory approaches can help create even more empowering and truth-telling environments for South Asian American LGBTQIA+ clients (Singh, 2016; Singh, 2020; Singh et al., 2020). Grounded in liberation psychology tenets from Martín-Baró (1994), liberatory practice can help refine some of the affirming work and foundations of competency with LGBTQIA+ communities (Singh et al., 2020).

There are four liberation psychology tenets that can help drive liberatory practice with South Asian American LGBTQIA+ clients: (1) concientización, (2) deideologizing psychology, (3) problematización, and (4) realism-critico.

1   *Concientización*—or consciousness-raising—is a liberation psychology tenet that seeks to "share out" information about the historical aspects of oppression with clients. For instance, exploring the history of white and western colonization of South Asia, the U.S., and of LGBTQIA+ identities with South Asian LGBTQIA+ clients can bring for the client abilities to speak back to this history and decide more openly (and with more accurate information) what they think, feel, and want to do related to this history of colonization. In doing so, South Asian LGBTQIA+ clients can begin to see their personal story of oppression is linked to a larger story—and also begin to identify what they would like their mental health to be (especially a good question is "What would your life be like as a South Asian LGBTQIA+ clients if white and western colonization had never happened?).

2   *Deideologizing.* A second tenet of liberation psychology is deideologizing psychology, which refers to the demystification of psychology practices. This is so important in work with South Asian LGBTQIA+ clients, as coming in to receive and access mental health services can be so challenging. A focus on deideologizing psychology means that mental health clinicians are sharing the links of current mental health practices to indigenous and South Asian roots of healing. For instance, there are likely stories in the families of South Asian LGBTQIA+ clients of people sitting in circles, talking through an issue at hand, and generating solutions. It may be a process that looks different in mental health today as it is practiced (which can make South Asian American clients hesitant to access mental health services)—but the roots of helping and psychology should be demystified in this way.

3   *Problematización.* A third tenet of liberating frameworks is problematización—or problematizing the oppression that South Asian LGBTQIA+ clients experience at the intersections of racism, sexism, heterosexism, and other interlocking oppressions. For instance, if a South Asian American, Punjabi intersex gay cisgender man has internalized self-hatred and rejection of his gender and sexuality while also experiencing

racism in U.S. society, then a mental health provider can start to problematize this internalization by asking "What if the real issue is the oppression of these systems that teaches you that you are less valuable? Why would these systems of white, straight, and cisgender oppressions want you to think, feel, and believe that you are inferior in these systems? How does that benefit them?"

4   *Realism-critico.* In the fourth liberation psychology tenet, realism-critico, is really naming the counter-stories to interlocking oppressions. For instance, if the interlocking oppressions of racism, sexism, heterosexism, xenophobia, and others exist for South Asian LGBTQIA+ clients and if these systems rooted in white, western colonization go unnamed, what have been the resilient, resistant, and ongoing counter-stories to these oppressive systems? Entering this exploration with cultural humility and being mindful of one's positionality as a mental health clinician can be extremely beneficial, asking questions such as "What are the counter-stories you see in South Asian LGBTQIA+ community that demonstrate joy, compassion, and love" and "Which South Asian LGBTQIA+ community members do you follow on social media who build out a story of empowered and self-loving South Asian LGBTQIA+ communities and practices?"

Case Study Discussion

In revisiting the opening case, Zoha (they/them) is 20-year-old, Nepali-American, Muslim, queer, nonbinary college student living in California who was assigned female at birth. Zoha was referred to therapy by their academic advisor, who was concerned about Zoha's low affect during a meeting. Zoha began therapy to address feelings of hopelessness and isolation. They reported that these feelings had begun 4 years prior after a high school teacher made continuous religious microaggressions about their hijab. Additionally, Zoha expressed persistent anxiety around coming out to their parents as both queer and nonbinary. When asked, Zoha denied any somatic symptoms or concerns. Prior to this, Zoha had never sought or been to therapy before.

Zoha's parents immigrated to the U.S. from Nepal when Zoha was only 2 years old. Zoha's parents immigrated shortly after the 2001 September 11 attacks, and Zoha reported that the entire family was a target of xenophobia, Islamophobia, and racism. Zoha grew up with two older brothers, both of whom only vaguely know about Zoha's sexual orientation. Zoha stated that although Nepal had legalized LGBT rights, a general sense of disapproval still exists. Zoha explained that their family has always "stuck together," and they were worried about causing a rift by coming out to their parents. Zoha was "out" as queer to the South Asian and Muslim communities at their college, which they stated was a "safe place" for them. Zoha was particularly enthused about their academics, stating that they "love to learn." However, they expressed concern about how others in the larger communities might respond to them as a queer, nonbinary person. Namely, Zoha did not have a safe and comfortable environment to express all of their identities.

On a personal level, Zoha had begun to experience joy in their liberation from the gender binary. Zoha reported that in their room at home, they had actually begun to feel euphoric because it felt like the one place where they could exist as they wanted to be out in the real world. This personal joy often fell into conflict with how people around Zoha perceived them. For Zoha, this led to a feeling of disempowerment and wanting to be freed from the gender impositions of society.

In understanding Zoha's feelings of hopelessness, isolation, and anxiety, it was first necessary to frame their difficulties through the family and systemic influences operating around them. Although Zoha seemed to be aware of Islamophobic sentiments growing up, this had intensified for them in high school. Furthermore, the prejudice experienced by their family upon arriving in the U.S. only strengthened the bond among the family members, who relied on one another for support. This is primarily why Zoha experienced anxiety around coming out. The possibility of experiencing rejection at home for their queer identity, whilst facing microaggressions at school for their Muslim identity led to a heightened concern about belonging. While Zoha had a support network with their South Asian and Muslim communities at college, they were forced to deal with systemic cis-sexism, especially since their college did not offer gender-neutral restrooms.

To assist with treatment planning, it was necessary to explore: What identities are most salient for Zoha? How is Zoha expecting their family members to respond to their sexual orientation and gender identity? How can Zoha seek support at college when facing microaggressions and discrimination? How can we draw from Zoha's feelings of liberation to empower them?

Zoha identified two goals for therapy: (a) address feelings of hopelessness and isolation, and (b) work through anxiety related to coming out to family. Since these symptoms had been persistent for 4 years, it was likely that Zoha was experiencing episodes of depression. To begin supporting Zoha, it was crucial to begin by using therapy as a space for processing their emotions, whilst addressing the ways in which Islamophobia and heterosexism played a role in their difficulties. Furthermore, it was important to provide Zoha with coping strategies that could help them work through the anxiety as we progressed further through treatment. Providing ways for Zoha to connect with individuals who share their identities would be particularly helpful in reducing feelings of isolation.

As clinicians, it is often intuitive to lean into similarities with clients as a way to strengthen the therapeutic relationship. However, it is important to remember the ways in which the client uniquely understands their problems, their relationships with family members, and their overall surroundings. In the case of Zoha, it would be critical to incorporate the importance of their family into their treatment plan in order to reduce their anxiety and feelings of hopelessness, specifically because they noted close family ties. Over the long-term, treatment also needed to include strategies to empower Zoha in the face of systemic oppression. By increasing Zoha's awareness of these systems, as well as the role of intergenerational trauma within their family, it would be possible to help them navigate difficult situations without internalizing it as a problem that lives within them.

Reflection Questions

There are many questions you can ask yourself in an ongoing manner as you work with Zoha—and clients like Zoha—or others under the South Asian American LGBTQIA+ communities. We discuss questions that can help you address content biases and expand clinical resources and support in work with South Asian American LGBTQIA+ communities.

Content Biases. As you are working with Zoha, you can ask yourself the following questions to identify and address any biases and assumptions you have that could impede or facilitate your clinical work:

- How do I define my own sex, gender, and sexuality? How has socialization impacted these definitions?
- How do I define my own racial identity and migration history? What did I learn about race and racism growing up? How many of these socialized messages impact my work with Zoha?

- What are my thoughts about affirmative and liberatory practice with South Asian LGBTQIA+ communities? Where do I still need to be learning and growing—as well as accessing consultation and supervision?

Clinical Resources and Support. Based on Zoha's case, there are the following clinical resources and support you can draw from as a mental health provider.

- Consult with mental health practitioners who utilize a liberation framework to facilitate healing in their clients
- Become familiar with community spaces that exist in Zoha's college and hometown
- Consider the ways in which your current clinical interventions draw from a liberatory framework
- In order to better support Zoha within the context of their family, consult academic literature pertaining to South Asian family structures

Summary

In this chapter, we have described how mental health clinicians can work from an affirmative and liberatory approach with South Asian American LGBTQIA+ communities in counseling. In doing so, we have named the ongoing impact of white and western colonization on both South Asia and the U.S. which fosters a restricted understanding of essential definitions and key terms related to South Asian American LGBTQIA+ communities and also sets these communities up for ongoing and persistent minority stress in society. However, mental health clinicians have the opportunity to help South Asian American LGBTQIA+ communities reclaim their LGBTQIA+ identities and foster self-advocacy within the many settings which they interact with in their everyday lives. In doing so, mental health clinicians disrupt both the South Asian and U.S. status quo of neglecting to name the impact of colonization and also begin to heal a larger narrative within our South Asian American families and communities that our South Asian American LGBTQIA+ communities are precious and valued members of our overall group.

Suggested Resources

Books

- Funny Boy by Shyam Selvadurai (1994)
- The Truth About Me: A Hijra Life Story by A. Revathi (2010)
- She of the Mountains by Vivek Shraya (2014)
- Moving Truth(s): Queer and Transgender Desi Writing on the Family by Aparajeeta Duttchoudhury & Rukie Hartman (2015)
- We Have Always Been Here: A Queer Muslim Memoir by Samra Habib (2019)

Movies

- *Arekti Premer Golpo* (2010)
- *Soongava* (2012)
- *Margarita With a Straw* (2014)
- *Aadat* (Short Film) (2019)
- *Funny Boy* (2020)

Asian Pacific Islander Queer Women and Transgender Community
http://apiqwtc.org/

Facebook Group: Desi Rainbow Parents and Allies
https://www.facebook.com/DesiRainbowParents/

NQAPIA—A Federation of LGBTQ Asian American, South Asian, Southeast Asian, and Pacific Islander Organizations
https://www.nqapia.org/

PFLAG (Parents and Families United with LGBTQ People)—Asian/Pacfific Islander Chapter
https://www.sangabrielvalleyapipflag.com/

Queer South Asian Network
https://queersouthasian.wordpress.com/

South Asian Sexual and Mental Health Alliance
https://www.sasmha.org/

Timeline of South Asian and Diasporic LGBTQ Community
https://en.wikipedia.org/wiki/Timeline_of_South_Asian_and_diasporic_LGBT_history

Trikone—South Asian LGBTQ+ Support Community and Magazine
https://www.trikone.org/

References

American Psychological Association. (2015). Psychological practice guidelines with transgender and gender nonconforming clients. *American Psychologist*, *70*(9), 832–864.

Bandyopadhyay, D. (2018). Protection of traditional knowledge and indigenous knowledge. In *Securing our natural wealth* (pp. 59–70). Singapore: Springer. 10.1007/978-981-10-8872-8_6

Crenshaw, K. (1991). Mapping the margins: Intersectionality, identity politics, and violence against women of color. *Stanford Law Review*, *43*, 1241–1299. 10.2307/1229039

Dave, N.N. (2011). Abundance and loss: Queer Intimacies in South Asia. *Feminist Studies*, *37*(1), 14–27.

Gopinath, G. (2005). *Impossible desires: Queer diasporas and South Asian public cultures*. Durham, NC: Duke University Press.

Gandhi, L. (2020). In many Asian languages, 'LGBT' doesn't translate. *Here's how to fill some of the gaps*. Retrieved from https://www.nbcnews.com/news/asian-america/many-asian-languages-lgbtq-doesn-t-translate-here-s-how-n1242314

Gupta, M.D. (2006). *Unruly immigrants: Rights, activism, and transnational South Asian politics in the United States*. Durham, North Carolina: Duke University Press.

Lefevor, G.T., Janis, R.A., Franklin, A., & Stone, W.M. (2019). Distress and therapeutic outcomes among transgender and gender nonconforming people of color. *The Counseling Psychologist*, *47*(1), 34–58. 10.1177/0011000019827210

Martín-Baró, I. (1994). *Writings for a liberation psychology*. Cambridge, Mass.: Harvard University Press.

Meyer, I.H. (1995). Minority stress and mental health in gay men. *Journal of Health and Social Behavior*, *36*, 38–56.

Meyer, I.H. (2003). Prejudice, social stress, and mental health in lesbian, gay, and bisexual populations: Conceptual issues and research evidence. *Psychological Bulletin*, *129*, 674–697. 10.1037/0033-2909.129.5.674

Needham, B.L., Mukherjee, B., Bagchi, P., Kim, C., Mukherjea, A., Kandula, N.R., & Kanaya, A.M. (2017). Acculturation strategies among South Asian Immigrants: The mediators of atherosclerosis in

South Asians living in America (Masala) study. *Journal of Immigrant and Minority Health, 19*(2), 373–380. 10.1007/s10903-016-0372-8

Novak, A. (2020). Transnational litigation against the mandatory death penalty and anti-sodomy laws: A new Commonwealth human rights strategy?. *Commonwealth & Comparative Politics,* 1–20. 10.1080/14662043.2020.1852678

Patel, S. (2019). "Brown girls can't be gay": Racism experienced by queer South Asian women in the Toronto LGBTQ community. *Journal of Lesbian Studies, 23*(3), 410–423. 10.1080/10894160.2019. 1585174

Ratts, M., Singh, A.A., McMillan-Nasser, S., Butler, S.K., & McCullough, R. (2016). Multicultural and social justice Competencies: Guidelines for the counseling profession. *Journal of Multicultural Counseling and Development, 44*(1), 28–48. 10.1002/jmcd.12035

Rochlen, M. (1977). Heterosexual questionnaire. Retrieved from http://higherlogicdownload.s3. amazonaws.com/NASN/e277e492-64b1-4f55-ac15-00857a7a5662/UploadedImages/Oregon %20Microsite/Documents/HeterosexualQuestionnaire.pdf

Sandil, R., Robinson, M., Brewster, M.E., Wong, S., & Geiger, E. (2015). Negotiating multiple marginalizations: Experiences of South Asian LGBQ individuals. *Cultural Diversity and Ethnic Minority Psychology, 21*(1), 76. 10.1037/a0037070

Scharrón-Del Río, M.R. (2018). Intersectionality is not a choice: Reflections of a queer scholar of color on teaching, writing, and belonging in LGBTQ studies and academia. *Journal of Homosexuality.* 10.1080/00918369.2018.1528074

Shariff, A. (2009). Ethnic identity and parenting stress in South Asian families: Implications for culturally sensitive counselling. *Canadian Journal of Counselling and Psychotherapy, 43*(1), 35–46.

Sillitoe, P. (2000). *Indigenous knowledge development in Bangladesh: Present and future.* Intermediate Technology Publications.

Singh, A.A. (2016). Moving from affirmation to liberation in psychological practice with transgender and gender nonconforming clients. *American Psychologist, 71*(8), 755–762. 10.1037/amp0000106

Singh, A.A. (2020). Building a counseling psychology of liberation: The path behind us, under us, and before us. *The Counseling Psychologist, 48*(8), 1109–1130. 10.1177/0011000020959007

Singh, A.A., Appling, B., & Trepal, H. (2020). Using the multicultural and social justice counseling competencies to decolonize counseling practice: The important roles of theory, power, and action. *Journal of Counseling & Development, 98*(3), 261–271. 10.1002/jcad.12321

Singh, A.A., Parker, B., Aqil, A., & Thacker, F. (2020). Liberation psychology and LGBTQ+ communities: Naming colonization, uplifting resilience, and reclaiming ancient his-stories, her-stories, and t-stories. In L. Comas-Dias & E. Torres-Rivera (Eds.), *Liberation psychology: Theory, method, practice, and social justice.* Washington, DC: American Psychological Association.

Singh, A. A., & dickey, l. m. (2016). Implementing the APA guidelines on psychological practice with transgender and gender nonconforming people: A call to action to the field of psychology. *Psychology of Sexual Orientation and Gender Diversity, 3*(2), 195–200. 10.1037/sgd0000179

Singh, A. A., & McKleroy, V. S. (2011). "Just getting out of bed is a revolutionary act": The resilience of transgender people of color who have survived traumatic life events. *Traumatology, 17*(2), 34–44. 10.1177/1534765610369261

Singh, A. A., Hays, D. G., & Watson, L. S. (2011). Strength in the face of adversity: Resilience strategies of transgender individuals. *Journal of Counseling & Development, 89*(1), 20–27. 10.1002/ j.1556-6678.2011.tb00057.x

Thresia, C.U., Srinivas, P.N., Mohindra, K.S., & Jagadeesan, C.K. (2022). The health of indigenous populations in South Asia: A critical review in a critical time. *International Journal of Health Services, 52*(1), 61–72. 10.1177/0020731420946588

Truong, N.L., Zongrone, A.D., & Kosciw, J.G. (2020). Erasure and resilience: The experiences of LGBTQ students of color. Asian American and pacific Islander LGBTQ youth in US schools. *Gay, Lesbian and Straight Education Network (GLSEN).* Retrieved from https://www.glsen.org/ sites/default/files/2020-06/Erasure-and-Resilience-Black-2020.pdf

Tulankar, D. (2020). Indigenous people in South Asia: Issues of identity and protection of cultural rights in a changing world. In *The Asian Yearbook of Human Rights and Humanitarian Law.* Leiden, The Netherlands: Brill | Nijhoff. 10.1163/9789004431768_011

Upadhyay, N. (2020). Hindu nation and its queers: Caste, Islamophobia, and de/coloniality in India. *Interventions*, *22*(4), 464–480. 10.1080/1369801X.2020.1749709

Velez, B.L., Watson, L.B., Cox, R., Jr., & Flores, M.J. (2017). Minority stress and racial or ethnic minority status: A test of the greater risk perspective. *Psychology of Sexual Orientation and Gender Diversity*, *4*(3), 257–271. 10.1037/sgd0000226

Zhasa, N.N., Hazarika, P., & Tripathi, Y.C. (2015). Indigenous knowledge on utilization of plant biodiversity for treatment and cure of diseases of human beings in Nagaland, India: A case study. *International Research Journal of Biological Sciences*, *4*(4), 89–106.

8 Religion, Spirituality, and Clinical Implications

Kinjal Panchal and Ahmed Alif

Case Overview

This case study involves the Sharma family who came to therapy involving issues related to communication and conflict. Problems began between family members after the sudden death of the eldest member of their family, their grandfather. The two children of the family include Maya (18 years old) and her brother Krish (20 years old), who are both second-generation South Asian Americans (SAA) and were born and raised in the United States. Both children deny any religious affiliation although the other members of the family hold religious views. Their mother, Anari Sharma, is a 45-year-old SAA who migrated from Mumbai, India as an adult. Anari was born into a Hindu family and continues to practice Hinduism. The father is Amar Sharma, a 68-year-old SAA who immigrated from Kerala, India as an adult. Amar was born into a Christian family, but he does not adhere to Christianity in terms of engaging in prayers or other rituals. The oldest present living member in the household is Sunita Sharma, Amar's mother and the widow of the deceased grandfather. Sunita identifies as a practicing Christian.

There were no preexisting religious conflicts among family members until the grandfather died. The children reported that they felt like their grandmother, Sunita, dismissed their beliefs and she was imposing her religious rituals of grief practices upon them. The children further conveyed that they felt like their parents did not protect them from Sunita and as a result, both children perceived their parents as not being supportive. Anari and Amar believe that their children have their own choices with respect to religion and spiritual practices; however, they did not intervene when Sunita imposed ideas of ritual prayers on the children.

Krish and Maya expressed that they missed their grandfather, and engaged in meditation rituals with him, an activity that they enjoyed regardless of religious beliefs. Maya reported that she and her grandfather would often discuss how most religions had spiritual practices that had an overarching and shared theme of meditation, and in turn, they were all connected to one another. Krish reported that his grandparents would often argue about rituals as his grandmother would insist on going to church for Christian holidays and their grandfather felt that you could celebrate at home. Krish noted that his grandfather often felt that church was more for socializing than for prayer and he was not interested in that. This case highlights the complex intergenerational differences in how religion is passed down from one generation to another in SAA communities. It also highlights the sensitive role the parents have to play to accommodate a grieving widow who is imposing religious values on their children and grandchildren. This case reflects the power dynamics between wife and in-law, in other words, when Anari, the mother of children did attempt to prevent the grandmother from imposing religious values on her children, she would end up complaining about it to Amar, her son, as a form of disrespect.

DOI: 10.4324/9781003081548-8

This would often result in arguments between Amar and Anari, which resulted in a failure of communication within the family dynamic.

Introduction

South Asian American (SAA) identities are interwoven with spiritual practices that are often passed down through ancestral folklore that have withstood historical erasure from centuries of oppression by organized religion and colonialist practices (Ramanujan, 1990). This chapter will provide a brief overview of the varying religious-cultural practices that bond SAA while celebrating the uniqueness of each region and locale and will provide insight around varying religions practiced by SAA, including influence from religious figures who often serve as advisors and counselors. As we delve in, it is important to keep in mind that religious and spiritual practices within the SAA community are not homogenous and it is the responsibility of clinicians to ask the client what their religion and spirituality means for them in theory and practice. Understanding religion and mental health must include exploring the intersection identities of SAA, including gender, colorism, and class. In this chapter, the case of the Sharma family will highlight interpersonal family systems as it relates to the practice of intergenerational transmission of religious beliefs. Similarly, smaller clinical stories will help the reader better understand the vulnerabilities and strengths of the SAA identity as it relates to the expression and interpretation of cultural idioms of distress.

Key Religions of South Asian Americans

The South Asian community is rich in diversity in culture, religion, and spiritual practices. There are aspects of culture and spirituality that transcend each region's sub-cultures. However, to understand the community, it is pertinent to first understand the versatility of the sub-cultures within the South Asian American (SAA) community.

There are 650 languages across South Asia, not including variants on each language based on region and local practice (Hock & Bashir, 2016). There are approximately six major religions that are practiced within the South Asian community: Hinduism, Islam, Sikhism, Buddhism, Christianity, and Jainism (Religions of South Asia, 2020), 2020). However, it is important to recognize that throughout history there have been various forms of indigenous religious practices within the South Asian American community, often forced to extinction due to colonization (Center for South Asia Outreach, 2020). Additionally, many SAA identify as religious but not practicing, often framed as spiritual (Fogelin, 2007). The term spiritual is often used to identify with the principles and beliefs of religion without connecting to the organization or any specific blueprint. Exploration of these beliefs can validate feelings of contradiction. These religious and spiritual practices are important to understand as they have direct connections to the cultural practices and norms that are passed through generations and are present today in our smaller SAA community. According to the Pew Research Center (2012), currently in the United States among the South Asian population, 51% identify as Hindu, 18% identify as Christian, 10% Identify as Muslim, 5% are Sikh, 2% are Jain and, 10% identify as unaffiliated. These are the practices that are often at the root of many questions and struggles around socio-cultural identity and religious affiliations. The Sharma family's case primarily focuses on the presence of Hinduism, Christianity, and other unaffiliated spiritual beliefs. A brief synopsis of each religion is provided for basic reference and to provide a snapshot of its practices. These synopses are geared to provide familiarity and to have some context of religious practices and differing cultural foundations. Further research is encouraged for those treating individuals that identify with the following religious practice to best work with your clients.

Hinduism

For most SAA, Hinduism is primarily based on their relationship to three core tenets of jnana (knowledge), karma (action), and bhakti (devotion) (Vivekananda, 1991), and to their local deity that was worshiped by their ancestors (Pillay et al., 2008). Some examples of these deities are; Brahma, Vishnu/Krishna, Shiva, Ganesha, and Ayyappan. Mainly deities are associated with the two major mythologies, The Ramayana (Ram's 14-year exile in the forest and the story of rescuing his wife, Sita, from the demon, Raven) and the Mahabharata (The history of the Bharat) (Pillay et al., 2008). Although Hinduism is perceived as a polytheistic religion, it is a monotheistic religion, where all deities are images of the supreme being which is formless known as Brahm (Pillay et al., 2008). Practitioners of Hinduism share similarities with other religious value systems of morality such as the concept of "dharma," which is the moral law of Hinduism and religious doctrine for Buddhism (Conze, 2014; Pillay et al., 2008). Likewise, the basis of Hinduism is to live a moral life based on the doctrine of karma (Bhagvad Gita). Much like all religions, believers of Hinduism may vary in their practice of the religion. For example, some individuals may engage in "darshan" during prayer "puja" and others may not (Pillay et al., 2008; Savarkar, 2021). People who are practicing Hindus, often have dedicated spaces in their homes where images, idols and or small temples are adorned for prayer and practice (Savarkar, 2021). Most Hindus use "The Bhagavad Gita," one of the 18 Puranas, which includes hymns, folklore, and rituals of worship (Pillay et al., 2008). These prayers are spoken during daily practice, and on special holidays (Savarkar, 2021). A Hindu client may cope with distress through prayer, this may include meditation with a "mala" similar to rosary beads, lighting diya's, and singing shlokas, hymns, and chants.

Islam

South Asia has the largest Muslim population in the world (Malik, 2020). Around 600 CE, the incursion of the Arab caliphate along the coastal region of India created a fissure to induct Islam into South Asia (Malik, 2020; Robinson, 2021). The intermingling of Arab Islamic practices and indigenous Indian practices gave rise to various Islamic empires and sultanates in South Asia, including the renowned Mughal empire (Malik, 2020; Richards, 1993; Robinson, 2021). The practice of Islam in South Asia became more divergent over time, often adapting various schools of practices such as Sufism, a form of Islam that focuses on the "inward" search for God ("Allah") (Karamustafa, 2007). Across all Islamic practices in South Asia, a common thread about resiliency, sacrifice, patience, and protection from evil (evil eye or spiritual possessions) began to emerge as a quantum belief that influenced how an individual celebrated life and coped with stressors within the South Asian Muslim community (Ahmed, 2011; Islam & Campbell, 2014; Malik, 2020).

Similarly, the willingness to sacrifice time and wealth, whether through praying five times a day or fasting during the month of Ramadan from sunrise to sunset, promotes the virtue of patience and self-determination (Malik, 2020). Knowing that you can survive through hardship and engage in delayed gratification becomes a protective factor that can be applied in various domains of life and mental health practices (Malik, 2020). The concept of patience and working hard in life as permitted by Islam (Halal) to attain "Jannah" (Heaven), can be applied in times of disdain and hardship such as the journey of recovery from substance use (Malik, 2020; Robinson, 2021). That is, if we can help a

Muslim client hone into their memories of when they could fast during Ramadan from food or other pleasures, that is the same trait they can use to refrain from illicit drugs and alcohol (Mackinem & Sporl, 2020). This form of resiliency may be exemplified by many clients and it is our responsibility to frame it from a strength-based framework and inquire about the practices through humility and empathy.

Jainism

The main directive of Jainism is to live a pious life, with Ahimsa "non-violence" as the center of it. This monotheistic religion focuses on a symbiotic relationship with the earth and the notion of self. Practicing Jains live to reach spiritual enlightenment through the detachment of worldly bonds (Long, 2009). Strict practitioners of this faith will only take what has been discarded from the earth vegetation and fruits are not pulled out from the ground or picked from trees only fruit and vegetables that have been released or have met the end of their life will be consumed by a Jain individual (Jaini, 1998). Through the years, this notion has changed into its contemporary practice of veganism and or vegetarianism where root vegetables are not consumed, or products taken from animals such as milk, honey, and cheeses are not consumed (Long, 2009). These sustainable practices create a sense of belonging with the earth, a crucial element for the development of self-actualization of one's and a form of a protective factor against negative mental health outcomes (Heylighen, 1992; Sumerlin, 1997).

Followers of the Jain faith believe that all life (plants, animals, insects, etc.) have a soul and should remain intentionally unharmed. The main prayer of the faith is known as "The Navkar Mantra." The "Navkar Mantra" acts as a reminder of the desire to end the birth and death cycle and as a way to show respect to those who have conquered the desire to be bound by earthly bonds. It is not a prayer to a god or divine being (JAINA, n.d.). Within Jainism, the notions of karma are thought to be universal, and noted to be true for not only those who identify as Jains but for non-Jains as well under the practices beliefs (Pechilis & Raj, 2013). Additionally, Jainism transcribes the pan-Indic belief of rebirth and transmigration of souls, which adheres to principles of protecting the realm of earth where the soul returns to, and as a result, this promotes a sense of belonging to the land (Pechilis & Raj, 2013; Turner, 2017).

Sikhism

Sikhism originated in South Asia about 500 years ago in Punjab, India as a new doctrine with the foundation for divine unity, civil service, and meditation (Nesbitt, 2018). The fundamental belief of Sikhism is that spiritual enlightenment and liberation are found through the individual's lifetime through duty, social responsibility, and inspirational action (Nesbitt, 2018).

Sikhism originated with the spiritual teacher known as Guru Nanak and the thoughts he had around religious practice (Nesbitt, 2018). He and his first five successors wrote the "Adi Granth," which is the text that is currently followed by Sikhs (Nesbitt, 2018). Tenets of karma and reincarnation are part of the practice along with prayers to Akal Purakh, the one and timeless God (Singh, 2011). Often the prayers take place in Gurdwara, a temple, where many Sikh individuals pray, connect with other community members, ask for forgiveness, and support. It is important for clinicians to explore with their clients what prayers in gurdwara means for them. That is, some people may attend the prayer as a form of diligence, whereas others may feel obliged by societal pressures. Similarly, protective factors such as informal social and financial support is often shared through people and programs in gurdwaras, an underlying philosophy that inner spirituality comes from service of humanity (Sewa) along with life of prayer (Simran) (Singh, 2011). The concept of "Sewa" and participating in events at gurdwaras creates a sense of communal safety, often serving a protective factor for mental health and socioeconomic support. However, if a client stops participating in such events abruptly, it may warrant further exploration as it can disconnect the individual from social support systems. Likewise, abrupt disruption from participation in communal temples and religious facilities after a client enters a new relationship, can often serve as a crucial indicator for intimate partner violence.

Social interaction at the gurdwara and religious attire such as wearing a turban serves as a salient trait in the Sikh community (Singh, 2011). The turban serves as a badge of honor, and the covering of the uncut hair is known as "kesh" (Singh, 2011). A clinician working with a Sikh individual should not impose their construct of beauty standards or hygiene maintenance on these issues, rather explore and learn through curiosity and compassion.

Christianity

Christianity (primarily Catholicism and Protestant) was brought to Kerala, South India in the 16th century AD. The origins of Christianity can be traced back 2,000 years and have a connection to Judaic and Hebrew traditions. (Nathan & Topolski, 2016). Christianity as a religious doctrine in South Asia mainly adheres to the Syro-Antiochene Rite, which follows the path of Saint James or Saint Thomas (Nathan & Topolski, 2016). Much like the teaching of Christianity in Europe and other parts of the world, the tenets of Christianity are that the Universe was created by God, and humanity is also created in God's own image. Additionally, the presence of the holy trinity, Father (God), Son (Jesus), and the Holy Spirit (Soul) are aspects of the religion included within the South Asian Christian practice (Guthrie, 1996). Although Christianity as a religion may be practiced among SAA's, Hindu cultural ethos and practices are often followed as well, including the caste system (Pechilis & Raj, 2013). As religious practices flourished, Catholicism grew in popularity with scripture becoming available in Tamil, Telugu, and Malayalam (Pechilis & Raj, 2013).

India has the second largest population of Catholics in Asia, which accounts for approximately 20 million people (Barrett & Johnson, 2004). Although there are many sects of Christianity being practiced in India, the Catholic Church remains the largest church India (Raj & Dempsey, 2012). Similar to the Cochin Jews, SAA Christian's will continue to follow traditions passed down through generations much like using foods of their ancestral region in connection with western practices (Nathan, & Topolski, 2016). Christianity in the SAA culture has taken on many factions, but all derive their faith practices from the disciple of Christ, Saint Thomas, or Saint James (Nathan, & Topolski, 2016; Yanger, 2017). The Christian factions in South Asia are broken into the Northists and Southists (Raj & Dempsey, 2012; Zhimomi, 2019). As clinicians, it is our duty to educate ourselves on the diverse practices of Christinaity within the South Asian community. An example of inquiry is to explore how the Christian religion was passed on from one generation, which may differ across regions. For example, a client with Knānāya, or "Southist" Christian faith may believe that religion is passed through the maternal line, connecting some of the beliefs and roots to Judaism, whereas a "Northist" may believe otherwise (Turek, 2011). However, the clinicians duty is to be authentic and curious about these aspects of religious history and practice without inflicting judgment (West, 2000).

Buddhism

Buddhism originated with Siddhartha Gautam and his journey to enlightenment (Gleig, 2019). "The Buddha," also referred to as Siddhartha Gautama, originally a Hindu prince, was born in the sacred area of Lumbini located in the Terai plains of southern Nepal (Berkwitz, 2012; Gleig, 2019). The concept of sacrifice or giving up worldly pleasure is a common thread that seeps through many South Asian religions but most prominently in the teachings of Buddhism. The foundations of Buddhism are based on the premise that all existence is unstable and Anicca "impermanence" and that the world and its existence are characterized by Dhukka "suffering" (Radhakrishnan, 1933). Buddhist followers sub-scribe to the classical Buddhist texts Jambudvipa, which identifies and explore the three realms of Buddhist cosmology: the "desire realm," "form realm" and "formless realm" (Conze, 2014). In addition to cosmic mythology, the life of the Buddha, and folklore also include Jatakanidhanakatha and the Tipitaka which are written in the Pali language (Conze, 2014).

"The Four Noble Truths" are a significant part of the teachings of Buddhism and include: the truth of suffering, the truth to cause suffering, the truth to end suffering, and the truth of the path that leads to the end of suffering (Sumedho, 1992). In other words, the practices of Buddhism are similar to concepts of fasting for Hindus and Muslims in an attempt to find their "true form" which is described as shedding worldly pleasure through a journey of suffering for the betterment of oneself and society (Sumedho, 1992). These practices are often felt through meditation or concepts of mindfulness, but it is more than a lifestyle for many Buddhist SAA as it embodies respect and empathy for the margin-alized, elderly, and vulnerable. Regardless of religion, these practices of helping the needy are themes that bring honor and meaning to families of SAA descent (Coleman, 2002). The ideas of sacrifice and suffering though a sociocultural perspective is not self-harm or loss of self, but rather to many SAA it is the beginning of finding one's self. Therefore, as clinicians we might have to sit with the discomfort of not knowing this process and collaborating with the client to learn through them by being honest and communicating concerns associated with risk of harm to self or others.

Zoroastrianism

The practice of Zoroastrianism is based on the teaching of the prophet Zoroaster, and focuses on the concepts of dualism and eschatology, and assumes a final destiny of entire humanity, where good is expected to overcome evil (Boyce, 1996). As detailed in the en-igmatic book of "Qissa-E Sanjan," the inclusion of Zoroastrianism in South Asia started somewhere between the 7th and 10th CE (Hodivala, 1920). It started through voluntary and involuntary migrations, through the trading routes and forced persecution by the Islamic Caliphate of Rashudun forced people who practiced Zoroastrianism to move along the mountains of Northern Persia through Afghanistan-Pakistan, and into the western coastal region of India (Ringer, 2011).

The descents of this ethnoreligious group are also referred to as "Parsis" in South Asia. According to the 2011 census of India, it is estimated that more than 57,000 Parsis are living in India, with a smaller population of over 3,000 people also living in Pakistan. Interestingly, the practice of Zoroastrianism is most closely related to the Vedic religion of ancient Hinduism, a connection to the Indo-Aryan bi-directional exchange of information that weaves the commonality of practice shared across Central Asia and South Asia (Boyce, 1996). The beauty of South Asian religions involves curation of values and morals from other cultures, including influence of reformed Zoroastrianism, which focuses more on the philosophy and less on the traditional ritualistic practices (Ringer, 2011). The influence of religion within the SA community changes with time, often adopting practices and ideologies from various religions to address contemporary issues of gender equity and social justice.

Family Systems

The experience of religious identity and cultural identity can feel conflicting between South Asian Americans (SAA) born and raised in the United States versus an individual who just immigrated recently based on factors such as assimilation, language proficiency, and familiarization with social systems (Ali, 2008). SAA could easily navigate the school and legal system more effectively due to familiarity of laws and proximity to such systems, whereas, a new first-generation South Asian immigrant, might be more prone to make mistakes and learn from the process how to navigate the school and legal system (Bhattacharya, 2000). Due to the blending of culture and religion in the U.S. when it comes to immigrants, there is often internalized confusion (Frey & Roysircar, 2006). Another example of this is the use of "yoga" within the U.S. as primarily meditative or health based practice without acknowledging the religious roots in Hinduism, Buddhism, and Jainsim. Similarly the concept of "karma" and "yoga" comes up during therapy sessions with SAA not only as a part of religion, but as an aspect of culture as well (Gengnagel et al., 2005). Going back to the case of the Sharma family, they struggle with intergenerational differences within the family with varying levels of acculturation and assimilation as it relates to gender, power, and cultural practices.

Oftentimes in South Asian culture, the concept of sacrifice of one's time and energy for their family is perceived as a form of care and love (Uberoi, 1998). Similarly, when an individual migrates to another country and labels it as a form of sacrifice, it also becomes a symbol of care and sacrifice for the family (Uberoi, 1998). In the case of the Sharma family, the sacrifice of the parents was leaving India for their children Maya and Krish to have a better future. If the children do not honor or recognize such sacrifices of their parents, the parents may feel invalidated for their sacrifice, and in turn not appreciated or loved by their children (Coleman, 2002).

> *I wish these kids knew how much sacrifice we made for them, they never took time to learn about my childhood or what it meant for me to live in a land where people often reject me for the color of my skin or the way I speak. The children take this for granted and it feels like the language, values and everything that our ancestors worked so hard to retain will be erased.*

—Amar

Likewise, when the children reject the parent's culture and religious practices, it could incite a form of resentment toward the children as the parents desire to preserve cultural traditions and the stories of ancestors are also erased by the children (Coleman, 2002). However, it is important to keep in mind that some traditions and religious practices are underlined with patriarchal roots, gender roles, and conservative practices and therefore it is important to explore how the practices influence the lives of the children. That is, the clinician should explore with the family how such practices are perceived across generations.

> *I worried about the limitations that I placed on myself because I knew that if I picked someone outside of my culture and religion my parents would not approve. But I also*

knew that there is a part of me that struggles with this as well. In the end, I chose to go against my family and even though it has been many years that still looms over our household.

—Anari

Mental health practitioners should be aware of the complexities of inter-racial marriage within the SAA community and address with clients if they identify it as a stressor. Identifying as a SAA can by itself bring forth a sense of obligation to uphold practices that for some first-generation SAA may consider outdated and arcane (e.g., marrying within one's caste) while simultaneously feeling guilty (e.g., marrying someone outside their caste) (Coleman, 2002). Some examples of these types of conflicts are, marrying within the same religion and culture, confession, entering a place of worship during menstruation, etc. There is a deep connection between religion, culture, and marriage that exists within the SAA community. Ceremonial marriages follow the tradition of the religion of the couple; however, culturally there are aspects of the ceremony that are universally associated with SA. For example, there are similarities in some rites by different SA religions, such as Hindu's, Sikhs, Jains and Muslims like the use of Henna to adorn the hands and feet (Hume, 2013). Although these examples are considered cultural practices, there are elements of religiosity and spirituality that are also present.

I'm not sure why there was so much discussion around the funeral and death rituals. Amar is the man of the house now and his word should be final. I feel very upset that Anari and the children don't show him that respect. This never happened in my home with my parents nor when Amar was growing up, when his father said something that was it.

—Sunita

Often religious death rites and the wants of the individual can be overshadowed by the desired religious needs of the family. As SAA attempts to respect individual wants, conflict can arise with older generations for whom death rites and grief can be a collective and familial process. In the case of the Sharma family, the children interpreted their grandfather's personality to be someone who might have desired a less rambunctious funeral, whereas the grandmother wanted the funeral ritual to encompass cultural practices that conflicted with the children's perception of funeral rituals, and more in compliance with religious norms. The goal of the clinician is to allow Sunita, the grandmother to communicate why these rituals are important and collaborate with the children in a constructive journey of learning, rather than labeling the children as defiant to wishes. For clinicians, this can be sensitive as the grandmother might perceive them as taking sides with the children. The clinician can actually help Sunita understand that children are curious and they want to understand and learn, and help reframe the perceived resistance from the children as an authentic opportunity for her to elucidate a collaborative moment of teaching and learning between them.

I don't know why their mother is not on my side and telling the children that they need to follow the values that I teach, it feels like she is ignoring me and disrespectful towards me. My son always listens and acknowledges what I have to say. When my son tells her that this is what my mother wants, she (his wife) completely disregards it. I used to always listen to my husband who was the man of the house, and now he has passed, which makes my son the head of the household, so why won't his wife listen to him.

—Sunita

For Sunita, her husband was the head of the household and now that role has been passed down to her son, Krish. Long-held beliefs of a "man's" role in the family as the patriarch can be problematic as it contributes to gender inequity and other problematic power dynamics (Das et al., 2012). The role of women being submissive to the man is prevalent in SA culture, which is not to say it defines the culture but acknowledges its problematic prevalence of it (Das et al., 2012; Procida, 2017). Newlywed women in SA and SAA cultures are expected to move into the husband's household with the in-laws, which can often create shifts in power dynamics where the wife may have to take on an extended role of the mother-in-law as homemaker (Procida, 2017). Additionally, some households are threatened with divorce if she does not comply with the rules and demands set by the in-laws often. This may lead to violence in some instances, housing, and financial insecurities for the wife who has left her family for the husband's family. Religious doctrines often support this system, for example "wives submit yourselves unto your husbands as the church is subject to Christ" (Ephesians 5:22 KJV) Likewise, the interplay of the generational gap between wife and in-laws can cause rifts within the household, where older gender norms could be used as an oppressive interpretation of cultural and religious obligation to coerce the wife into servitude. As clinicians, it is important to educate ourselves on such occurrences and explore if such experiences may impact the client's mental health. Additionally, as clinicians, it is important to truly navigate fully through the family dynamics without pre-judgment of an existing dynamic.

> *I want to be the best mother to my children and a supportive wife and daughter-in-law ... but I feel helpless and alone, scared and nervous. My father-in-law was always there for me to communicate with and to buffer between my mother-in-law and me. He did not subscribe to the gender roles I was raised in and it was refreshing. He was a man who cooked, cleaned and really empowered my mother-in-law, my daughter and myself to fight against sexist notions. He used to quote the Bible and the Gita, always noting the passages that promoted equality. His passing has caused a ripple of depression and anxiety in my family. My husband has been avoiding talking about the loss, and my mother-in-law can't stop talking about it and I'm busy trying to support everyone. I feel lost in my own sadness.*
>
> —Anari Sharma

Afterlife

Where do we go when we die? This is a significant question layered by religion and spirituality. As we delve into the struggles brought up by the Sharma family as it relates to grieving and saying goodbye to their grandfather. The different religious beliefs around death rituals play a significant role in the disconnection the family is experiencing. As clinicians, we must honor how our clients use religion to cope with the ambivalence of the afterlife. For example, the Sharma family practiced Hindu, Christian, and spiritual beliefs within their home. What does this look like when it comes to death rites?

> *My dadu wasn't a religious man, in fact, if you sat with him he was really very spiritual, I used to joke with him that he was more of a Buddhist than a Christian, and he would laugh, and say that it all came from the same place. My Dadi really wanted to have a full Christian funeral for him, so that's what we did ... I don't think he wanted that, he wanted to be cremated and put back into the earth, I don't know how to talk to anyone in the family about it. Mom's family grew up Hindu and she's been really quiet the last 13 days, Not sure what to do, but no one's really talking to each other. There is just this big void.*
>
> —Maya

A clinician should address Maya's feelings around her grandfather's death and the desire by her grandmother to have a "proper" funeral as dictated by her own religion as a process of both letting go and the need to let go in a specific manner (Hoy, 2013). Assessing the individual's concept of death and the afterlife can be done through self-report interventions. In the Sharma family's case creating a space for members of the family to express their concerns and also validate the individual's grief experience. As a mental health clinician, the integration of religious rites is important to understand whilst treating grief and loss.

In Maya's case, there is confusion around death rites and rituals given the desire of her deceased grandfather while also appeasing the religious views of the rest of the family. A mental health clinician may explore the beliefs around a loss from each family member by asking questions such as:

1   When you think of death, what is it that you believe?
2   How does your faith/belief help you with coping with death?
3   What is something you can do as a family that respects the beliefs of the deceased as well as your own?

Additionally, the mental health clinician can provide examples of universal ways of saying goodbye. For example one universal show of peace is diya lighting, or candle lighting which is found in each religion addressed. When working with children the utilization of art can be used with prompts such as "Draw me a picture of where your grandfather is." In addition to these interventions there is the assessing attitude toward Hinduism: the Santosh–Francis Scale (Francis et al., 2008). Along with a series of self-report assessments that assess attitudes toward a given religion. They have one for Christianity, Hinduism, Judaism, and Islam.

Looking into SAA concepts of death, it is important to recognize that all religions from South Asia are accompanied by death rituals (Hoy, 2013). For example, in Anari's case, she observes "Teravin" which is the Hindu death ritual done by the family of the deceased to sit for thirteen days of mourning (Gengnagel et al., 2005). The rite is important because it allows the soul to linger and then be set free. The importance of these death rituals are directly connected to the individual and families' ability to grieve their loved one, although they do differ for each individual, the clinician should explore this with the clients in order to process the client's grief journey. A similar ritual exists within Judaism known as "Shiva." The 13-day ritual shows respect for the body of the deceased and spirit/soul assuring proper transport and arrival to the afterlife (Hoy, 2013). Although Anari often felt alone in the journey of Teravin, she also reported feeling a sense of validation through therapy and working with the therapist around finding her own voice within her grief journey.

This can be limiting for clinicians as the concept of how to grieve becomes more scripted to fulfill the spiritual norms of their religion. As a therapist, we there is a need to let go of some control and sit with the complexities of grief as dictated by the client's spiritual beliefs, without imposing our expectations which is necessary for the therapeutic alliance

Additional Clinical Stories

Safina is a 25-year-old Bangladeshi-American female who grew up in an abusive household, where religion was often used to suppress her rights. She immigrated to the United States when she was 14-years-old with her family and was later forced into an arranged marriage when she turned 18-years-old. She was referred to come to therapy as a mandated client, after having her child separated from her by the Children's Protective Services due to an incident of domestic violence. She was falsely accused by her ex-partner as the perpetrator of violence and as a result her child was removed from the home and her custody. She works as a home-aide where she would provide childcare and housekeeping services. More often than not, many SAA will enter therapy for the first time as a mandated client and it is our role as clinicians to understand their trepidation with therapy as it relates to stigma. And at the same time, honor their value systems and create a therapeutic alliance that promotes psychotherapy as a protective tool against gender-based violence and systemic oppression.

> *I felt like an outcast, like it was my fault that I could not hold on to my child when it was my husband who would abuse me. When I finally did seek help, he said I hit him and this is when they removed my child from me. Even my own family would use religion, the misinterpretation of Islam, to shame me for not being able to hold on to the marriage. Sadly, you are the only person that ever cared to even listen, even my own siblings have shamed me for the divorce.*

> —Safina

Safina came to the first therapy session experiencing shame from her own parents and siblings for divorcing her abusive partner. Unfortunately, her family members used false religious interpretation to limit her freedom as a woman. Therefore, it is crucial for clinicians to assume that religion is a protective factor for clients, and instead inquire how religion is perceived by the client. As Safina would frame it, "my parents would knit pick whatever they desired from Islam and frame it in a way that is wrong and misrepresentation of Islam."

When Safina lost her father at a young age, her grieving process involved religious and cultural influences. Mourning is a practice encouraged in Islam, often verbalize by making statements like "I don't want to live without him." These statements may not mean crisis or statements associated with suicide but a greater understanding of culture, religion, and behavior. Instead, the degree to which women mourn was influenced more by locality than traditional Islamic practice (Eyetsemitan, 2021; Ökten, 2007). In this region, families were often encouraged to hire professional "grievers" (Eyetsemitan, 2021; Klass & Goss, 2003). Not surprising that this practice has been so openly encouraged to the extent that many families would hire professional griefers who would grieve exuberantly, with loud chants and crying, to honor the dead. In Islam, there is no mandate for someone to cry over their loved ones with the understanding that death is not the end of life and the afterlife is the eternal one. Even though these two women practiced completely different religions, certain rituals, often associated with local practices allowed them to bond over the ritualistic grieving process often practiced by many SAA.

Building Rapport

> *Eid, I enjoy Eid, I really enjoy cooking during Eid, I make the best egg karma, it's my signature dish, the fragrance and aroma of that dish is so comforting.*

Candor, humor and curiosity can be utilized by clinicians to build rapport and assist with assessment of strengths and limitations as described from the client's perspective. A simple open-ended question, such as "what is your favorite cultural holiday," can help break barriers and create a sense of curiosity and reliability, which in turn will create a strong therapeutic alliance.

Superstition

A major part of SAA culture that draws on local folklore, language, and teachings are the many mystical and superstitious beliefs that have been passed down through ancestral lore. An example would be the story of a "churel," a witch, who will haunt the in-laws and their forthcoming generation upon her death, if the in-laws abuse or hurt her (Kakar, 1991). These stories warn of behaviors that are evil and have moral consequences. They are typically passed on through the generations by oral tradition; they have survived the historical erasure from colonization and imperialism. One example of this sort of lore involves an ancient tale of the indigenous peoples of the Chittagong Hill Tracts in Bangladesh called the "The Legend of the Dragon Lake," a beautiful story that highlights the importance of honoring the land and the animals through kindness and rituals that protect the people and the land that they live in. These theories transcend religion and are more spiritual beliefs that exist within South Asian culture and not any specific religious faction.

Astrology and Numerology often play an integral role when considering religion and spirituality in the lives of many South Asians and SAAs. It is believed that the positions and movements of the planets have an effect on the lives of individuals and their moods. Numerological superstitions across SA religions are noted to impact the individual, couple or family's fortune, and even mental health status. For example, the removal of the 13th floor in many buildings to avoid bad luck can be traced to ancient Christianity and the number's association with Judas, the betraying apostle. Additionally, according to Hindu lore and the Cochin Jews the 13th day in the death ritual signifies the release of souls and therefore should be left alone (Jayasuriya, 2000.) Astrological predictions are also used to plan major life events to ascertain auspicious dates and are used to predict natural and environmental occurrences (Jayasuriya, 2000). In addition, astrology and numerology are also used to identify supernatural occurrences and even the possession and birth of *Dakinis* or Witches. As Dwyer (2003) notes, Dakinis are born at an inauspicious time, may have been possessed by a malevolent spirit in their youth or possibly consumed impure substances during childhood, particularly feces and urine. Because they are inherently malevolent, they have no control of the evil power that constantly emanates from their eyes. As such, whatever they look at is negatively affected by their gaze. It becomes evident then that witchcraft is closely linked to the concept of *Nazar* or "evil eye." (Dwyer, 2003) Nazar is primarily the belief that someone can project harm or create adversity employing an envious gaze (Dwyer, 2003). This belief is found among most SA and SAA cultures. The power of Nazar is an attack on those in a place of transition and vulnerability (i.e., newly married, babies, and young children). Abu-Rabia (2005) adds to this by stating that the young, the wealthy, and the beautiful, are also vulnerable to Nazar attacks as it is an attack of envy. Preventative measures against Nazar are mainly stipulated by the smudging of the outer eye or a dab behind the ear with kajal, which is made of kohl (soot from the burning of candles mixed inside a coconut shell castor oil). In some households, a tiny knife may also be pinned to the clothing to protect the individual by cutting the evil (Maloney, 1975). Along with Nazar, other superstitions around luck are also associated with the eyes. Twitching is widely interpreted with good or bad luck. For example, in Maharashtra and in most of north India, when your left eye twitches it means good luck as it is connected to the heart line (Spiro, 2005). When your right eye twitches it means that bad luck is upon you. The same superstition exists in the Middle East and South India with a slight distinction. They believe that the woman's left eye twitching is a sign of good luck and for men it is the right eye twitching (Spiro, 2005).

Community and Vulnerability

Charity serves as an important tool to build and alleviate socioeconomic stressors in the SAA community, which in turn serves as a protective factor for mental health. Often practiced in Islam and Sikhism, charity serves as a cornerstone for promotion of cross-cultural relationships within SAA community (Nadzri et al., 2012; Singh, 2011). The obligatory act of engaging in charity (Zakat) as required by the five pillars of Islam can help people find "meaning" to life, a cause for the greater good. In other words, it helped promote self-efficacy as it supported one's ability to not only help themselves but the larger community, especially with the underprivileged (Bandura, 2010; Nadzri et al., 2012). The vulnerability of South Asian immigrant women intersecting with patriarchal systems of oppressive powers often suppresses the religious practices of Zakat or kindness (Zakar et al., 2012). As a result, we often see toxic patriarchal beliefs override resilience established by religion and indigenous practices that empower South Asian American women. As indicated by Safina who was unemployed and temporarily staying with a friend and her husband,

> the friend was nice, I met her in high school a while back, but she had to ask her husband's permission of whether I could stay with her and they appeared generous as they didn't even ask for rent or food expenses … they were also religious and my friend treated me as a sister, but whenever my friend was away, let's say she was in the kitchen and I was alone with the husband, he would gaze at me and make remarks about my beauty and body.

Limitations of Religious Beliefs

> *I don't believe in God or any being. I'm an atheist. My parents have been trying to get me to change my mind, but they blindly believe. I mean lighting a candle and saying some words isn't going to bring my grandfather back. All my life growing up Ammi, Papa, and Nani always used God as a way to scare us into doing things, but Dadu never did, he was so chill about people having their own beliefs.*
>
> —Krish

At times, religion and spiritual beliefs can leave a long-lasting impact on children and their mental health, where they lose their ability to choose and autonomy (Koenig, 2013). However, it can also be a very positive influence, fostering community, meaning, and serving as a form of coping. In the case of the Sharma family, the children could feel triggered later in life if someone imposed religion on them like their grandmother did, which resulted in a negative family dynamic. Often religion and certain guides provided by religious doctrine can be used to scare, shame, and harm individuals (Koenig, 2013; Previn, 1995). The internalization of religious expectation and, at times, the inevitable disappointment can create a pattern for a decreased sense of self and unworthiness (Dugassa, 2021). The son from the case study, Krish, expresses his disdain for the religious practices and their use as a way to punish and scare and his experience of this. As a clinician, one must work to understand how religious practices and beliefs impact the family system as a whole. Does one member of the family impose religious doctrine on the other through their own oppressive interpretation? If so, is that really religion or manipulation? Encouraging the client to put forth these honest narratives is important when it comes to clinical intervention.

Although Amar and Anari as a couple talked about their vulnerabilities and emotional stressors, when it came to mourning the loss of Amar's father, Amar would often isolate himself in a manner that created a fissure in the communication chain between the couple. As clinicians, it is important to recognize and assess the unique attachment Amar had with his father, even as his anxiety was often masked in toxic masculinity, coming, as he did, where male vulnerability was shamed. That is, even though Amar was vulnerable with his wife, the loss of his father served as a trigger for him to "honor" what his father might have liked, which is a stoic sense of self that shamed vulnerability. It is the client who must not only grieve, but also process how they honor their parents, even within the complexities of intergenerational expression of love and trauma.

As a part of his mourning, the son Krish identifies losing an elder in the family that was open to his way of thinking. He noted that his grandfather created a safe space for him to question religious beliefs and even state that he was an atheist. Krish noted that when he would bring up similar questions with his mother, father, and grandmother he would be dismissed. Krish's experience of being dismissed and its impact on his interpersonal relationship with his family allowed for a broader conversation around how religious beliefs and, at times, blind faith can cause ruptures within relationships that remain unaddressed. Oftentimes, second- generation SAA who have assimilated into their new environment avoid addressing their true beliefs as a way to keep the peace. It seems that "keeping the peace" with elders in the family often felt "easier" and helped to avoid conflict. However, in the long run, it also creates disconnection and false identities. This is another conflictual dynamic that should be addressed with ease and patience with the understanding that there may not be a resolution that feels positive at first but will be helpful in the long run (Ishara, 2018). Additionally, many SAA transmit their parents and grandparent's religious beliefs and positively use religion as a form of coping and to ascribe meaning to the journey of life.

Reflection Questions

- What are some religious practices that I believe in as a clinician that might conflict with my ability to engage in authentic curiosity and cultural humility?
- How do intergenerational beliefs conflict with our own contemporary understanding of society and environment?
- How can I engage my client in a meaningful dialogue around their beliefs without stereotyping them based on media and internal stereotypes?
- What can we do as clinicians for our clients in an ability to empower them by their culture whilst drawing attention to some limitations?

Summary

The overview of key religions shed light on concepts that emerge in mental health settings that require authentic curiosity. Authentic curiosity in practice with SAA includes open-ended questions the client educates the clinicians about their beliefs, values and rituals. The Sharma case study delves into the complexities of family systems that exist across SAA communities, with specific insight into intergenerational conflict of beliefs and practices. More importantly, this chapter highlights the religious practices, not as a form of criticism to any religion, rather to prepare a clinician for prevalent themes of socio-emotional distress that often emerge in therapy with SAA clients. The themes of afterlife and additional clinical stories sheds light on scenarios that are common across SAA communities in respect to religion as a form of protective factor and stressor. It is important that clinicians use caution and engage in cultural humility when interpreting a client's religious practice as a form of defense mechanism. In this context, cultural humility involves caution from the clinician who engages in reflective listening and summarization of client's thoughts without imposition or judgment. However, radical honesty through reflective listening is much needed for the client to recognize their defenses and justification for harm they may be responsible for. On the other hand, the clinicians should highlight the client's strengths and religious values and practices in navigating therapy and resiliency in their lives. Religion and spirituality are often valuable tools to enable the client to function normally and adaptively.

Suggested Resources

Agnihotri, V., & Agnihotri, V. (2017). Hinduism, Jainism, and Sikhism. In *Better health through spiritual practices: A guide to religious behaviors and perspectives that benefit mind and body.* (pp. 29–42), ABC-CLIO.

Francis, L.J., & Lewis, C.A. (2016). Internal consistency reliability and construct validity of the Astley–Francis Scale of Attitude toward Theistic Faith among religiously unaffiliated, Christian, and Muslim youth in the UK. *Mental Health, Religion & Culture, 19*(5), 484–492.

Francis, L.J., Santosh, Y.R., Robbins, M., & Vij, S. (2008). Assessing attitude toward hinduism: The Santosh–Francis Scale. *Mental Health, Religion and Culture, 11*(6), 609–621.

Francis, L.J., Athwal, S., & McKenna, U. (2020). Assessing attitude toward Sikhism: The psychometric properties of the Athwal-Francis scale among Sikh adolescents. *Mental Health, Religion & Culture, 23*(3–4), 234–244.

Jain, J. (2017). Converging paths in Indian meditational system and Jainism. *IAHRW International Journal of Social Sciences Review, 5*(2), 296–299.

Najam, K.S., Khan, R.S., Waheed, A., & Hassan, R. (2019). Impact of Islamic practices on the mental health of Muslims. *International Dental & Medical Journal of Advanced Research, 5*(1), 1–6.

Reddy, M.S. (2012). Psychotherapy-insights from bhagavad gita. *Indian Journal of Psychological Medicine, 34*(1), 100–104.

References

Abu-Rabia, A. (2005). Indigenous practices among Palestinians for healing eye diseases and inflammations. *Dynamis: Acta Hispanica ad Medicinae Scientiarumque Historiam Illustrandam, 25,* 383–401.

Ahmed, I. (Ed.). (2011). *The politics of religion in South and Southeast Asia.* Taylor & Francis.

Ali, S. (2008). Understanding acculturation among second-generation South Asian Muslims in the United States. *Contributions to Indian Sociology, 42*(3), 383–411.

Bandura, A. (2010). Self-efficacy. In *The Corsini Encyclopedia of Psychology*, Vol. 4, John Wiley & Sons, Inc. Retrieved from http://onlinelibrary.wiley.com/doi/10.1002/9780470479216.corpsy0836/abstract

Barrett, D.B., & Johnson, T.M. (2004). Annual statistical table on global mission: 2004. *International Bulletin of Missionary Research, 28*(1), 24–25.

Berkwitz, S.C. (2012). *South Asian Buddhism: A survey.* Routledge.

Bhattacharya, G. (2000). The school adjustment of South Asian immigrant children in the United States. *Adolescence, 35*(137), 7. https://search.ebscohost.com/login.aspx?direct=true&db=a9h&AN=3089830&site=ehost-live&scope=site

Boyce, M. (Ed.). (1996). *History of Zoroastrianism: The early period (Vol. 1).* Brill. Centers for South Asia, 2020.

Coleman, J.W. (2002). *The new Buddhism: The western transformation of an ancient tradition.* Oxford University Press.

Conze, E. (2014). *Buddhist texts through the ages.* Open Road Media.

Das, A., Mogford, E., Singh, S.K., Barbhuiya, R.A., Chandra, S., & Wahl, R. (2012). Reviewing responsibilities and renewing relationships: An intervention with men on violence against women in India. *Culture, Health & Sexuality, 14*(6), 659–675.

Dugassa, B.F. (2021). The public health significance of religious imposition: The Experience of oromo people in ethiopia. *Journal of Religion and Health, 60*(2), 974–998.

Dwyer, G. (2003). *The divine and the demonic: Supernatural affliction and its treatment in North India.* Routledge Curzon.

Eyetsemitan, F.E. (2021). *Death, Dying, and Bereavement Around the World: Theories, Varied Views and Customs.* Charles C Thomas Publisher.

Fogelin, L. (2007). History, ethnography, and essentialism: The archaeology of religion and ritual in South Asia. *The Archaeology of Ritual, 3,* 23–42.

Frey, L.L., & Roysircar, G. (2006). South Asian and East Asian international students' perceived prejudice, acculturation, and frequency of help resource utilization. *Journal of Multicultural Counseling and Development, 34*(4), 208–222.

Gengnagel, J., Hüsken, U., & Raman, S. (Eds.). (2005). *Words and deeds: Hindu and Buddhist rituals in South Asia (Vol. 1)*, Deutsche Forschungsgemeinschaft (German Research Council), University of Heidelberg.

Gleig, A. (2019). *American Dharma: Buddhism beyond modernity.* Yale University Press.

Guthrie, S. E. (1996). Religion: What is it? *Journal for the Scientific Study of Religion,* 412–419.

Heylighen, F. (1992). A cognitive-systemic reconstruction of maslow's theory of self-actualization. *Behavioral Science, 37*(1), 39–58.

Hock, H.H., & Bashir, E. (Eds.). (2016). *The languages and linguistics of South Asia: A comprehensive guide.* De Gruyter.

Hodivala, S.H. (1920). The Qissa-i Sanjan. *Studies in Parsi History, 3*(6), 94–117.

Hoy, W.G. (2013). *Do funerals matter?: The purposes and practices of death rituals in global perspective.* Routledge.

Hume, L. (2013). *The religious life of dress: Global fashion and faith.* A&C Black.

Ishara, M. (2018). Women, religion and spirituality in South Asia "one does not have to be a man in the quest of truth", *Anthropology and Ethnology, 1,* 000109.

Islam, F., & Campbell, R.A. (2014). "Satan has afflicted me!" Jinn-possession and mental illness in the Qur'an. *Journal of Religion and Health, 53*(1), 229–243.

Jaini, P.S. (1998) [1979]. *The Jaina Path of Purification.* Motilal Banarsidass. ISBN 978-81-208-1578-0.

Jayasuriya, K.S. A Comparative (2000). Study of the origins of the lakshmi concept in Sri Lanka, numerological sources in Sri Lanka and India.

Kakar, S. (1991). *Shamans, mystics and doctors: A psychological inquiry into India and its healing traditions.* University of Chicago Press.

Karamustafa, A.T. (2007). *Sufism.* Edinburgh University Press.

Klass, D., & Goss, R. (2003). The politics of grief and continuing bonds with the dead: The cases of maoist China and wahhabi Islam. *Death Studies, 27*(9), 787–811.

Koenig, H.G. (2013). *Is religion good for your health?: The effects of religion on physical and mental health.* Routledge.

Long, J.D. (2009). *Jainism: An introduction.* Macmillan.

Mackinem, M.B., & Sporl, C. (2020). A Primer on substance use and Islam. In A. Bagasra, & M. Mackinem (Eds.). *Working with Muslim Clients in the Helping Professions* (pp. 23–39). IGI Global.

Malik, S. (2020). Influence of family violence on the marital quality in Pakistani muslims: Role of personal factors. *Religions, 11*(9), 470.

Maloney, C. (1975). Religious beliefs and social hierarchy in Tamil Nadu, India. *American Ethnologist, 2*(1), 169–191.

Nadzri, F.A.A., Rahman, A., & Rashidah & Omar, N. (2012). Zakat and poverty alleviation: Roles of zakat institutions in Malaysia. *International Journal of Arts and Commerce, 1*(7), 61–72.

Nathan, E., & Topolski, A. (2016). *Is there a Judeo-Christian tradition?: A European perspective.* de Gruyter.

Nesbitt, E. (2018). Sikhism. *The International Encyclopedia of Anthropology, 1,* 1–12.

Ökten, N. (2007). An endless death and eternal mourning. *The Politics of Public Memory in Turkey,* (pp. 95–113), Syracuse University Press.

Pechilis, K., & Raj, S.J. (Eds.). (2013). *South Asian religions: Tradition and today.* Routledge.

Pew Research Center. (2012). Chapter 7: Religious Affiliation, beliefs and practices. Pew Research Center's Social & Demographic Trends Project. Retrieved July 21, 2022, https://www.pewresearch.org/social-trends/2012/06/19/chapter-7-religious-affiliation-beliefs-and-practices/

Pillay, Y., Ziff, K., & Bhat, C.S. (2008). Vedanta personality development: A model to enhance the cultural competence of psychotherapists. *International Journal of Hindu Studies, 12*(1), 65–79.

Previn, M.P. (1995). Assisted suicide and religion: Conflicting conceptions of the sanctity of human life. *Georgetown Law Center, 84*, 589.

Procida, M.A. (2017). *Married to the empire.* Manchester University Press.

Raj, S.J., & Dempsey, C.G. (Eds.). (2012). *Popular Christianity in India: Riting between the lines.* SUNY Press.

Radhakrishnan, S. (1933). The teaching of Buddha by speech and silence, *Hibbert Journal, 32*(a).

Ramanujan, A.K. (1990). Who needs folklore?: The relevance of oral traditions to South Asian studies. *Center for South Asian Studies, School of Hawaiian, Asian, and Pacific Studies.* University of Hawaii at Manoa.

Religions of South Asia. Center for South Asia Outreach. (n.d.) Retrieved July 21, 2022. https://southasiaoutreach.wisc.edu/religions/

Richards, J.F. (1993). *The Mughal Empire (Vol. 5).* Cambridge University Press.

Ringer, M.M. (2011). *Pious citizens: Reforming Zoroastrianism in India and Iran.* Syracuse University Press.

Robinson, F. (2021). *The muslim world in modern South Asia: Power, authority, knowledge.* SUNY Press.

Savarkar, V. (2021). *Hindu rashtra darshan.* Prabhat Prakashan.

Singh, N.G.K. (2011). *Sikhism: An introduction.* Bloomsbury Publishing.

Spiro, A.M. (2005). Najar of bhut – evil eye or ghost affliction: Gujarati views about illness causation. *Anthropology and Medicine, 12*, 61–73.

Sumedho, A. (1992). *The four noble truths.* Retrieved July 22, 2022. http://buddhism.lib.ntu.edu.tw/BDLM/toModule.do?prefix=/search&page=/search_detail.jsp?seq=139982

Sumerlin, J.R. (1997). Self-actualization and hope. *Journal of Social Behavior and Personality, 12*(4), 1101.

Turek, P. (2011). Syriac heritage of the Saint Thomas Christians: Language and liturgical tradition. *Orientalia Christiana Cracoviensia, 5*–16.

Turner, T.P. (2017). *Belonging: Remembering ourselves home.* Her Own Room Press.

Uberoi, P. (1998). The diaspora comes home: Disciplining desire in DDLJ. *Contributions to Indian sociology, 32*(2), 305–336.

Vivekananda, S. (1991). *The complete work of Swami Vivekananda,* Volume 2, Kartindo.com

West, W. (2000). *Psychotherapy & spirituality: Crossing the line between therapy and religion.* Sage.

Yanger, A. (2017). The Impact of christian missions and colonization in northeast India and Its role in the tribal nation-building movement (Doctoral dissertation, Southwestern Baptist Theological Seminary).

Zakar, R., Zakar, M.Z., Faist, T., & Kraemer, A. (2012). Intimate partner violence against women and its related immigration stressors in Pakistani immigrant families in Germany. *Springer Plus, 1*(1), 1–14.

Zhimomi, K. (2019). Northeast India. In K.R. Ross (Ed.). *Christianity in South and Central Asia.* (pp. 156–167). Edinburgh University Press.

9 South Asian American Marriages and Dating

Harpreet Malla, Nita Tewari, and Sheharyar Hussain

Case Overview

Anjali* is a 34-year-old, Telugu, Hindu, Indian-American woman presenting to treatment for help managing her relational anxiety. She comes from a very traditional family background and has two older sisters (39, 36) who are already married, but Anjali is the only American-born sibling in her first generation immigrant family. Growing up, she dreamt of having typical experiences like her peers such as dating, going to prom, and bringing home a boy to meet her family. In her early teens, however, she began to see differences in her friend Stella's (Italian American) experience and her own. Anjali discovered that her parents were very against dating and expected their daughters to follow the model of a traditional Indian family who arranged the matches of their daughters. Anjali's family held true to this tradition for her eldest sister, however when her middle sister got married they allowed her to maintain control of her own shaadi.com (a South Asian and South Asian American dating and marriage website which translates to marriage.com in Hindi) profile which gave her much more freedom in the arranged marriage process as she was able to message matches on her own. Anjali, too, was able to maintain her own profile but when she brought home her "perfect match" named Karan* her parents complained of his height, complexion, and caste, along with the fact that he "was a northerner (North Indian region)." Anjali and Karan announced their decision not to go through with the match, however as this was Anjali's best relationship in years, she decided to continue dating Karan in secret without their parents' knowledge. Anjali and Karan decided to allow their parents to continue seeing matches for them, declining them and dating in secret until they felt ready to announce a formal engagement. They planned to work through issues regarding communication, trust, and strengthening their own bond by allowing themselves a secret "courtship" stage that their families wanted to rush in finding a match.

Introduction

South Asian Americans represent a unique subset of Asian Americans that share the vast continent of Asia. Despite the shared cultural commonalities of South Asian Americans, there are regional and interregional differences based upon one's South Asian country of origin and interregional differences that make for a rich and varied expressions and perspectives on dating and arranged marriages. In this chapter we will explore approaches to working with South Asian American marriages and dating in therapy based upon existing research and clinical experiences to give the reader an understanding of general approaches to marriage and dating in the South Asian community. We begin our exploration with definitions of both arranged and free-choice marriages for us to examine the cultural

DOI: 10.4324/9781003081548-9

values that underlie South Asian traditions. Traditional Hindu ceremonies and Islamic ceremonies are contrasted as the predominant religious traditions across South Asia, and some unique medical considerations are presented. We also explore dating in the diaspora as well as intercultural exchanges in modernizing, remixing, and playing with long-held cultural traditions and values.

Arranged Marriage and Free-Choice Marriage

The idea of arranged marriage tends to elicit a broad range of reactions, often dependent upon one's knowledge of or adherence to traditional South Asian values, customs, and level of acculturation. Reactions by South Asian Americans and non-South Asian Americans alike can include contemplating what a modern-day arranged marriage entails, the degree of choice in the arranged process, and whether or not they are a good model for matchmaking at all. Before we elaborate further upon arranged marriage, our working definitions are the following: Arranged marriages are those in which an individual's spouse is selected by family elders, matchmaking services, or the larger community. Free-choice marriages are those in which individuals select their own spouse, commonly after a period of courtship or dating and perhaps cohabitation. People's preferences for one marital selection method over another relate to adherence to traditional cultural norms, level of progressivism, trust in their family's knowledge of their individual identity, preferences for idealized western romance, individual level of acculturation, and perceived power to say no.

Of the three million Asian Indian American, the majority of Asian Indian American are foreign-born with only 13% of Indian-Americans being born in the U.S (U.S. Census Bureau, 2010). This is relevant since the cultural beliefs and worldviews from first-generation immigrants differ from descendants of the South Asian diaspora, often resulting in intergenerational and acculturative distress within families (Tummala-Narra et al., 2016). Acculturative distress is commonly experienced in the adjustment process of negotiating between Western and other nondominant value systems. For many South Asians who come from traditional families, these conflicts may center around career choice, marriage, duty to family, and other cultural expectations.

With regard to marriage, 64% of Indians view marriage as one of the "most important things" in their lives, as compared to just 34% of all Americans polled in a study on Asian-Americans (Pew Research Center, 2012). This statistic indicates the importance of marriage as a primary focus in South Asian culture, with families talking about the marriage process with their children as soon as they are able to have a conversation about what kind of match to seek when the time comes. In a veritable "melting pot" of American cultures in the diaspora, marital arrangements vary cross-culturally and there can be conflict regarding whether families choose the traditional arranged route or modernize with free-choice marriages in which their children select their own partners. Although research largely focuses on Indians since Indians are one of the largest ethnic groups to continue the practice of arranged marriages today (Banerji et al., 2013; Chaudhuri et al., 2014; Das & Kemp, 1997; Hodge, 2004), many cultures have historically espoused this method of partner selection including Chinese, Arab, and Jewish cultures to name a few.

Arranged marriages continue to occur in the South Asian diaspora, however many myths about the practice of arranged marriage persist in the ever-evolving tradition. Arranged marriage connotes a variety of images: bright, colorful, melanges of saris and gagras (traditional feminine Indian clothing), days-long celebrations, intricately decorated mehndi (henna) hands, and a couple that may be meeting for the first time at the mandap (Hindu altar) or for their *nikaah* (Muslim wedding ceremony). Courtship has evolved from dating to "swipe" culture (where options are available at your fingertips for instant "hookups" or dating by swiping on a match instantly) in America, so has arranged marriage. Unlike the matches arranged between families at their children's birth, today modern arranged marriages differentiate themselves from western marriages in the way a spouse is chosen as well as values that uphold this tradition. Today, these can include matchmaking websites, professional matchmaking bureaus or matchmaker services, the informal "aunty network" of non-blood related elders, and one's family connections suggesting a good match for an unmarried youth.

Historically, arranged marriages involve having one's life partner chosen by elders or matchmaking services (Sastry, 1999; Shachar, 1991; Singh & Bhayana, 2015). This is drastically different from western romances that evolve into marriages based on personal compatibility and love (Acevedo & Aron, 2009; Xiaohe & Whyte, 1990). Dr. Nita Tewari highlights the interplay between the ideas of love and marriage in both cultures as such: "in the American culture, you marry the person you fall in love with versus with traditional arranged marriages, you fall in love with the person you marry" (N. Tewari, personal communication, March 3, 2020). This notion underscores that while love may not the basis for a successful marriage in South Asian cultures as it is in the west, it is often an expected outcome of a successful marriage partnership.

The values that underlie an arranged marriage are complex and multifaceted, including marrying to fulfill familial obligations, procreate, maintain one's culture, and typically to preserve traditional gender norms (Madathil & Benshoff, 2008; Medora et al., 2002; Sastry, 1999; Shukla & Kapoor, 1990). Matchmakers, whether they be elders in the "aunty network" (elders are affectionately termed aunty or uncle despite not having actual blood or relative ties in South Asian culture) or members of a professional marriage bureau, base their decision on practical factors such as age, religion, subsistence skills, wealth, family status, health, astrological compatibility, and interpersonal relationships among the families of the bride and groom (Contreras et al., 1996; Medora et al., 2002; Myers et al., 2005; Sastry, 1999; Singh & Bhayana, 2015; Xiaohe & Whyte, 1990). Such decisions are also based on matching geographic regions of family birth, dietary preferences (vegetarian vs. non-vegetarian), and educational attainment with a belief in the similarity hypothesis indicating the greater the similarity of the match, the lesser chances of conflict with dissimilarity. Because of the importance of the extended family in collectivist cultures, how well in-laws get along can impact the suitability of one partner for another, thus the saying, "a marriage is not between two people, but two families" (N. Tewari, personal communication, March 3, 2020).

In contrast, western marriages often endorse practices such as dating, marrying for mutual compatibility, shared interests, intimacy, affection, and love (Madathil & Benshoff, 2008; Medora et al., 2002; Sastry, 1999; Shukla & Kapoor, 1990). Partner selection in free-choice marriages is based on mutual attraction and romantic love, whereas partner selection in arranged marriages may be based on finding partners who fulfill traditional gender roles and enhance relationships between in-laws and their larger community (Acevedo & Aron, 2009; Buss et al., 1990; Sastry, 1999; Singh & Bhayana, 2015; Strohschein & Ram, 2017; Verma, 1989). Marriages in which western, or free-choice criteria, are used for South Asian matches are often referred to as "love marriages" (Yelsma & Athappilly, 1988). Therefore, we use the term "free-choice marriage" in defining this type of marriage in not conflating the idea that arranged marriages do not involve love in using the colloquial term "love marriages" yet want to distinguish these marital arrangements from those in which spouses did not select their own partners.

Distinguishing these marital types helps to better understand the cultural motivations underlying the pairing of two partners in identifying the types of stress experienced by those attempting to fit into one model over the other. For example, someone who dates may not be concerned with family acceptance immediately, but may struggle to define the relationship and its intended course- whether it be casual, recreational dating, or a more meaningful, goal-oriented courtship meant to lead to marriage. In contrast, someone engaging in an arranged marriage may not have to worry about pre-screening a match or what to wear on a date, though they may have to contend with familial disagreement regarding a match and whether there is conflict between their taste and their parents'. In the diaspora, intergenerational conflict and level of acculturation may further complicate the matchmaking process. Similarly, a couple engaging in a love marriage in India may face further stigma than a couple who undergoes the same process abroad where it is the cultural norm (Weigel & Ballard-Reisch, 1999).

Case Study Discussion

Anjali's family has been making comments about how relieved they are to leave Karan in the past, and are beginning to push harder for other matches. They send her *biodatas* (informational sheets about potential matches which include information about age, job title, height, health history, weight, salary, skin complexion, etc.) via e-mail regularly. In addition, Anjali's sisters are pushing her to be more involved in the process, with her middle sister sharing advice on how to better screen her Shaadi matches. They center qualities like willingness to raise a large family, salary, and closeness to family. Anjali, meanwhile, wants to allow herself to experience romance, courtship, and feeling doted on or wooed in the dating process as she sees this effort as something that will ultimately translate to her future husband's efforts in their marriage. Though Anjali has never felt more comfortable or excited with another partner she dated, she and Karan have not yet decided whether they want to go through with re-announcing their intentions to their parents. Anjali is beginning to grow anxious about Karan's lack of commitment though she also understands his uncertainty. In a phone conversation after work that went from joking about their parents' poor understanding of what they found attractive, Anjali became jealous that Karan's matches may be actual marriage possibilities in his mind and that she was being compared to these other women.

Anjali was hurt, stressed, and anxious after her tiff with Karan but had to attend a weekly family dinner immediately afterward. Her family prodded about her "sour face," with her father chiming in that she would never be able to find a match if she was so "moody all the time." Anjali felt so incensed by her father's comment and so frustrated by the situation that she decided to take her friend's suggestion to seek counseling. After reading some more about Indian marriages, we will revisit Anjali's case below.

Marital Satisfaction

Marital satisfaction is a vital factor in maintaining marriages, and is also linked with overall life satisfaction and health regardless of marital type (Celenk & van de Vijver, 2013; Hatfield & Rapson, 1993; Kim & Hatfield, 2004; Levenson et al., 1993; Sastry, 1999). Oftentimes, there is a stigma about couples in arranged marriages discounting their happiness in order to appease family and community, however it is well-established that marital satisfaction is possible in both arranged and free-choice marital types (Gupta & Singh, 1982; Madathil & Benshoff, 2008; Myers et al., 2005; Yelsma & Athappilly, 1988). Scholars have suggested that people in arranged marriages tend to begin marriage with lower expectations than do people in free-choice marriages (Medora et al., 2002; Myers et al., 2005; Sastry, 1999; Shukla & Kapoor, 1990). Romanticism, or belief in love in lieu of a pragmatic approach to male-female interactions, has been linked with "unrealistic standards for marital relationships," (Medora et al., 2002, p. 155). These can include depictions of Hollywood or Bollywood romances in which there is a cinematic conflict that is ultimately resolved by the power of love and results in a "Hollywood ending" with the couple riding off into the sunset rather than communicating about their differences and finding a resolution that results in meaningful change and growth. When such standards are imposed, they have been linked with disappointment, higher levels of conflict, and even divorce (Baucom & Epstein, 1990; Glenn, 1991, as cited in Medora et al., 2002). These differences in initial expectations of a marital partner may underlie why marital satisfaction can vary in arranged versus free-choice marriages, at least in early marriages soon after the wedding.

Furthermore, among people in arranged marriages, marital satisfaction is predicted by more interpersonal factors such as having children and level of family involvement in the marriage (Baucom & Epstein, 1990). Among people in love marriages, intrapersonal factors such as passion and sexual satisfaction are better predictors of marital satisfaction (Epstein et al., 2013). Valuing of interpersonal versus intrapersonal factors related to marital satisfaction may be due to the South Asian tendency to orient themselves in terms of the groups to which they belong rather than orienting to themselves in an individualistic fashion. Essentially, finding out what marriage model is ideal for Anjali versus her sisters and parents involves assessing how she defines herself and what her expectations of marriage are. An assessment of these factors will help Anjali navigate her relationship and conversations with her family regarding her uncertainty about Karan.

In therapy, identifying what works best for whom is a far worthier pursuit than trying to validate one model of marriage over another. In practice, working with South Asian American clients around their marriages can be difficult as clinicians cannot assume which values orientation their clients ascribe to, and marital type no longer distinguishes one's values in the same ways it did decades ago as major cultural shifts are currently occurring. The following sections will help illustrate the various values and dynamics that serve as a basis for clinical considerations in working with South Asian brides and grooms including dowry, divorce, caste and skin complexion.

Dowry

Dowry refers to property or monetary value brought into a marriage from the wife's side, often given by parents of the bride. In older or traditional South Asian communities, dowry was historically seen as a way to balance familial investments from the parents: the bride's side provided a large dowry to start off the couple, and the groom's side provided the education and foundation for him to be a strong earner and maintain the new family's finances. The bride's family, much of the time, gave the inheritance of the bride to her and her new groom on their wedding day as that was the point of transfer for South Asian women to leave their families of origin and join their in-laws' side, symbolized by her changing her last name.

While the dowry process made sense in the context of historical realities about earning potential, it no longer functions in the same way as gaps in earning potential closed between genders. As women are earning independently in diaspora and in South Asia, they are becoming less dependent on their husbands to support them financially. Recently, generations have upheld the dowry tradition, but it was considered a "gift" from the bride's side to the groom's. This value of this dowry gift has been linked with the bride's worth in exchange for the groom's long-term financial security of family or protection, which further makes the currently illegal process of dowry negotiations emotional for brides and their families. For example, a family with a groom who was a doctor (high earning potential), fair or light-skinned, and in shape, may demand a higher dowry. This can be inflated further if the bride in question was overweight, older, darker-skinned, or otherwise seen as undesirable as determined by the groom's family. The "negotiating power" of a family has been linked to skin color, caste, and class (Philips, 2004). Such beliefs over these problematic practices have led to dowry being formally outlawed in the Dowry Prevention Act of 1961. In some parts of South Asia, families have found ways around "voluntarily gifting" to grooms' families who believe the tradition should persist (Sukumar, 2017). Recently, a table in Vox news was created as theoretical sampling to demonstrate the fluctuating possibilities of dowry amounts to be paid by the bride based upon her characteristics. See Table 9.1 as an illustration of the randomness of how dowry amounts may or may not be determined.

Table 9.1 Attempt at Making Sense of Dowry Variability

Haggling over Dowry

How much dowry can a women expect to pay? How much can a man expect to receive? It depends on a lot of factors, including the language you speak at home, your caste, skin tone, age, horoscope, and family's social and economic status.

These factors affect brides and grooms differently. Over the years, I have tried to understand how all these variables interplay. Fill in the blanks below with your information to see a distilled version of my understanding of this institution which still confounds me.

I am _____ years old and _____ tall. I _____ after studying _____.
I have _____ brothers and _____ sisters, and my family _____ wealthy.

You can change your information to see how each factor increases of decreases your dowry, or sometimes affects it in more complex ways.

Bride	Groom

Image from: Sukumar (2017, February 6). Dowries are illegal in India. But families—including mine—still expect them. Retrieved March 29, 2021, from https://www.vox.com/first-person/2017/2/6/14403490/dowry-india-bride-groom-dilemma

Current South Asian society is evolving as feminism is taking hold, earning potentials are closer to equalizing, men have become more egalitarian in their attitudes, and women have become more outspoken. Many young couples are experiencing "dowry ambivalence" (Diamond-Smith et al., 2019) which describes the mixed, complex feelings of those who are unsure of whether to go against centuries of tradition and perhaps their own families' wishes or whether to let go of a practice that no longer serves them or aligns with their values. In Nepal, the researchers studied 20 triads of brides, their grooms, and their mother-in-laws to draw conclusions about how dowry conversations functioned in an ever-evolving marital landscape. They described how changing conditions in Nepal had led to shifts in practices (e.g., change in female agency within marriage, pre-marital conversations or courtship, household dynamics), but not necessarily attitudes. Oftentimes couples in the study would express shame (*sharam, sigghu*) upon disclosing that they had gotten to know one another prior to marriage. This trend existed in Christian Nepali couples in the sample as well.

In collective South Asian cultures, appearances are often important and indirect communication may be the norm, thus making it important for clinicians to identify numerous factors such as dowry expectations before conceptualizing clients' values orientation regarding: individual preferences, whether or not the couple has negotiated and come to a compromise regarding their values, degree of influence in-laws and extended family have, extended family's values, and lastly, the perceived risk of disobeying elders' wishes regarding marriage.

Divorce

Cultural taboos and stigmas against separation have a large influence on marital satisfaction as well. The effort put forth into conflict resolution is assumed to be higher because separation may not be a viable option (Donley & Wright, 2008; Markus & Kitayama, 1991; Oyserman et al., 2009; Sastry, 1999; Yelsma & Athappilly, 1988). In traditional families, the extended family may intervene to advise and guide the couple since divorce is not believed to be an option for more traditional Indian couples due to strongly held beliefs about unity and the importance of the family structure (Donley & Wright, 2008; Markus & Kitayama, 1991; Oyserman et al., 2009; Sastry, 1999; Yelsma & Athappilly, 1988). Indians generally believe that divorce affects the entire family, not just the individuals in the marriage, and thus must be avoided at all costs (Ariplackal & George, 2015; Yelsma & Athappilly, 1988).

India has a lower national rate of domestic violence in marriage and lower divorce rates than does the U.S., with current rates of divorce at 1 of 100 marriages compared to the United States' 1 of 2 marriages that end in divorce (Ariplackal & George, 2015; Donley & Wright, 2008; Sassler, 2010; Yelsma & Athappilly, 1988). These rates may be a reflection of the high cultural value placed on marital commitment and harmony. DuPree et al. (2013) also cited explanatory factors such as adherence to traditional gender roles, level of acculturation, and the influence of the extended family as reasons that commitment is upheld. Although couples may stay married, inferences regarding the quality of the marriages cannot be made as the level of marital satisfaction has not been determined in these studies. It is essential, however, that clinicians be aware that the perceived risk of becoming a divorcee is heightened in South Asian American communities and that the impact of facing shame in the community, along with conflict, abuse or even role reversal (women being the breadwinners) may be strong motivating factors to remain married despite disconnection within the marriage.

Caste

The intricacies of the caste system in India are complicated and discussed in further detail in another chapter pertaining to casteism here in America. However, we will briefly discuss the impact of the caste system on the marriage market in South Asia. Broadly defined, the caste system is an ancient social hierarchy which reflected the way in which people made their livelihoods in India. The social stratification was seen at first as providing order, but has since become problematic and regressive as it does not allow one to move beyond the class or social strata they were born into.

There have been numerous attempts at bringing fairness back into the caste equation such as affirmative action policies, renouncing the caste system, etc. however South Asian identity can still be tied to one's "place" in the social hierarchy, and traditional families allow these stratifications to persist. Due to social stigma and the notion of "log kya kahenge" (What will people think?), some old-fashioned or traditional families discourage marrying "beneath" one's caste, and oftentimes push to marry within the same caste or even subcaste (Philips, 2004). Though legal restrictions have diminished the power of the caste system, families pass down information about their "roots" in the caste system, and factors such as dietary preference, hometown, and last name often give clues to one's caste to the trained eye or ear.

While tensions regarding caste-sliding or inter-caste marriages may have diminished over the years, it is important for clinicians to recognize that casteism tends to exist in older generations who often have a strong say in determining the fit of a match. Family discord about suitability may serve as a major roadblock for young couples. These couples may have to defend against stereotypes or justify their partner's or their own worthiness depending on their generational or immigration contexts. Assessing whether casteism is an issue or empowering clients to identify with their own values regarding caste and suitability, as well as encouraging them to navigate family opinions with confidence and humility, are likely to be more effective interventions than simply setting individualistic boundaries or courageously defying family depending on the client's level of connection to their family and their family's level of traditionalism. Furthermore, considering immigration histories, second generation and third generation of South Asians born in the US from the first wave of 1965 Naturalization and Immigration Act immigrants are more likely to find caste irrelevant and unretained by many American citizens of Indian descent. This further illustrates how imperative it is for clinicians to determine casteism saliency for South Asian clients.

Complexion

Colorism also maintains saliency in the South Asian community with lighter skin being perceived as more beautiful, handsome, and valued. In determining marriage partners, skin complexion continues to impact the marriage market heavily as those who are lighter-skinned are still considered more desirable (Philips, 2004). Listing skin tone is a common descriptor in South Asian biodata and in online marriage profiles. For families who value skin color, family members are told to avoid sunlight and outdoor activities in order to maintain their complexion and not darken in the sun. Depending on the saliency of skin color among the family, some grandparents may also see marrying a dark skinned individual as "risky" in the chance of also producing dark skinned offspring. See the chapter on Colorism for further information on this topic. Normalizing colorism in the role of attractiveness and desirability would likely be empowering for clients—once this reality is acknowledged, they can both focus on delving deeper into larger values regarding selecting a life partner.

Case Questions for Consideration

- What are Anjali's values in looking for a husband? How do they align or differ from her family's?
- What complicates Anjali & Karan's match (complexion, region, caste, age, gender, etc.)?
- How can Karan and Anjali clarify their relationship readiness to their parents?
- What intergenerational conflicts are likely?
- What will make Anjali's reveal of her relationship with Karan easier/harder?
- What communication/reassurances will be helpful in Anjali and Karan navigating the arranged matchmaking process while dating each other?
- How does acculturation level impact the family's approval of Karan? (on Anjali's side? Karan's?)
- How will her age and gender impact Anjali's matchmaking journey?
- In what ways are Anjali's cultural roots and values maintained in her relationship with Karan?

Hindu and Muslim Wedding Events

Pakistani Muslim weddings, like Indian Hindu weddings are celebrations with traditional music, clothing, vibrant colors, and marriage itself is a major central focus in Pakistani and Muslim culture. Pakistani parents usually consider it their responsibility to find a suitable match for their children and arrange their marriage, when societal expectations deem successful completion in raising their children. In addition to arranging the match, parents play a vital role in organizing most wedding events, beginning from the proposal leading to the wedding day.

While Pakistani parents may feel a sense of pride and fulfillment for organizing their children's weddings, the bride and groom who are socialized in the US may experience frustration for having little control over their wedding planning. This may cause a sense of loss for brides and grooms in the South Asian American diaspora who have grown up watching elaborate bridal showers, "yes to the dress" moments, and other western traditions in which the bride and groom are agentic and central to wedding planning decisions. Brides and grooms describe the feeling of just having to "show up" almost as if they were guests in their own wedding, with all the preparations, wedding colors, and guest lists arranged by their parents.

Counselors working with South Asian and South Asian American clients preparing for marriage may find it beneficial to understand South Asian wedding terms by asking their clients to describe the events they will be participating in and can reference the brief summary charts below. Oftentimes, the differing events elicit a combination of stress, excitement, sadness, fun or even anger. For example, in considering the case of Zeenat (bride), she has heard her parents repeatedly discuss how after marriage she will become a part of Ahmed's (groom) family and that she will no longer be the responsibility of her parents. Having attended Rukhsati's previously, she is uncomfortable with the tearful or sobbing display of emotions commonly exhibited from the bride's side. On the other hand, Ahmed and his family look forward to the Baraat, when he, his family and friends arrive in a lively procession to greet his soon-to-be bride. Thus, it is important for clinicians to understand the nuances, the traditions and the meanings behind the events as it pertains to the couple's individual feelings leading up to the marriage and thereafter. See Tables 9.2 and 9.3 for a comparison of the different Pakistani and Hindu wedding events.

As a comparison, we will also include information about Hindu weddings below for clinician reference when discussing important marital events in the South Asian community:

Table 9.2 Pakistani Muslim Wedding Events

Marriage proposal	A marriage proposal is formalized when the groom's parents and other family members (usually elders) pay a formal visit to the bride's house to ask for her hand in marriage and families agree on the match.
Engagement (*mang-ni*) party	The bride- and groom-to-be exchange rings, while family members exchange gifts including jewelry, clothing, and sweets. A customary prayer is also held.
Dholki* or *Dholak	Named after the percussion instrument *dholki,* female relatives gather to sing traditional songs and dance to celebrate the occasion as the *dholki* drum is played.
Rasm-e-henna	Henna is a reddish-orange dye made by crushing the leaves of *lawsonia inermis* plant, which is then applied onto bride's hands and feet in intricate henna designs. These henna patterns symbolize love, joy and luck.
Baraat	the groom arrives at the wedding venue with his family and friends for the official wedding ceremony.
Nikaah	The *nikaah* is considered the most important part of the Islamic wedding ceremony. In the presence of a religious scholar known as an *imam,* both families agree on their terms and conditions of the wedding agreement. The bride and the groom then give their consent to marry each other three times and sign the official marriage contract known as *nikaah-nama.*
Rukhsati	the act of "departing" or "leaving." Usually, *rukhsati* is filled with tears and sadness as the bride bids farewell to her family and leaves with the groom to start a new chapter of life.
Valima	to "gather" or "assemble." It is a concluding event in which the newly married couple arranges a lunch or dinner for their relatives to express their gratitude and joy toward the union of two individuals and families.

Table 9.3 Hindu Wedding Events

Rishta (match) Meeting	This is a series of meetings with prospective matches in which both families meet to determine fit and discuss family values and possible wedding details.
Formal Engagement	Family members exchange gifts of clothing, gold, and sweets to represent good will between future-in-laws, and the bride- and groom-to-be exchange rings and announce. their plans to marry. Oftentimes, a wedding date is chosen at this point (typically well within a year).
Kanyadaan	A religious ceremony in which the bride's side gives her to the groom's family as a gift for which they receive good karma from the Divine. This transferal process is officially completed in the *vidaai.*
Mehndhi Ceremony	Henna or mehndhi is applied to the bridal party's hands and feet, with the bride's plant-based design sometimes going from her elbows to her fingertips. The darker the temporary plant dye is, the more "in love" the couple is said to be. Modern families include the groom with a simple design.
Sangeet	Although all events include some elements of singing and dancing, this night is the main "party" night in which there is lots of merrymaking, mingling, and friendly family competition in outdoing one another with choreographed dance performances.
Haldi Ceremony	Days before the wedding, the bride and groom and ceremonially bathed in a holy yellow powder called puspu or haldi, which purifies skin and removes impurities. This is a way for family to further bless the couple before the auspicious day.
Wedding Ceremony	Oftentimes based on the couple's vedic astrology charts, an auspicious time is chosen and pujas, or prayers, are conducted amid a host of symbolic rituals that can last from 30 minutes to 2 and a half full hours with the final step involving the couple walking for 7 rounds around the fire to symbolize their commitment for 7 lifetimes. A wedding necklace is traditionally tied by the groom around the bride, and flower garlands are exchanged.
Vidaai	The bride symbolically, and literally, leaves her family of origin to join her husband's side as she traditionally takes on his last name. Traditionally a somber and tearful occasion, modern families celebrate this with joy knowing that the "separation" is ceremonial.

Consanguineous Marriages and Thalassemia in the Pakistani Community

Muslim South Asian populations include both clinical and medical implications in marriages, particularly consanguineous marriages. A consanguineous marriage is a marriage between close relatives, usually first or second cousins (Shaw & Charsley 2006). Such marriages are a commonplace practice among Muslim communities and Pakistan is no exception (see Afzal et al., 1994) as maintaining family values and wealth is of utmost importance in Pakistani culture. It is estimated that nearly 50% of marriages in Pakistan are between first or second cousins (Merten, 2019), with some studies reporting such marriages to be as high as 66% (Chauhan et al., 2020). While these marriages might make sense for a number of reasons, they can also create serious medical concerns for children resulting in thalassemia and other hereditary disorders. According to Ahmed et al. (2002), an estimated 5–7% of the population (approximately 10 million Pakistanis) are carriers of thalassemia genes. This high carrier rate combined with a high number of inter family marriages dramatically increase the likelihood of transferring thalassemia to the next generation.

Thalassemia is a genetic medical condition passed on genetically and causes defective hemoglobin production in children (Dahlui et al. 2009; Wacharasin et al., 2015). It is a serious public health concern (Maheen et al., 2015) with a very high prevalence in developing countries, particularly in Asian and Mediterranean countries (Weatherall, 2005). Pakistan is one of the highest risk countries for thalassemia, with a prevalence of every 1–4 infants per 1,000 in Pakistan currently suffering from thalassemia (Alwan & Modell, 1997; Langlois et al., 2008). Compared to Pakistan, thalassemia in the US is quite rare; the World Health Organization (2008) estimates that only 2,000 people in the US are living with thalassemia. Some of the challenges that children with thalassemia experience include delays in physical and sexual growth, diabetes, thyroid failure, hypogonadism, hyperparathyroidism, myocardial infarction, arrhythmia, hyperparathyroidism, and liver damage (Arian et al., 2018). Previous studies have also documented that many children with thalassemia experience psychological, social, and spiritual difficulties on a regular basis (Weatherall, 2005). They are also twice as likely to receive a diagnosis for psychiatric disorders (Sadowski et al., 2002). Although much of the research on thalassemia cited here specifically applies to Pakistanis residing in Pakistan, it is also relevant to the Pakistani American diaspora.

The Sundas Foundation, one of the few non-profit organizations working with children suffering from thalassemia in Pakistan, emphasizes the importance of genetic testing before inter family marriages to reduce the likelihood of transmission of the disease, as stated by Tariq Rashid, one of the administrators at Sundas Foundation (T. Rashid, personal communication, January 10, 2020). Although the older generation of Pakistanis prefer marriages within their extended families, many younger Pakistani Americans who are more assimilated into American culture may strongly oppose this practice. For mental health professionals working with Pakistani Americans, it is likely they will come across a client who has married someone or is considering marrying someone within their family due to a multitude of reasons. It is crucial for mental health professionals to adopt a non-judgmental and supportive stance that displays an understanding of this cultural norm and its context so that clients may freely discuss their concerns rather than shut down due to fear of judgment. It is also critical for clinicians to educate themselves about thalassemia and how genetic testing can help clients make informed decisions about their offspring.

South Asian/South Asian American Marital Expectations

In eastern cultures characterized by collectivism, conflict avoidance, reverence for elders, group cohesion, modesty in expression especially for women and youths, and pride in one's background are considered essential factors promoting integration into society (Hofstede, 2001; Myers et al., 2005; Sastry, 1999; Shukla & Kapoor, 1990; Verma, 1989; Yelsma & Athappilly, 1988). In many eastern cultures, marital partnerships are arranged by elders and love is expected to develop over time rather than precede marriage (Myers et al., 2005; Verma, 1989). Therefore, South Asians are more likely to adjust to their marital circumstances rather than entering it with preconceived expectations (Contreras et al., 1996; Myers et al., 2005; Sastry, 1999; Shukla & Kapoor, 1990). In eastern cultures, clearly defined gender roles for each partner in the marriage as well as the shared endorsement of these gender roles results in a match between expectation and reality regarding the division of labor related to child rearing, homemaking, and breadwinning (Madathil & Benshoff, 2008; Sastry, 1999; Shukla & Kapoor, 1990). Additionally, familial support during marital conflict buffers against negative outcomes such as marital dissatisfaction or divorce by facilitating more open communication among family members and between married couples (Yelsma & Athappilly, 1988).

Other research suggests that the collectivistic, group orientation of South Asians leads couples to view themselves as a single unit rather than as two separate but united individuals (Sassler, 2010; Shukla & Kapoor, 1990). If so, couples' expectations are that their new family dyad is the core, and will protect that against outside influences, including extended families. This may prove especially true for those in the diaspora who are not part of established immigrant communities as the distance serves as an implicit boundary.

Individuals in collectivist settings view themselves as embedded into their society, as they themselves are simply extensions of their families of origin (Markus & Kitayama, 1991). Thus, Verma (1989) proposes that marital satisfaction may also depend on relationships with family members. If extended family is close by, couples may set the expectation for themselves that they will remain connected to their families as they would have in their countries of origin.

Research on western couples suggests family members can exacerbate problems that couples experience within their marriages (Snyder et al., 2007). Indian Americans may similarly clash with their families, especially since intergenerational conflict is a well-established part of interactions particularly in first-generation immigrants (Stuart & Ward, 2011; Tummala-Narra, 2013; Tummala-Narra et al., 2016). In-laws in particular are cited as a stressor of Indian marriages (Madathil & Benshoff, 2008; Sassler, 2010; Shukla & Kapoor, 1990; Yelsma & Athappilly, 1988) as they often heavily influence decision-making and day-to-day life in couples who uphold family hierarchy as a collectivist value. For Indian couples that have either immigrated away from their family of origin in India or who have acculturated and have less enmeshed family relationships, it is possible that they experience "the best of both worlds" (Barker, 2015; Contreras et al., 1996; Madathil & Benshoff, 2008; Negy & Snyder, 1997).

Since mate selection is an active process for westerners, individuals in diaspora may end up being disappointed when a suitable partner does not meet the ideal partner that an individual may start imagining in adolescence (Contreras et al., 1996; Myers et al., 2005; Sassler, 2010). The flipside of this is that western models of romance may minimize eastern premarital matching on finances, values around children, and whether in-laws get along. Factors such as premarital sex with multiple partners and cohabitation have also been cited as possible contributors to marital distress as these practices may minimize the "special" status and privilege endowed by the traditional institution of marriage (Abraham, 2002; Donley & Wright, 2008; Sassler, 2010) and South Asian families can be conservative regarding living together before marriage and premarital sex.

For South Asian Americans who participated in arranged marriages and are living in the United States, a more complex, multidimensional explanatory approach is necessary, as their cultural practices are not the norm in their country of residence. It may be difficult for these individuals to explain the circumstances of their union, and exhausting for them to defend against stereotypes and assumptions made about the way in which they were selected for one another. In fact, disclosure of a couple's participation in an arranged marriage is often rare outside of South Asian contexts, with many couples opting to simply explain to those outside the culture that they "met through mutual friends" or family connections. The dissonance between their lived experience and outward image may cause an internal struggle between value systems, with few spaces to discuss their issues as openly as they would have preferred. Additionally, wives may take on western gender roles and maintain jobs while still utilizing the conflict resolution, communication, and deference skills characteristic of traditional Indian couples. These changes culminate to create a more balanced partnership in which the husband and wife are working together to achieve success in their new homeland (Shukla & Kapoor, 1990).

Marital Satisfaction and Models of Love

One predominant theory is that marital satisfaction develops on a different timeline for arranged marriages than it does for free-choice or "love" marriages (Epstein et al., 2013; Myers et al., 2005). Love increases as the couple gets to substantially know one another better, and the timeline for this varies in arranged versus free-choice marriages. As couples who have the opportunity to date prior to walking down the aisle (or sitting under the mandap!), those in free-choice marriages often begin the courtship process earlier and thus also develop a "spark" and glide into the honeymoon phase earlier than do arranged spouses—who begin that process after their wedding day. Rather than marrying the person you fall in love with, those in arranged marriages fall in love with the person they marry. Though love may not occur in these marriages, there may be compatibility or family goals that are valued over "love." Whereas romantic love is the necessary basis of a free-choice or of course, "love" marriage, it is simply a result of a successful arranged marriage. Jeff Mio, Ph.D. eloquently conceptualizes the differences "(in the west) Weddings are viewed as the culmination of a love affair; whereas in the east, arranged marriages are viewed as the beginning of the love affair" (J. Mio, personal communication, October 27, 2021).

In a study on cross-cultural perceptions of romantic love (Levine et al., 1995), the major trend that emerged was that cultures that were more economically developed, westernized, and individualistic tended to emphasize romantic love more than countries that were collectivistic, traditional in their values, and less economically developed. It is vital that clinicians decenter their notions of what makes couples happy and successful, as western ideals of romantic love may not resonate with their clients. Despite the Beatles' assertion that "love is all you need," South Asian communities often push more practical factors and conceptualize love differently.

Regardless of how people from different ethnicities conceptualize romantic love, there are other aspects to relationships and their maintenance. Sternberg's triangular theory of love posits that there are three components of love in relationships, which combine in different ways to form various types of intimate relationships. The three components of love include: 1) passion, 2) intimacy, and 3) commitment and are conceptualized in research as passionate love, companionate love, and commitment, respectively (Sternberg, 1986; Sternberg & Weis, 2006). Passion is the word we use to describe intense feelings about one's partner and is dependent upon one's physical arousal. Intimacy is described as the level of security, trust, and mutual interests that partners share, as well as their tendency to spend time together and share their secrets. Commitment, on the other hand, describes one's goal that their relationship will last and their dedication to put forth effort to make it work. These types of love are not mutually exclusive, and each relationship can have combinations of the three to varying degrees. Recent research has shown the three factors in Sternberg's theory are distinct and predictive of relationship satisfaction (Lemieux & Hale, 2000).

These preferences can also evolve over time, as research indicates that passion and intimacy decline with the length of the relationship, while commitment increases (Acevedo & Aron, 2009; Rhyne, 1981; Sumter et al., 2013). Reasons for this decline include the processes of habituation, conflict inherent in interdependency, and familiarity (Acevedo & Aron, 2009). That is, one's level of passion and excitement for their partner is mitigated by their compounded experiences of conflict and by simply getting used to them over time. It stands to reason then, that in a collectivist culture that does not emphasize the happiness of the individual, more practical maintenance factors of love such as intimacy and commitment are prioritized over passionate, fiery romantic love which tend to ebb and are thus not always a strong foundation for marital relationships on their own. Research supports that companionate love is linked with overall life satisfaction across cultures, whereas passionate love is linked with extreme positive and negative emotions (Hatfield & Rapson, 1993; Kim & Hatfield, 2004). That is, those who primarily experience companionate love report being more satisfied in their day-to-day lives.

Religious and Astrological Considerations in Matchmaking

In many traditional South Asian American families, religious and astrological considerations are a major part of finalizing or determining a match's fit. The primary religions of South Asia include, by population: Hinduism, Islam, Buddhism, and Christianity, with Hindu-originating religions such as Buddhism, Sikhism, and Jainism included (Sawe, 2018). Much importance is given to religious-matching, as families strive to maintain their culture and way of life by ensuring that both spouses have similar views.

Beyond this, most South Asian religions do not dictate much of how marital arrangements are made. In fact, in Buddhism marriage is considered a secular affair and monks may bless a couple but not perform the marriage rite. The primary consideration in Islam is that active consent is obtained from both parties at the time of marriage, regardless of how the match was found (by the spouses themselves or by the community). There are some considerations that impact how couples are selected for one another in Hinduism, however.

One such aspect is the notion of vedic astrology in Hinduism, which, unlike western astrology, prioritizes lunar cosmology over Sun signs. Vedic astrology has its origins in Hinduism, however it should be noted that it has become popularized among nonreligious South Asians as well. In many matchmaking bureaus or traditional families, each partner's chart is required to be compared against the other's in order to determine compatibility. In many families, a poor result can ruin an otherwise worthy match's chances of marrying one's son or daughter. Vedic astrology is considered "old-fashioned" by many South Asian families who no longer rely upon chart-matching, however per suggestion of a Hindu *panditji* or priest, matchmaker, or family elder, oftentimes these charts are consulted and become at least a consideration in the matchmaking process. This can be true for couples who select their own spouse as well, with extended family demanding that they ensure minimal compatibility by having their charts read.

While there is scant psychological research available about these astrological processes, there is a rich history of charts being used to confirm or deny a match (Narayanan, 2018) among those who adhere to such beliefs. An individual birth chart is referred to as a *janam kundli*, and the two pairs of kundli are assessed to obtain a point value out of 36 points or *gunas*. Anything above 18 is considered acceptable, with matches above 24 or 26 (depending on who you ask!) being considered exceptional. These gunas reflect sexual chemistry, emotional, fertility, lifespan, and other aspects of compatibility which are considered in determining spousal fit. Beyond the gunas, there are special astrological considerations for some—such as those rare few who are born under the strong influence of the planet Mars and are referred to as *manglik*. These individuals are considered to have unfavorable or inauspicious periods of their lives that could be disastrously transferred to their partners. Mangliks then must either marry other mangliks who are immune to influence or must rid of their manglik energy by marrying a tree prior to marrying their spouse, who then becomes their second marriage. Though this procedure may seem odd in the west, it is commonly viewed as a harmless way to overcome one's misfortune by finding absolution in nature and even those as wealthy and popular as Bollywood's Aishwarya Rai, formerly Miss World 1994 and current spouse to Bollywood royalty Abhishek Bachchan, have done it (Razdan, 2006).

It is imperative that the religious and cultural practices of South Asians are examined on an individual basis, as meaning-making often determines how one interprets a particular belief. The concept of determinism can be either fatalistic for someone who feels that they cannot escape their expectations, or soothing to someone who views their difficulties as inevitable and is therefore comforted by the lack of culpability (Patel, 2015).

Younger generations of South American Asians, and certainly South Asians in diaspora, are attempting to form their own relationships to the traditions of their culture, family, and hometowns by honoring parents' wishes while contending with their level of belief in the superstitions and traditions that they follow. Others still are using a return to tradition and text to upend regressive thought patterns. Millennials and the generations behind them in the Islamic diaspora have begun to cite the Quran, the holiest book for Muslims, as a rationale for allowing interracial marriages between people of the same faith and further, to combat colorism within the community (Grewal, 2009). Hindus have pointed toward gender fluidity in revering *hijras* (transgender, intersex, or eunuch individuals) who are often invited to weddings to bless the union, as well as in holy depictions of Ardhanarishvara, who is a composite of the male Lord Shiva and his celestial wife Goddess Parvati as examples of their Hindu roots being more progressive than their Hindu present.

Same-sex marriages, similarly, have also been re-gaining favor in the community as the colonial influence of British occupation is slowly shedding its hold on Indian morals and beliefs. The repeal of Article 377 in 2018 was no doubt the sharpest turning point in this movement, as it decriminalized same-sex unions in India (Tan, 2019). As there is another chapter in this book specifically focusing on queer relationships, the lens we will explore in this section is how the focus on marriage and having children supersedes the desire to constrain sexuality in South Asian populations (Dhillon, 2018) so much so that there are even matchmaking bureaus for queer couples. As Dhillon eloquently puts it, "in an odd kind of way, gay marriage might end up being more socially acceptable in conservative India (whenever homosexuality is legalised (sic), of course) than in more liberal countries … Marriage is, after all, the bedrock of Indian life." This attitude allows for couples to modernize old traditions and customs to fit their unique partnerships, and for the institution of marriage to evolve along with its return to pre-colonial values and more open mindsets (Khan, 2011). The Media Corner below includes several TV shows and movies that showcase this evolution.

Dating and Singlehood

Dating is particularly contentious in the South Asian community as arranged marriage is the norm and the expectation, and even in families that do not plan on having an arranged match, South Asian society's judgments of families that break the norm prevent them from being open about allowing their children to date. The intense stigma against dating and fear of "log kya kahenge" (what will people think?) which permeates every aspect of South Asian dating and marriage make it difficult for people to be open about the process of finding a match and prioritize the end result of an engagement and wedding.

Intergenerational conflict and level of acculturation can intensify anti-dating sentiments in diaspora, particularly for women (Zaidi et al., 2016) as they do not want to go against their families. While women are held to higher standards regarding maintaining their chastity and purity, men struggle more with pressure to become strong earners which begins with academic pressure and evolves into pressure to strive for more in career and salary (Rahman & Witenstein, 2014). This results in close monitoring of youth by elders in the family, which restricts how they spend their free time and diminishes the opportunity to date or to "get into trouble." Premarital sex is a major fear in South Asian and South Asian American communities, specifically religious ones that value family honor, chastity, and restraint and consequently forbid dating, although very recently those in upper classes and who live in more urban areas are becoming more permissive (Majumdar, 2018). Research shows that although romantic interest may be equally high in South Asian countries of origin and in diaspora, South Asian diaspora may have more access to opportunities to date due to increased autonomy from their parents in their host culture, friends who foster "permissive" expectations that favor casual dating, and lastly greater cross-sex network composition which affords them the opportunity to be around those of the opposite sex in casual ways that are often prevented in South Asian countries of origin (Dhariwal & Connolly, 2013). Secrecy then becomes an integral part of the dating process for many South Asian youth, an inevitability for those wanting to explore courtship on their own without parental pressures to marry or meet one another's families.

One major concern for South Asian American youth who enter the dating circuit is that they do not have anyone to guide them through interactions, flirtations, and conflict that arise while dating a member of the opposite sex as their parents either did not date themselves, or because they have to keep their dating lives a secret from their families altogether (Manohar, 2008). Intergenerational differences contribute to how relationships are approached, and in many cases, South Asian American youth relied exclusively on their peers and extrafamilial support to navigate dating. Oftentimes, these sources of advice and support contradict the South Asian value systems and messaging daters hear at home which deepens their intrapsychic and bicultural conflict. However, recently several virtual communities have popped up which allow for diaspora to connect with one another and share their secretive dating experiences with one another to gain support, a sense of belonging, and advice without risking losing their anonymity in their immediate physical communities. The founder of this author's favorite such community BrownGirlTherapy (est. 2019), and the first and largest mental health community for children of immigrants, Sahaj Kohli eloquently summarizes,

> For South Asians and children of immigrants, self-care is often about finding the agency we have within the systems we live in. It's not uncommon for this to look like 'lying' to our parents to protect our own mental health and well-being. Sometimes this is secretly pursuing our dreams or romantic partners because we fear disappointment and rejection from our family, and other times it's hiding the fact that we're in therapy to learn how to communicate our choices and needs to our families.
>
> S. Kohli Kaur, personal communication, February 26, 2021

When South Asian youth are ready to reveal their relationships to family, it often happens in stages. Perhaps an older sibling or more progressive aunty is the first to hear of or meet an individual's partner, and they help scaffold a digestible story and meeting for older, more conservative family members. It is not uncommon for a couple to have several different storylines and timelines of how and when they met by the time they marry, especially if they are interracial or queer. It is vital that clinicians not pathologize this as "dishonesty" or encourage clients to come out or be open regarding their relationships as this behavior is in fact protective in the South Asian community and allows for an important twofold process: for the individual to navigate their own preferences in dating and determine their individual readiness to progress the relationship, and also to allow the family processing time in stages.

In addition to dating disrupting arranged marriage norms, the decision to stay single or not to date may also be difficult for South Asian families to digest. The pressure to marry begins, as stated previously, from a very early age and is persistent in most South Asian families. In a society that prioritizes marriage and family above all else, choosing to stay single late in life is oftentimes equated with failure. Literature suggests that South Asian women who remain unmarried in the community, are at higher risk for developing low self-esteem and depressive symptoms as a result of being shunned by their community (Joseph et al., 2020). In some families, the focus on women over men is deliberate, as men may have agency to make their own career and life decisions even if they are unmarried while women are continuously monitored by their families of origin in order to maintain honor and "protect" them. In other families, women in Asia and in the United States are delaying marriage. Such women may be more acculturated, be more educated, be financially independent or do not view marriage in the same way as previous generations. These women may also not adhere to the traditional notions of arranged marriage and have the choice of finding a match compatible with their worldview, maybe someone as acculturated, or someone who shares their values and notions on marriage. Either way, clinicians working with clients who choose to remain unmarried or who consider themselves asexual need to be mindful of the expectations to marry and procreate within a South Asian context.

Dating in Pakistani American Muslim Community

Just like the term "dating" consists of a broad spectrum of sexual and romantic activities (Bogle, 2008), there is a wide range of practices and beliefs about sexual behavior that exist in the Muslim community. The Quran explicitly forbids premarital sex and sexually intimate relationships before marriage. Islam places a strong emphasis on marriage because it sees family as the most important building block of society (Alshugairi 2010; Lo & Aziz 2009). Consistent with Islamic teachings, many Muslim parents prohibit their children from dating or having sexual relationships before marriage and emphasize marriage over dating. In this section, we discuss how Islamic religious views impact attitudes about dating and marriage in Pakistan and Pakistani Americans, as 97% of the population are practicing Muslims (Mahr et al. 2015).

Navigating dual identities may be challenging in one's struggle to balance both American and Pakistani ideals while feeling caught in between both cultures and their conflicting values. Their American self may place a considerable amount of pressure on them to participate in dating culture, while their Pakistani self may be struggling to meet familial expectations of a traditional courtship through arranged marriage.

The anthropological accounts of Muslim American women on US college campuses illustrates this point (Mir, 2014). In a qualitive study conducted with Muslim American women undergraduate students at Georgetown and George Washington Universities in Washington, D.C., Muslim students reported feeling alienated because they were not dating, while their non-Muslim peers dated on a regular basis. One Muslim student described that she found it stressful to live in a culture in which most people were dating. Another Pakistani Muslim woman, Sarah, was often infantilized by her non-Muslim friends Jennifer and Chelsea for refraining from engaging in sexual behaviors and viewed her Pakistani American identity with resentment. After Sarah expressed a mild interest in a male student, her friends began pestering her to approach him and she finally gave into their pressure. While alienation and lack of belonging contributes to the feeling of being othered, there are consequences to consider when going against one's culture and dating as well.

Seeking a romantic partner and dating, on the other hand, may directly conflict with one's religious beliefs, family mores, and social values, causing intrapsychic and familial discord. Pakistanis may experience a considerable amount of shame and fear of rejection or abandonment by family members, as being disowned is a common threat within families to prevent their children from ruining a "good family name." One "solution" to this conflict between culture and self is to simply hide aspects of one's identity. Many date secretly without telling their families and sometimes friends about their relationships. This results in Pakistani Americans living parallel lives; one in which they pursue romantic relationships while their families have little to no knowledge of it, and another in which they have to constantly perform traditionalism to be considered a "proper" child that resists the influence of the west within their family. The tension of keeping these two lives separate may lead to substantial stress and anxiety of being found out at any moment and facing adverse consequences.

It is also important to highlight the gendered expectation and consequences of dating for Pakistani American girls and women, as men are often not punished as severely nor are their reputations as fragile as women's seem to be. Mir (2014) argues that for many immigrant girls and women who are often monitored by tight-knit communities and are raised in strictly gendered communities in which they rarely interact with the opposite sex, the consequences of openly expressing their sexuality are dire. These consequences could include damaging the family's honor and diminishing the prospects of any future marriage proposals, including for younger siblings in the family as the family name is "tainted." Thus, mental health professionals working with Pakistani Muslim Americans should value the lived experiences of their clients and not attempt to prescribe western ideals of "boundary-setting" against their families due to cultural complexities. Close attention should also be placed on the nuanced identities that clients have to navigate daily and assisting clients to integrate their fragmented selves into a continuous narrative of who they are would likely be helpful.

Evolution and Revolution

In working with South Asian Americans, clinicians must have a base understanding of the fundamental definitions and distinctions within the culture, and how traditionalism, religion, family opinions, and acculturation can impact the marriage process. Helping individuals identify their values and how they can make room for them in a collectivist culture is difficult, but rewarding work as couples eventually find their own rhythm and place within their larger cultural and extended family network. Another noteworthy aspect is how the wave of progressivism is impacting South Asia and its diaspora in this process.

This is a unique cultural time for South Asia, as it is experiencing a revolution of sorts in which long-held beliefs and values about marriage and marital practices are being reworked and reimagined in sometimes playful ways and sometimes with transgressive delight. The rise of globalization, media portrayals of romance in both Hollywood and Bollywood (India's film scene which is the most prolific producer of feature length films in the world), and a feminist wave in South Asia are shaking up gendered norms and assumptions about courtship and marriage. What especially reinforces these waves are online communities in which memes are shared and participants can anonymously post, share content, and support one another without risking their family's name in the process. South Asian cultural messaging is no longer solely in the hands of elders, and the youth has a lot to say.

Suggested Resources

Given the diversity of South Asia Americans, with its myriad of marital traditions, foods, languages, and customs, it is difficult to capture the breadth of marital and dating considerations. We suggest becoming familiar with South Asian culture through both formal education and popular media sources. See media suggestions for movies and shows below for additional resources to gain knowledge:

Movies/Shows

Wedding Season (Netflix)
The Big Day (Netflix)
Indian Matchmaking (Netflix)
Family Karma
Meet The Patels
Mismatched (Netflix)
Made in Heaven (Amazon Prime)
Never Have I Ever (Netflix)
Four More Shots Please (Amazon Prime)
Arranged
Married At First Sight
Karan Johar's What the Love

Reflection Questions

- How can you help orient your client to therapy? What might be helpful in setting treatment expectations?
- How can you destigmatize your client's help-seeking and highlight the value of processing emotions and the past while respecting cultural values?
- How can you reinforce confidentiality for wary clients? What reassurances can be repeated or made clearer?
- What can you do to create an environment in which your client can critique or assess their family without feeling as though it is a betrayal?
- How will you know when consultation is the best option, and where can you connect with consultation sources?
- What exercises, activities, or discussions can you use to help your client differentiate their values from that of their culture's or family's?
- How can you encourage your client to find sources of support within their family?
- What online support resources are you aware of for South Asians? How can you encourage your client to connect with valuable outside resources?
- What are your own biases regarding topics like courtship, secrecy, premarital sex, etc?
- What literature and media sources can you find to help you more fully understand South Asian culture?
- South Asians may prefer directive styles of therapy, but how can you still make space for your client to disagree with you or let you know when they may not want to follow a certain course of treatment?
- How can you ensure a safe environment in which your client can acknowledge cultural differences in the room rather than overlook them? What conversations can you bring up early in treatment to showcase your commitment to learning with and for your clients?
- How can you keep the level of acculturation at the forefront of your treatment plan, and when would it be appropriate and inappropriate to incorporate a client's family into your treatment plan?
- When might it be appropriate to refer to southasiantherapists.org rather than treating a case yourself?

References

Abraham. (2002). *Attitudes of second -generation Asian-Indians toward dating and arranged marriage: An exploratory study*. ProQuest Dissertations Publishing.

Acevedo, B.P., & Aron, A. (2009). Does a long-term relationship kill romantic love?. *Review of General Psychology, 13*(1), 59–65. 10.1037/a0014226

Afzal, M., Ali, S.M., Siyal, H.B., & Hakim, A. (1994). Consanguineous Marriages in Pakistan [with Comments]. *The Pakistan Development Review, 33*(4), 663–676. 10.30541/v33i4IIpp.663-676

Ahmed, S., Saleem, M., Modell, B., & Petrou, M. (2002). Screening extended families for genetic hemoglobin disorders in Pakistan. *New England Journal of Medicine, 347*(15), 1162 1168. 10.1056/NEJMsa013234

Alshugairi, N. (2010). Marital trends in the American Muslim community: A pilot study. *Journal of Muslim Mental Health, 5*(3), 256–277. 10.1080/15564908.2010.551275

Alwan, A., & Modell, B. (1997). *Community control of genetic and congenital disorders*. WHO Regional Office for the Eastern Mediterranean. EMRO Technical Publications Series.

Arian, M., Mirmohammadkhani, M., Ghorbani, R., & Soleimani, M. (2018). Health-related quality of life (HRQoL) in beta thalassemia major (β-TM) patients assessed by 36-item short form health survey (SF 36): a meta-analysis. *Quality of Life Research, 28*(2), 321–334. 10.1007/s11136-018-1 986-1

Ariplackal, R., & George, T.S. (2015). Psychological components for marital distress and divorce in newlywed Indian couples. *Journal of Divorce & Remarriage, 56*(1), 1–24. 10.1080/10502556.2014. 972210

Banerji, M., Martin, S., & Desai, M. (2013). Are the young and the educated more likely to have "love" than arranged marriage? *A study of autonomy in partner choice in India*. Working Paper Series (pp. 1A'43). NCAER.

Barker, G.G. (2015). Choosing the best of both worlds: The acculturation process revisited. *International Journal of Intercultural Relations, 45*, 56–69. 10.1016/j.ijintrel.2015.01.001

Baucom, D.H., & Epstein, N. (1990). *Cognitive behavioral marital therapy*. New York: Bninner/Mazel.

Bogle, K.A. (2008). *Hooking up: Sex, dating, and relationships on campus*. NYU Press.

Buss, D.M., Abbott, M., Angleitner, A., Asherian, A., Biaggio, A., Blanco-Villasenor, A., Bruchon Schweitzer, M., Ch'U, H.-Y., Czapinski, J., Deraad, B., Ekehammar, B., El Lohamy, N., Fioravanti, M., Georgas, J., Gjerde, P., Guttman, R., Hazan, F., Iwawaki, S., Janakiramaiah, N., …Yang, K.-S. (1990). International preferences in selecting mates: A study of 37 cultures. *Journal of Cross-Cultural Psychology, 21*(1), 5–47. 10.1177/0022022190211001

Celenk, O., & van de Vijver, F.R. (2013). What makes couples happy? Marital and life satisfaction among ethnic groups in the Netherlands. *Journal of Cross-Cultural Psychology, 44*(8), 1275–1293. 10.1177/0022022113486003

Chaudhuri, S., Morash, M., & Yingling, J. (2014). Marriage, migration, patriarchal bargains, and wife abuse: A study of South Asian women. *Violence Against Women, 20*(2), 141–161. doi:10.11 77/1077801214521326.

Chauhan, B.G., Yadav, D., & Jungari, S. (2020). Association between consanguineous marriage and child nutritional outcomes among currently married women in Pakistan. *Clinical Epidemiology and Global Health, 8*(1), 38–44. 10.1016/j.cegh.2019.04.003

Contreras, R., Hendrick, S.S., & Hendrick, C. (1996). Perspectives on marital love and satisfaction in Mexican American and Anglo-American couples. *Journal of Counseling & Development, 74*(4), 408–415. doi:10.1002/j.1556-6676.1996.tb01887.

Dahlui, M., Hishamshah, M.I., Rahman, A.J.A., & Aljunid, S.M. (2009). Quality of life in trans-fusion dependent thalassaemia patients on desferrioxamine treatment. *Singapore medical journal, 50*(8), 794–799.

Das, A.K., & Kemp, S.F. (1997). Between two worlds: Counseling South Asian Americans. *Journal of Multicultural Counseling and Development, 25*(1), 23–33. 10.1002/j.2161-1912.1997.tb00313.x

Dhariwal, A., & Connolly, J. (2013). Romantic experiences of homeland and diaspora South Asian youth: Westernizing processes of media and friends. *Journal of Research on Adolescence, 23*(1), 45–56. 10.1111/j.1532-7795.2012.00803.x

Dhillon, A. (2018, February 23). In India, even gay people want an arranged marriage. *The Sydney Morning Herald*. https://www.smh.com.au/world/asia/in-india-even-gay-people-want-an-arranged-marriage-20180219-p4z0t5.html

Diamond-Smith, N.G., Dahal, M., Puri, M., & Weiser, S.D. (2019). Semi-arranged marriages and dowry ambivalence: tensions in the changing landscape of marriage formation in South Asia. *Culture, health & sexuality*, *22*(9), 971–986. 10.1080/13691058.2019.1646318

Donley, A.M., & Wright, J.D. (2008). For richer or for poorer: The impact of state-level legislation on marriage, divorce, and other outcomes. *Sociological Spectrum*, *28*(2), 133–159. 10.1080/027321 70701796239

DuPree, W., Bhakta, K.A., Patel, P.S., & DuPree, D.G. (2013). Developing culturally competent marriage and family therapists: Guidelines for working with Asian Indian American couples. *American Journal of Family Therapy*, *41*(4), 311–329. 10.1080/01926187.2012.698213

Epstein, R., Pandit, M., & Thakur, M. (2013). How love emerges in arranged marriages: Two cross-cultural studies. *Journal of Comparative Family Studies*, *44*(3), 341–360. 10.3138/jcfs.44.3.341

Glenn. (1991). The Recent Trend in Marital Success in the United States. *Journal of Marriage and Family*, *53*(2), 261–270. 10.2307/352897

Grewal, Z.A. (2009). Marriage in colour: Race, religion, and spouse selection in four American mosques. *Ethnic and Racial studies*, *32*(2), 323–345. 10.1080/01419870801961490

Gupta, U., & Singh, P. (1982). An exploratory study of love and liking and type of marriages. *Indian Journal of Applied Psychology*, *19*(2), 92–97.

Hatfield, E., & Rapson, R.L. (1993). *Love, sex, and intimacy: Their psychology, biology, and history*. HarperCollins College Publishers.

Hodge, D.R. (2004). Working with Hindu clients in a spiritually sensitive manner. *Social Work*, *49*(1), 27–38. 10.1093/sw/49.1.27

Hofstede, G. (2001). *Culture's consequences: Comparing values, behaviors, institutions and organizations across nations*. Sage publications.

Joseph, A., Jenkins, S.R., Wright, B., & Sebastian, B. (2020). Acculturation processes and mental health of Asian Indian women in the United States: A mixed-methods study. *American Journal of Orthopsychiatry*, *90*(4), 510–522. 10.1037/ort0000465

Khan, F.A. (2011). Powerful cultural productions: Identity politics in diasporic same-sex South Asian weddings. *Sexualities*, *14*(4), 377–398. 10.1177/1363460711406789

Kim, J., & Hatfield, E. (2004). Love types and subjective well-being: A cross-cultural study. Social *Behavior and Personality: An international journal*, *32*(2), 173–182. 10.2224/sbp.2004.32.2.173

Langlois, S., Ford, J.C., Chitayat, D., Désilets, V.A., Farrell, S.A., Geraghty, M., … & Wyatt, P. (2008). Carrier screening for thalassemia and hemoglobinopathies in Canada. *Journal of Obstetrics and Gynaecology Canada*, *30*(10), 950–959. 10.1016/S1701-2163(16)32975-9

Lemieux, R., & Hale, J.L. (2000). Intimacy, passion, and commitment among married individuals: Further testing of the triangular theory of love. *Psychological Reports*, *87*(3), 941–948. 10.2466/pr0.2000.87.3.941

Levine, R., Sato, S., Hashimoto, T., & Verma, J. (1995). Love and marriage in eleven cultures. *Journal of Cross-Cultural Psychology*, *26*(5), 554–571. 10.1177/0022022195265007

Levenson, R.W., Carstensen, L.L., & Gottman, J.M. (1993). Long-term marriage: Age, gender, and satisfaction. *Psychology and Aging*, *8*(2), 301–313. 10.1037/0882-7974.8.2.301

Lo, M., & Aziz, T. (2009). Muslim marriage goes online: The use of internet matchmaking by American Muslims. *The Journal of Religion and Popular Culture*, *21*(3), 5. 10.3138/jrpc.21.3.005.

Madathil, J., & Benshoff, J.M. (2008). Importance of marital characteristics and marital satisfaction: A comparison of Asian Indians in arranged marriages and Americans in marriages of choice. *The Family Journal: Counseling and Therapy for Couples and Families*, *16*(3), 222–230. 10.1177/10664 80708317504

Maheen, H., Malik, F., Siddique, B., & Qidwai, A. (2015). Assessing parental knowledge about thalassemia in a thalassemia center of Karachi, Pakistan. *Journal of genetic counseling*, *24*(6), 945–951. 10.1007/s10897-015-9830-z

Mahr, F., McLachlan, N., Friedberg, R.D., Mahr, S., & Pearl, A.M. (2015). Cognitive-behavioral treatment of a second-generation child of Pakistani descent: Ethnocultural and clinical considerations. *Clinical child psychology and psychiatry*, *20*(1), 134–147. 10.1177/1359104513499766

Majumdar, C. (2018). Attitudes towards premarital sex in India: Traditionalism and cultural change. *Sexuality & Culture*, *22*(2), 614–631. 10.1007/s12119-017-9486-y

Manohar, N. (2008). "Sshh … !! Don't Tell My Parents": Dating among Second-Generation Patels in Florida. *Journal of Comparative Family Studies*, *39*(4), 571–588. 10.3138/jcfs.39.4.571

Markus, H.R., & Kitayama, S. (1991). Culture and the self: Implications for cognition, emotion, and motivation. *Psychological Review*, *98*(2), 224–253. 10.1037/0033-295X.98.2.224

Medora, N.P., Larson, J.H., Hortascu, N., & Dave, P. (2002). Perceived attitudes towards romanticism: A cross cultural study of American, Asian Indian, and Turkish young adults. *Journal of Comparative Family Studies*, *33*(2), 155–178. 10.3138/jcfs.33.2.155

Merten, M. (2019). Keeping it in the family: consanguineous marriage and genetic disorders, from Islamabad to Bradford. *BMJ: British Medical Journal* (Online), 365. 10.1136/bmj.l1851

Mir, S. (2014). *Muslim American women on campus: Undergraduate social life and identity*. The University of North Carolina Press.

Myers, J.E., Madathil, J., & Tingle, R.L. (2005). Marriage satisfaction and wellness in India and the United States: A preliminary comparison of arranged marriages and marriages of choice. *Journal of Counseling & Development*, *83* (2), 183–190. 10.1002/j.1556-6678.2005.tb00595.x

Narayanan, S.A. (2018, January 15). What Are 36 Gunas in Hindu Marriage. *Times of India*. Retrieved March 15, 2021, from https://timesofindia.indiatimes.com/astrology/relationshipsmarriage/what-are-36gunas-in-hindu-marriage/articleshow/68205861.cms

Negy, C., & Snyder, D.K. (1997). Ethnicity and acculturation: Assessing Mexican American couples' relationships using the Marital Satisfaction Inventory—Revised. *Psychological Assessment*, *9*(4), 414. 10.1037/1040-3590.9.4.414

Oyserman, D., Sorensen, N., Reber, R., & Chen, S.X. (2009). Connecting and Separating Mind Sets: Culture as Situated Cognition. *Journal of Personality and Social Psychology*, *97*(2), 217–235. 10.1037/a0015850

Patel, A.K. (2015, December 10). The Heart Said Yes; the Horoscope Said No. *The New York Times*. https://www.nytimes.com/2015/12/13/fashion/the-heart-said-yes-the-hinduhoroscope-said-no.html

Pew Research Center. (2012). *The Rise of Asian Americans*. Retrieved from https://www.pewresearch.org/social-trends/2012/06/19/the-rise-of-asian-americans/

Philips, A. (2004). Gendering colour: Identity, femininity and marriage in Kerala. *Anthropologica*, *46*(2), 253–272. 10.2307/25606198

Rahman, Z., & Witenstein, M.A. (2014). A quantitative study of cultural conflict and gender differences in South Asian American college students. *Ethnic and Racial Studies*, *37*(6), 1121–1137. 10.1080/01419870.2012.753152

Razdan, P. (2006, November 28). Ash To Marry Tree First. *Hindustan Times*. Retrieved March 15, 2021, from https://www.hindustantimes.com/india/ash-to-marry-tree-first/story-9IAdyRZhe8l2btiq3Bx3jO.html

Rhyne, D. (1981). Bases of marital satisfaction among men and women. *Journal of Marriage and the Family*, 941–955. 10.2307/351350

Sadowski, H., Kolvin, I., Clemente, C., Tsiantis, J., Baharaki, S., Ba, G., Lee, C., & Taylor, B. (2002). Psychopathology in children from families with blood disorders: a cross-national study. *European Child & Adolescent Psychiatry*, *11*(4), 151–161. 10.1007/s00787-002-0257-3

Sassler, S. (2010). Partnering across the life course: Sex, relationships, and mate selection. *Journal of Marriage and Family*, *72*(3), 557–575. 10.1111/j.1741-3737.2010.00718.x

Sastry, J. (1999). Household structure, satisfaction and distress in India and the United States: A comparative cultural examination. *Journal of Comparative Family Studies*, *30*(1), 135–152. 10.3138/jcfs.30.1.135

Sawe, B.E. (2018, August 16). Religious composition of South Asian countries. Retrieved March 15, 2021, from https://www.worldatlas.com/articles/religious-composition-of-the-countries-of-south-asia.html

Shachar, R. (1991). His and her marital satisfaction: The double standard. *Sex Roles*, *25*(7), 451–467. 10.1007/BF00292534

Shaw, A., & Charsley, K. (2006). Rishtas: adding emotion to strategy in understanding British Pakistani transnational marriages. *Global Networks*, *6*(4), 405–421. 10.1111/j.1471-0374.2006.00152.x

Shukla, A., & Kapoor, M. (1990). Sex role identity, marital power, and marital satisfaction among middle-class couples in India. *Sex Roles*, *22*(11–12), 693–706. 10.1007/BF00292055

Singh, M.D., & Bhayana, R.M. (2015). Straddling three worlds: Stress, culture, and adaptation in South Asian couples. *Contemporary Family Therapy: An International Journal*, *37*(1). 45–57. 10.1 007/s10591-014-9319-1

Snyder, D.K., Baucom, D.H., & Gordon, K.C. (2007). *Getting past the affair: A program to help you cope, heal, and move on–Together or apart*. Guilford Press.

Sternberg, R.J. (1986). A triangular theory of love. *Psychological Review*, *93*(2), 119–135. 10.1037/ 0033-295X.93.2.119

Sternberg, R.J., & Weis, K. (2006). *The new psychology of love*. Yale University Press.

Strohschein, L., & Ram, U. (2017). Gender, marital status, and mental health: A test of the sex role hypothesis in India. *Journal of Family Issues*, *38*(13), 1899–1922. 10.1177/0192513X16680090

Stuart, J., & Ward, C. (2011). Predictors of ethno-cultural identity conflict among South Asian immigrant youth in New Zealand. *Applied Developmental Science*, *15*(3), 117–128. 10.1080/1 0888691.2011.587717

Sukumar, K. (2017, February 06). Dowries are illegal in India. but families - including mine – still expect them. *Vox*. Retrieved March 29, 2021, from https://www.vox.com/firstperson/2017/2/6/ 14403490/dowry-india-bride-groom-dilemma

Sumter, S.R., Valkenburg, P.M., & Peter, J. (2013). Perceptions of love across the lifespan: Differences in passion, intimacy, and commitment. *International Journal of Behavioral Development*, *37*(5), 417–427. 10.1177/0165025413492486

Tan, N. (2019). Was 1992 a turning point for homosexuals in contemporary India? *Sexuality & Culture*, *23*(1), 142–153. 10.1007/s12119-018-9548-9

Tummala-Narra, P. (2013). Psychotherapy with South Asian women: Dilemmas of the immigrant and first generations. *Women & Therapy*, *36*(3–4), 176–197. 10.1080/02703149.2013.797853

Tummala-Narra, P., Deshpande, A., & Kaur, J. (2016). South Asian adolescents' experiences of acculturative stress and coping. *American Journal of Orthopsychiatry*, *86*(2), 194–211. 10.1037/ ort0000147

U.S. Census Bureau. (2010). 2010 Census shows Asians are fastest-growing race group: 2012. Retrieved from http://www.census.gov/newsroom/releases/archives/2010_census/cb12-cn22.html

Verma, J. (1989). Marriage opinion survey and collectivism. *Psychological Studies*, *34*(3), 141–150.

Wacharasin, C., Phaktoop, M., & Sananreangsak, S. (2015). A family empowerment program for families having children with thalassemia, Thailand. *Nursing & Health Sciences*, *17*(3), 387–394. 10.1111/nhs.12201

Weatherall, D.J. (2005). Keynote address: The challenge of thalassemia for the developing countries. *Annals of the New York Academy of Sciences*, *1054*(1), 11–17. 10.1196/annals.1345.002

Weigel, D.J., & Ballard-Reisch, D.S. (1999). All marriages are not maintained equally: Marital type, marital quality, and the use of maintenance behaviors. *Personal Relationships*, *6*(3), 291–303. 10.1111/j.1475-6811.1999.tb00193.x

World Health Organization. (2008). Management of haemoglobin disorders: Report of a joint WHO-TIF meeting, Nicosia, Cyprus, 16–18 November 2007.

Xiaohe, X., & Whyte, K. (1990). Love matches and arranged marriages: A Chinese replication. *Journal of Marriage and the Family*, *52* (3), 709–722. 10.2307/352936

Yelsma, P., & Athappilly, K. (1988). Marital satisfaction and communication practices: Comparisons among Indian and American couples. *Journal of Comparative Family Studies*, *14*(1), 37–54. 10.3138/ jcfs.19.1.37

Zaidi, A.U., Couture-Carron, A., & Maticka-Tyndale, E. (2016). 'Should I or Should I Not'?: An exploration of South Asian youth's resistance to cultural deviancy. *International Journal of Adolescence and Youth*, *21*(2), 232–251. 10.1080/02673843.2013.836978

10 Considerations for South Asian American Parenting and Families

Neha Navsaria and Razia F. Kosi

Case Overview

To underscore important therapeutic elements, a fictional case study is presented high-lighting themes commonly reported in South Asian American (SAA) families. The themes include: intergenerational expectations, family secrets, bullying, cultural bias and how clinicians can build therapeutic alliances, surface their assumptions, and serve as culture brokers or guides both during therapy and navigating systems outside of therapy. The case study focuses on the Shah family and therapist Jasmine Kapoor. The Shahs, which are composed of by a father, Anand (39), mother, Seema (36), and son, Taj (10), have lived in the United States (US) for over 13 years and are first generation coming from India. The family is middle-class with both parents working in the Information Technology (IT) in-dustry. They have extended family in the US and their parents come from India for ex-tended visits. The therapist, Jasmine Kapoor (33), is a Licensed Clinical Social Worker (LCSW) and has been working in the field for 9 years. The setting for the case study is a suburb with predominantly White families near a metropolitan city.

Introduction

There is an extensive amount of literature that focuses on parenting children and ado-lescents in the US which provides clinicians and researchers with important insights on US based parenting styles and beliefs. The act of parenting represents a convergence of varied influences residing within the parent and values informed by community and societal expectations. One such set of influences is the cultural contexts that shape parent behaviors and expectations of childhood. However, the exploration of culture and parenting is limited as data obtained from parenting populations is characterized by a lack of diversity in the samples. This leaves little understanding about parenting practices and underlying processes from other cultures and less researched informed service work addressing par-enting needs in minoritized communities. The SAA population is a minimally researched cultural group.

The countries comprising South Asia have one commonality across the cultures, re-ligions, and ethnic groups, that is the value of family. As people from South Asia im-migrated to the US the high value placed on family remained, however the influence and support of the extended family lessened. Young adults became parents in a new land, and it became essential for South Asian parents to intentionally practice traditions that they believed would root their children in their culture of origin, while helping them thrive in an unfamiliar new land. While that narrative holds true for many first-generation families, new stories have unfolded for SAA families. There are similar challenges in retaining aspects of South Asian cultural identity within a majority culture, managing models of

DOI: 10.4324/9781003081548-10

parenting passed down from the previous generation and consideration of new opportunities to reconceptualize the role of a South Asian parent in the US. There has been little emphasis on the way in which research, clinical, and social service work address how SAA parents can engage in effective parenting practices to promote healthy child and family functioning. The "South Asian American" parent is one that conjures up images of hierarchy, tradition, and strict discipline. What defines a "South Asian" parent today? What traditions and practices do SAA parents value? How can mental health professionals create culturally relevant spaces for discussing and providing guidance on parenting and supporting families?

Chapter Contents

Parenting and family are important values in SAA cultures. With families leaving countries of origin, parenting and family life become influenced by both traditions and expectations of the South Asian countries and that of the newer home country. This chapter begins with an overview of current research on SAA parenting and families, shares findings from the voices of SAA parents across the nation, offers considerations for parenting in therapeutic interventions with SAA, and lastly offers an SAA perspective in the context of parenting on critical topics that often surface in therapy with SAAs. Key topics in working with SAA families include, surfacing clinician assumptions, building therapeutic alliances, assessing parenting goals, working with the family context, and understanding how acculturation informs parenting beliefs and goals. Lastly, the chapter reviews interventions that engage parents and the community for bridging understanding and increasing support for SAA parents. Future directions and suggested resources are presented.

This chapter provides guidance on SAA parenting with a focus on parenting of SAA young and school-age children. Given the limited literature on this specific group, the authors acknowledge the need to expand the literature review to different age groups, countries, and generations. Relevant data and themes from literature on parenting and SAA adolescents are also presented. An understanding of outcomes for SAA adolescents may help inform parenting strategies that implemented at an earlier developmental stage becomes a preventive approach. In addition to research from the US (United States), existing research on South Asian parenting in the United Kingdom (UK) and Canada are summarized. This further broadens and enhances the understanding of common elements in South Asian parenting across the diaspora. Lastly, studies on various generations of South Asian parenting are reviewed as there is a tendency for studies to combine data from new immigrants, 1.5 generation and second generation South Asian parents into one sample. Studies on parents who live in South Asia are excluded from the review as contexts of immigration and acculturation uniquely shape parenting behaviors and family functioning for the South Asian diaspora.

Current Knowledge about South Asian American (SAA) Families and Parenting

Collectivism and Orientation to Family

South Asian culture is characterized by collectivism. Collectivist cultures organize values, identity, and behaviors around one or more collectives, such as a kinship network, religious group or country, with group values emphasized over individual independence (Maiter & George, 2003; Triandis, 1994). One such collective is the family. Specifically, parenting and the parent-child relationship being salient features of family and community processes. Reflecting the collectivist orientation in these parenting processes, SAA parents have expressed that a goal of child rearing is to create communities and not individuals (Paiva, 2008). Additionally, SAA family life is embedded in the extended family system (Deepak, 2005), highlighting the intricate and complex nature of these collectives.

There are general family characteristics attributed to SAAs that include primacy of the family over the individual, harmony between hierarchical roles, filial piety, structured family roles and relationships, sense of duty to family, and protection of honor and "face" of family (Tewari et al., 2003). Obedience to parental rules, respect, and acceptance of the decisions of elders are a few values that have been attributed to South Asian parents (Maiter & George, 2003). In contrast, a "good" parent from Westernized perspectives encourage children's growth toward eventual independence by allowing for individual decision-making, personal space, and privacy (Deepak, 2005). There is a perception by SAAs that this promotion of independence can lead to deterioration in family structure. Many SAAs hold a belief that American families are fragile, conflict-ridden, and usually ending in divorce (Deepak, 2005). Therefore, due to these attributions placed on Westernized families, many SAA parents prioritize their parenting around preserving family structure. These concerns also play a role in SAA parents' decision-making around child care and approaches to supervision. For example, some SAA parents report having their parents come to the US to take care of their young children, rather than consider the option of day care (Deepak, 2005). Additionally, these family and collectivist characteristics can be viewed as cultural developmental domains for South Asians leading to healthy development for South Asian children (Iqbal & Golombok, 2018). From this perspective, competency attainment in these domains is likely to inform parenting goals and behaviors in SAA parents.

The orientation toward family and community has been shown to have positive and protective effects on SAAs. SAA adolescents identify that connections to family, community and heritage increased their cultural pride, emotional closeness, and reliability in relationships (Tummala-Narra et al., 2016). This family cohesion and community support also play a protective role in the psychological well-being of SAAs when managing acculturative stress (Lueck & Wilson, 2010) and coping with discrimination (Tummala-Narra, et al., 2012). At the same time, while the family and community system can be viewed as a form of security and source of support, the family and gender role adaptations, generational conflicts and societal pressures can be major sources of stress for SAAs (Farver et al., 2007; Tewari, et al., 2003; Tummala-Narra et al., 2016). Overall, the family context and greater collective has a foundational, yet complex role in the development of a SAA child and is vital in the understanding of the trajectory of SAA parenting.

Acculturation and Parenting

Acculturation describes the cultural shifts that occur as a result of contact between two or more cultural groups and involves the incorporation of beliefs and behaviors from a new dominant cultural context into a heritage culture (APA 2012). The challenges accompanying acculturation are known as *acculturative stress* (APA, 2012). Families cope with the constraints and possibilities experienced through the process of migration by accepting, rejecting, accommodating, and reformulating these demands in ways that can either strengthen family relationships or increase the stress on the family system (Deepak, 2005). Understanding the stresses and possibilities specific to the South Asian acculturative experience is essential to culturally competent practice with families.

There is considerable research highlighting the negative effects of acculturative stress on mental health outcomes among SAAs (Inman et al., 2014; Tummala-Narra et al., 2016). For SAA children and adolescents, identity formation while acculturating can be particularly challenging. The resulting struggle to navigate conflicting identities and to establish a healthy sense of self, as well as an ethnic identity that encompasses their bicultural experience may lead to increased family conflict, heightened anxiety, low self-esteem, and poor school performance (Farver et al., 2007). This acculturative stress is found to be experienced both at home and school (Tummala-Narra et al., 2016). Parents of these children may not be well informed on how to support their children on these issues or even be aware of the specific origins of their children's emotional struggles in the context of acculturation and identity development. The case study provides examples of how children and families navigate the bicultural experience. The parents chose the nickname, Taj, for their son under the advice of teachers that his formal name would cause difficulties in school. Taj's parents prioritize the teaching of some religious and cultural practices at home. Influenced by what he sees in his peer environment, he rejects some practices based on his observation that other children do not engage in these activities.

For SAA parents, the psychological impact of immigration and acculturation on adult behaviors, that influences child-rearing practices, thus impacting developmental outcomes and family environment. Both Deepak (2005) and Inman et al. (2007) report that South Asian parents in the US hold real fears of the perceived culture of the US, such as teen sexual activity, pregnancy, experimentation with drugs and alcohol, sexually transmitted diseases, sexual and physical child abuse, rape, and divorce. The effect of these fears can result in SAA parents being wary of their children interacting with American children and their families, restricting children's social contact with non-South Asian children (Deepak, 2005) and disapproving of their children's adoption of Westernized values and behaviors (Inman et al., 2007; Tummala-Narra et al., 2016). Parents may communicate to their children that they are disrespectful to their elders and their native culture. Therefore, in the interest of maintaining harmony, children are expected to avoid confrontation, conform to rules, respect others and avoid open conflict. However, the resulting family discord can impact family relationships and functioning as SAA adolescents describe experiencing familial stress concerning their connection to mainstream culture (Tummala-Narra et al., 2016). In the case study with the Shah family, the avoidance of open communication about stressors and the hiding of emotions contribute to familial stress and ultimately surface in the school setting.

As part of navigating acculturative stress and the impact on children and parents, SAA families cope in a variety of ways. One strategy used by second-generation SAA youth is to manage their lives differently inside and outside the home (Deepak, 2005) where they develop a dual sense of self (Inman et al., 2007; Tummala-Narra et al., 2016). SAA adolescents have also identified specific mechanisms that improved their coping: appreciation of their parents' struggles and new opportunities in the US and, seeking peer support and seeking help from other adults, not necessarily mental health professionals (Tummala-Narra et al., 2016). This knowledge of SAA adolescents' coping styles can inform guidance to SAA parents on discussions related to acculturation and family disagreements. From the SAA parent perspective, how parents interpret what it means to be South Asian American in the US affects the choices they make about living their lives, from childcare to expectations of their children (Deepak, 2005; Inman et al., 2007). This interpretation is part of the acculturation process for SAA parents that shape their identity and impact family functioning. For example, SAA parents who possess have an integrated or assimilated acculturation style, and therefore a lessened acculturation gap between them and their children, report less family conflict and adolescents with higher self-esteem and less anxiety compared to less assimilated parents (Farver et al., 2007). The findings suggest that ways in which SAA parents relate to their culture of origin, as well as to the host culture, has direct effects on SAA children's psychological outcomes and family functioning.

Inman et al. (2007) observed that many SAA parents invested considerable efforts to hold onto cultural values and practices. However, it was clear that they maintained a bicultural and compartmentalized identity that shifted based on context. Furthermore, these parents believed that a bicultural approach in parenting enhanced relationships with their children by adjusting parenting practices, such as taking children's view into consideration, and helped to facilitate children's bicultural adjustment. Deepak (2005) demonstrates the complex way in which SAA mothers and daughters work together to develop acculturation styles resulting in new interpretations of the traditional communication and family structure. Mothers and daughters described dynamic and supportive relationships in which communication was strong, although not always open. Daughters would monitor their own public behaviors for the sake of protecting parents, while parents would sometimes defend their daughters' lives and choices to their communities. Mothers would advise and guide their daughters' behavior, sometimes strategizing with them on the best way to communicate and function within the parameters of community expectations.

Overall, the observations and findings on the role of acculturation in SAA parenting demonstrate that it is a fluid process with no "right way" to manage it. It consists of complex layered negotiations occurring between parent and child (Deepak, 2005). When it comes to child-rearing, SAA parents may combine different cultural elements together in a way that best promotes family adaptation that is dependent on the context (Farver et al., 2007). These results support the critical need for clinicians to explore and raise awareness on concepts of generational and acculturative differences as they work with SAA parents and families. Later in this chapter, the case study with the Shah family will explore aspects of acculturative differences.

YOUNGER CHILDREN

Much of the literature on SAA parenting is derived from experiences raising adolescents. Research on practices of SAA parents in early childhood is scant. This developmental period typically represents infancy to early school-age. The research that does exist outlines themes related to understanding of the role of play, literacy, and early education from a lens of South Asian parenting. Play is an action that occurs across cultures; however, there are cultural differences in the frequency and content of play as well as caregiver—child interactions (Jent et al., 2011). Some families may value academic components of play (Farver & Shinn, 1997), while others may emphasize individualism and self-reliance, preferring more child-directed play. For collectivistic families, early choice making may be discouraged due to the emphasis on child obedience and respect (Johnston & Wong, 2002). These dynamics could lead to seemingly restrained play that is more parent driven. Furthermore, collectivistic societies often rely on the extended family or community to engage children in play activity (Navsaria & Hong, 2016). These parents may appear to place less importance on one-to-one playtime, when in reality, they expect the child to have other adults and children involved in their play.

South Asian immigrant families view preschool programs as venues for teaching conduct and academics and do not understand the use of play as a learning strategy (Joshi, 2005). Parmar et al. (2004) compared the play beliefs of Asian (including South Asian) and Euro-American parents of preschoolers in the US. The Euro-American parents were found to believe that play is an important vehicle for early physical, social, emotional, and cognitive development. In contrast, the Asian parents did not value play in the development of preschool children. They did not believe play helps children get ready for school. On the other hand, the Asian parents believed more strongly that an early start in academic training is important for cognitive development in the preschool years. Another study found that a substantial number of SAA mothers of young children strongly agreed that it is more important for their child to have good academic skills than to play well with other children (Navsaria, 2011).

Beliefs about the role of play in early childhood also inform SAA parents' decisions around the provision of resources to their child and the way in which they engage their children in activities. Parmar et al. (2004) found that Asian parents bought fewer toys for their children, and those they selected were typically more educational. Euro-American parents facilitated their children's play by playing with their children themselves, whereas the Asian parents served as their children's teachers and academic coaches at home to promote cognitive development. In general, South Asian Americans parents view instruction as one of their main parenting strategies (Paiva, 2008). SAA mothers of young children have shared that they are not sure if they should go along with their child's pretend play, and would prefer to read with their child than play with them (Navsaria, 2011). These dynamics could lead to inaccurate conclusions about play that appear to deviate from the norm and give rise to interpretations that the SAA parent places less importance on playtime.

Although research on SAA parenting of young children is emerging, these preliminary findings are informative. They suggest that play is a culturally mitigated construct and SAA parents hold and act on clear beliefs on the emphasis on academics in early childhood. The research findings identify the precursors to parenting styles and values that emerge in the later years and are useful to future assessment and prevention. For example, the case study briefly highlights the parent's questioning the use of playing games in the therapeutic context with her son. These parental opinions on play may have formed during early childhood and set a foundation for the extent to which play is emphasized and used at home for learning and relationship-building. During the early years, parents play an important role in shaping a child's skills for emotional regulation, problem-solving, autonomy, exploration, and self-control (Dallaire & Weinraub, 2005; Deater-Deckard et al., 2005). Therefore, it is a reminder for clinicians to understand family patterns, acculturations, and, parenting goals when addressing SAA parenting during the early years rather than hold an assumption it is more relevant to later developmental stages based on existing research. For these important reasons, more studies need to explore the realm of SAA parenting and young children.

PARENTING STYLES

At first glance, SAA parenting appears to hold characteristics of less warmth and over-control of children. This is commonly referred to as an authoritarian style of parenting and historically considered to be damaging to children's well-being. In contrast, an authoritative style is defined as communicating warmth and praise to children and setting clear expectations with moderate limits (Van Campen & Russell, 2010). This approach is typically associated with Westernized parenting and psychological well-being. However, categorization into these styles and child outcomes can be too simplistic and mask complex layers of knowledge and parenting mechanisms that could assist those in helping relationships with SAA families. It is important to understand that parenting in the US and UK is often guided by Westernized beliefs about parenting and parent-child interactions with a focus on what it means to be parents and what parent-child relationships are supposed to look like (Van Campen & Russell, 2010). How well these current models fit South Asian populations, particularly South Asians in the diaspora, has also been questioned in the research literature with contradictory findings (Sorkhabi & Mandara, 2013). Further examination of the literature is needed to better understand what it means for SAA parents to support and discipline their children.

Iqbal & Golombok (2018) examined characteristics of British-born Indian, Pakistani, and White mothers of 5- to 7-year-olds. All mothers demonstrated appropriate levels of warmth, control, and mother-child interaction which was associated with positive child adjustment. Higher levels of overt discipline (the extent to which a parent loses temper or raises voice) were found in both the Pakistani and Indian mothers. Taken together with the positive adjustments for all the children, but differences in discipline styles, the authors suggest that there are different pathways for parents to achieve positive outcomes. These findings also raise the questions on whether high discipline should always be associated with lack of warmth. Inman et al. (2007) observed that South Asian parents in the US often used authoritative parenting styles. They describe growing with and learning from their children. However, given their cultural influence and their own upbringing, often SAA parents seemed to blend their new attitudes toward parenting with some familiar aspects of authoritarian parenting. It can be inferred that parenting styles are not fixed categories and can be blended with other styles based on parents' adaptation to their current environment.

Garg et al. (2005) found high percentages of perceived authoritative parenting by Asian-Indian adolescents in Canada. This parenting style was associated with higher levels of parent concern and family cohesiveness. There were no differences in adolescents' academic outcomes due to parenting style. The lack of relationship between parenting style and academic competence raises the question on whether there are specific mechanisms or pathways that specifically capture the pattern of emphasis on academics as it relates to parental warmth and discipline style for SAA families. An alternative parenting style, *training*, has been proposed by Chao (1994) to better capture and validate Asian parenting, taking into account the meaning behind control and discipline behaviors. Training is defined as high levels of parental control and involvement to guide children, physical closeness, and concern for educational success. It has been endorsed in research studies on Chinese Americans (Chao, 2000), British-Pakistani (Iqbal & Golombok, 2018) and Indian American families (Farver et al., 2007). The pattern of training also seems to hold constant, regardless of acculturation style (Farver et al., 2007). The exploration seems to provide a more robust explanation of aspects of SAA parenting and is deserving of further study and consideration when working with SAA families.

In summary, research on SAA parenting styles suggests that established conclusions about parenting styles may not fit all families. It is possible for there to be multiple pathways leading to optimal development for SAA children and adolescents. These studies also reflect the differences in how warmth, control, and support are operationalized for South Asian versus more Westernized cultures and how different parenting approaches serve as mechanisms to achieve culturally mitigated parenting goals for South Asians.

Parenting Goals

Most SAA parents who live in the US hold a unique set of ideologies with respect to child rearing goals (Joshi, 2005). These goals and ways in which they are transmitted to children are influenced by their cultural values, beliefs, and norms, but also mediated by social and environmental factors that they encounter (Maiter & George, 2003). A summary of three major goals derived from qualitative studies on SAA parents will be presented. The studies include interviews with South Asian parents (primarily mothers) in the US (Deepak, 2005; Inman et al., 2007; Rasool & Zhang, 2020; Walsh, 2007), Canada (Maiter & George, 2003) and the UK (Paiva, 2008), ranging from parenting young children to school-age children to young adults.

Imprinting Identity around Culture and Religion

A significant goal for SAA parents centers around helping children develop a sense of identity around culture and religion. This results in parenting becoming organized around the shaping of a cultural identity from early childhood into young adulthood. South Asian American parents often feel that if their children don't have knowledge of their culture, they will not have a sense of belonging, connectedness, or a sense of community resulting in negative effects on their identity development (Maiter & George, 2003). For many SAA parents, maintaining continuity of culture was reflected in being involved with South Asian and South Asian American friends and associations, maintaining vegetarianism, knowing the native language, and marrying a South Asian (Inman et al., 2007).

Although the extent to which religion is practiced by SAA parents, it is agreed that religion is a significant transmitter of culture (Maiter & George, 2003) and used as a form of identification by South Asians (Inman et al., 2007). Some parents also feel the need to adhere more strictly to religious rituals than they did in their country of origin, because they felt that otherwise their children would not have sufficient knowledge of their religion or see their religion practiced (Maiter & George, 2003). For example, South Asian Muslim mothers in the US describe that their parenting emphasizes the wish for their children to develop an understanding about Islam, Islamic practices, lifestyle, and values and encourage participation in religious activities for young people organized by the local mosques (Walsh, 2007). In speaking about the importance of religion and spirituality, Hindu parents reported going to the temple with their children, teaching prayers and hymns, observing important religious holidays, and engaging in religious discussions (Inman et al., 2007). Although the focus on cultural religious identity is paramount to South Asian parents, it is important to highlight that Inman et al. (2007) noted that parents recognized the ongoing challenges in transmitting facets of cultural and religious identity within a different culture and found themselves questioning whether they were correct in emphasizing these values that were important to them or whether they should have encouraged values that would help their children adapt to the new society. This questioning and reflection led parents to develop an approach that balanced active flexibility with traditional values.

Accepting and Taking Responsibility

Another theme that emerged was the burden and responsibility mothers felt in their child's outcomes, resulting in a more intense emphasis in their parenting methods. In South Asia, the extended family often assists with child-rearing and parental decision-making. South Asian American immigrant parents acknowledged that it was no longer possible to get an entire family to parent a child and feel they must make do with a two-parent model. Many parents experience this absence of the extended family as a significant loss (Inman, et al., 2007; Paiva, 2008) with the responsibility of parenting fully upon them (Deepak, 2005). Immigrants to the US or other countries often feel more isolated in their responsibility for transmitting their cultural values and norms in a new environment (Inman et al., 2007; Maiter & George, 2003). For some SAA parents, migration distanced them from extended family and community expectations, which allowed them to make parenting decisions more independently than they might have if they were living in the same country with extended family. This freedom was experienced as an exciting challenge despite the lack of instrumental and emotional support (Deepak, 2005).

These ideals of responsibility guide their parenting approaches. For example, SAA parents do not often leave children with babysitters or go on their own trips (Maiter &

George, 2003). Some indicated that they had quit their jobs when their first child was born and did not work outside the home again until their children entered primary school. Parents report being closely involved with their children in activities to improve their level of academic achievement. Such activities included the discussion of learning activities at school, assisting children with homework, time management, enforcing social media and screen time, and monitoring socializing with friends (Rasool & Zhang, 2020). When it came to responsibility in religious education, parents would consciously work hard to assure exposure and following of religious practices (Walsh, 2007). For example, South Asian American Muslim mothers shared their efforts in socializing with coreligionists, facilitating participation of children in religious education classes, developing religious education classes, and offering services as teacher assistants (Walsh, 2007). Overall, the mothers knew that there was a reliance on them for their children's outcomes and cultural knowledge.

INSTILLING THE FOUNDATION FOR SUCCESS

South Asian American parents describe that the purpose of migration was for their children's future (Walsh, 2007). They describe that their children define their life and there is also a sense of taking full responsibility for their future, achievements, successes, and failures (Maiter & George, 2003; Walsh, 2007). Concerning this theme, parents have also shared that the parental role is a key to the success of their children (Rasool & Zhang, 2020). A significant theme centered around the goal of instilling skills for success in life (Maiter & George, 2003; Walsh, 2007) and personal qualities to develop one's character (Maiter & George, 2003). Much of the intent of parents' approaches were grounded in helping their child succeed in society. Mothers wanted their children to gain the necessary education and life skills to enable them to lead a good quality of life (Walsh, 2007). Most participants agreed that earning higher degrees could lead to a successful career and more comfortable lifestyle (Inman et al., 2007; Rasool & Zhang, 2020). Cultural and familial values were viewed as having benefits because it was believed that they can help children be useful and productive citizens of their new country which will ultimately lead to success (Maiter & George, 2003).

There were also mechanisms by which parents pursue the goals of character formation. An emphasis on aspects of cultural and religious values was considered by mothers to be essential for positive and healthy development. Research on British Pakistani families, suggest that an upbringing in Islam, allows parents to pass on values of morality and discipline (Iqbal & Golombok, 2018). In addition to drawing from religion and culture, mothers often used personal examples to emphasize character development (Maiter & George, 2003; Walsh, 2007). They wanted to set a good example for their kids to deter unacceptable behaviors in their children and reduce disciplinary actions. Along with participation in cultural and religious activities, extended family connections and community support also provide ways for parents to achieve parenting goals of character formation (Maiter & George, 2003). In summary, the common themes across the research regarding SAA parenting are (a) elevating the importance of identity with both culture and religion and (b) owning and taking responsibility to raise children with the cultural and religious values, and (c) building the children's foundation so they enter adulthood ready for career success.

Considerations When Addressing South Asian American (SAA) Parenting in Therapy

Given that parental conflict and parent-child relations are important factors in the development of stress and psychological symptoms in SAA children and adolescents, an understanding of parenting goals and approaches is important for prevention of negative outcomes and the development of culturally sensitive interventions for SAA parents, children, and families. These practices should combine unique cultural beliefs while preventing or reducing the negative impact on families. Parenting factors can be explored in a number of contexts: parenting education programs, parenting interventions, family therapy, child therapy, couples therapy, and school counseling. To illustrate these practices within some of these contexts a case study will first be presented, followed by discussion of various therapy considerations and how they relate to the case study.

Case Study

A group private practice in a suburban area completed an intake from a 36-year-old woman, Seema Shah, who was seeking family therapy for her 10-year-old son, Taj, who was getting into fights at school. The private practice recently hired a therapist who identified as South Asian, and the mother specifically asked for this individual. This clinician, Jasmine Kapoor, is a second generation South Asian American, whose parents immigrated to the US from India, however her parents had lived in Bahrain for several years prior to immigrating. Ms. Kapoor was raised in an area of the US that had very few South Asians and did not come into contact with other South Asians outside her family until college.

Mrs. Shah came to the first session with Taj and stated her husband, Anand Shah, could not leave work in time to attend the session. Mrs. Shah immediately asked the clinician where she was from, and if she was a doctor. The therapist shared that she was a board certified clinician who specialized in family therapy and that she could refer to her as Jasmine, or Ms. Kapoor, whichever she felt more comfortable with, and Taj could call her Miss Jasmine. Ms. Kapoor then asked why the mother was curious about where she was from, to which the mom asked if she was Indian. Understanding this might be important to bridging therapeutic alliance, the therapist did identify her Indian ancestry and then warmly acknowledge they shared their country of origin.

After the exchange acknowledging the shared cultural background and expansion of the therapist's qualifications to lead the sessions, the mother was able to proceed with the intake questions. Mrs. Shah went on to say her son is a good boy and had been getting good grades, but recently he has become "naughty" and the school said she should bring him for counseling. Taj, responded to questions when asked, but remained quiet in the session. He said he did not want to be in counseling and thought it was unfair that the other kids did not get in trouble like he did. While hesitant to be in family therapy, Mrs. Shah did acknowledge she needed help with her son's behavior. Mrs. Shah offered a brief family history of coming to the US 13 years ago, after she and her husband married. He had already been working in the US and returned to get married. Their marriage was not fully arranged, but both families were involved in the introductions, wanting them to marry within the religion and culture. Mrs. Shah described the years of the marriage as warm, but lonely with Mr. Shah working long hours. They have relatives in the US, but not close by. Mrs. Shah made friends in the local Indian community and after the birth of Taj their parents started to come from India for visits on a regular basis. After Mrs. Shah's visa status changed; she started to work in the IT industry, but chose a part-time position so she would have more time for child-rearing. The mom stated she felt it was important for her to pass on cultural traditions to her son, and home, only spoke to him in Gujarati, and taught him how to do pooja. The only Hindu temple was an hour away, so the family was able to attend the temple, but not as regularly as they would have liked. During the session, Mrs. Shah texted her husband about adjusting sessions to the evenings so he could attend without missing work. He agreed to attend, and sessions were scheduled for the next few weeks.

The first few sessions Ms. Kapoor noted the parents both asked questions about her own upbringing, the language she spoke, and her ties to her culture. She navigated the boundaries by giving broad examples of her experience growing up in the U.S. but was cautious to not share her own feelings of being an outsider among other Indians or having cultural experiences more prevalent in areas with a higher population of South Asians. While Ms. Kapoor was building trust with the parents, she was not sure if she was gaining trust with Taj. When she had individual sessions with him, he would respond, but gave minimal answers. He did enjoy playing Uno or checkers with her, while talking, but both parents would state that they did not see why they were coming to sessions for Taj to play with her.

At the start of the family therapy, the parents reported that the goal for the session was to have Taj focus on schoolwork and to not fight with the boys at school if they teased him. Both parents stated they did not spank Taj, like they had been disciplined as children, so they did not understand why he was getting into fights at school. The therapist realized she had expected the Shahs would have believed in spankings as a form of punishment, as her own parents had. Upon realizing this assumption, she went back to the intake and her session notes to reflect on other assumptions she made with this family so she could either counter her own stereotypes or raise questions in the session that would benefit the family. The parents also explained that they practiced meditation at home and when Taj was younger they taught him yoga and meditation as a part of their religious practice. They thought he enjoyed doing it with them, but more recently he stopped joining his parents, saying it was stupid and none of the other kids did those things.

The parents continued to share how they both doted on Taj, being the first-born grandson in the family and felt great pride in his paternal grandparents coming to the US for his birth and even naming their son. When this was shared, Ms. Kapoor noticed Taj became agitated and asked to leave the room. The parents again seemed perplexed as to why Taj was upset. When Taj rejoined, Ms. Kapoor asked why he wanted to leave the room. This is when Taj blurted out that he hated the name his grandfather gave him. When asked why he did not like the name Taj, he said, "not that one, the real one." This is when the parents explained Taj's given name was Shitij, which means sky. The grandfather wanted his first grandchild to have no limits and selected this name. The Shahs had not grown up in the US and were from traditional families in India and accepted the name. When they registered him for school the teachers immediately told them the name would cause a great deal of teasing among the students, so the family asked that he be called Taj in school. The documentation in school had his formal name, but Taj was indicated as his preferred name. The family had gotten into the habit of calling him Taj and did not realize their son was upset about his given name.

At the start of this school year, Taj's teacher unexpectedly took a leave of absence because of a medical issue and different substitute teachers were monitoring the class until a long-term substitute was secured. At this time, the substitute teachers were calling the name Shitij- and pronouncing it Shit-ij, which caused all the children to laugh and further taunt him during recess. One student said Shitij and his skin were both the color of "'shit." This revelation was surprising to both parents as the school and Taj had not said anything about the racist comments. Taj stated that he did not want to be a "snitch" and face more harassment from this person. The parents were angry at Taj for not saying something before and for him not reporting this to the teacher and principal. Ms. Kapoor, drawing on her own cultural knowledge in U.S. schools, went on to explain the term "snitch" to the parent and how the peer pressure to not speak out could have prevented Taj from reporting the student. Taj also said he didn't really think it was a racial slur because it was not like the "n" word, or someone pulling their eyes back to mimic features of his friend from Korea. The therapist helped the family discuss how to report this to the school staff to end the harassment from the aggressor. When the parents asked Taj why he had not shared this with them, he said he did not want to make them upset when he knew how sad his parents had been for the past few years.

In the next few parent sessions, Mrs. Shah admitted that she had suffered several miscarriages over the past years and both she and her husband were grieving over the losses. Shah also expressed guilt over the loss of the pregnancies, and thought she was not being as faithful in her religious practices. While Mr. Shah never blamed his wife for the miscarriages, he did not know how to process the grief and was staying at work longer to avoid facing the grief. The parents also stated they did not share this medical history because of the shame in losing the pregnancies and did not see the relevance to what was happening with their son. They also revealed they did not talk about this with anyone, which also made it difficult when well-intentioned family and friends continuously asked when they were having another child.

As Ms. Kapoor continued to work with the family, she found grief support groups in the area, and even one for parents who suffered miscarriages. Both Mr. and Mrs. Shah said they were not comfortable with this but agreed to talk with Taj about this. The parents had gained enough trust with Dr. Kapoor's expertise in the counseling sessions to bring this painful subject into the discussion. During the sessions, the therapist sometimes asked Taj to draw pictures and she asked him to bring in a picture about what he thought his parents were sad about. Taj drew a large sky with large teardrops engulfing his parents. He was not in the picture. His mom asked him why he was not in the picture, and he said he was the sky, making his parents sad. Taj had thought his parents were sad because they only had him, and they wanted other children. He said he tried to pray in the pooja room at home to be an obedient son. He knew he failed when he hit the boy who teased him and that was when he stopped trying to be obedient. The mother and father were able to express their feelings with their son and share how proud they were of him and their wanting another child was also about having siblings for him.

In a subsequent session, the family stated they wanted to report the harassment and Ms. Kapoor discussed with both the parents and Taj ways they could do this. The family decided to have a discussion with the school counselor and principal. They felt the school was responsive and teachers were more aware of intentionally teaching and sharing about racism, cultural identities, for both adults and students. The parents and Taj decided the goals for therapy had been met with Taj's grades back on track and the teasing about his name had subsided. The parents shared that the grandparents were coming to spend a few months with them. The Shahs had decided to share with Mr. Shah's parents about the struggles they faced the last few years. The mom asked how Taj felt about his grandfather calling him Shitij, and Taj replied he always liked the way his family had said his name, and it made him proud that his grandfather gave him his name.

Clinicians' Assumptions

First and foremost, it is important for clinicians to be aware of their own assumptions and biases when working with SAA families. This is important for both clinicians who identify as SAA and as different racial and ethnic identities. As previously stated in this book, the term "South Asian" includes seven countries, at least seven major religions, and numerous languages and cultures from the countries of origin. Anti-Muslim sentiment in the US post 9/11 has affected Pakistani, Bangledishi, and Indian-Muslims differently than Hindu families (Nath, 2005) with specific impacts on the parenting practices of Muslim parents (Iqbal, 2014; Walsh, 2007). Greater awareness from clinicians of their own stereotypes and biases, and actively countering those stereotypes outside of the sessions will be important to successful interventions. In the case study, the therapist surfaced assumptions about the parents' views on discipline and corporal punishment, and while the therapist didn't overtly acknowledge it, she held assumptions about how much the family would trust her if she revealed her own feelings of being an outsider within the Indian culture. While the experiences of SAA are diverse, reading literature, articles, and blogs written by SAA authors voicing the experiences and issues relevant to SAA is a starting point to understand their perspectives in a broader context.

THERAPEUTIC ALLIANCE

Research on best practices and interventions for SAAs is scarce at this point in time. Studies from Canada and England offer insight into engaging with families of South Asian origin. A qualitative study with South Asian British families found that for these families the quality of therapeutic alliance was viewed as greater than any specific cultural interventions (Pandya & Herlihy, 2009). Specifically, six factors were found to increase therapeutic alliance. As with most therapeutic relationships, safety and trust were essential to create the environment for family therapy. Safety was described as having discussions about topics not related to therapy to provide opportunities for the families to see the therapist as caring and trusting, which was the second quality for therapeutic alliance. Third, the flexibility of the therapist as to how they interacted with the family was identified as important. An example of flexibility from the therapist is their role in the session. The participants acknowledged if the parents are older or first generation, then they want the therapist to have an expert role in the session, offering advice and recommendations. Whereas, with younger family members, often second generation, preferred a collaborative approach to the family sessions, which followed Western expectations in therapy (Pandya & Herlihy, 2009). Lastly, equality in the sessions and a shared sense of purpose were also identified. Reflecting on the case study, what were some intentional steps Dr. Kapoor took to build a therapeutic alliance? How did she demonstrate safety, trust, flexibility, and a shared sense of purpose?

ASSESSING PARENTING GOALS

LeVine (1980) noted that although parents share common goals for parenting, there are also cultural differences in this realm that must be taken into consideration in understanding the meaning of "effective parenting" for parents. It is important for a therapist to understand how parenting goals, values, and beliefs can influence the behaviors that move toward the goals. For example, SAA parents often have goals focused on emphasizing cultural values. It is also important to have conversations with parents about their decision-making around goals. Maiter and George (2003) assert that providers need to be aware that for South Asian American parents' social contexts with potential to have negative consequences for their children impact the way in which they think through their approaches to parenting.

Often, based on SAA parents' minimal response to traditional school and community engagement strategies, it is assumed that these parents are not interested in learning about parenting their children. However, when reviewing goals specific to South Asian parents (see section on parenting goals), the reality is that most South Asian families care deeply about their children's education, health, and future. They may keep their distance from school and community agencies out of respect for educators, limited English proficiency, work schedules, and discomfort in those interactions. To meet these challenges within the case study, Dr. Kapoor worked to address the issue of Taj fighting in school, but as the sessions progressed, in what ways could Dr. Kapoor assess and explore the parenting goals with the family?

WORKING WITHIN THE FAMILY CONTEXT

Due to the emphasis on collectivism and the family for SAA, the family context must be considered. Tewari et al., (2003), suggest routine use of a genogram to understand the immigration history and pathways, family structure, alliances in the extended family and community network. A goal of the genogram is to elicit information on acculturation levels, religious affiliations, communication, role socialization, education, and Socioeconomic Status (SES). The use of narrative has also been shown to be effective with SAA families to explore the family context (Tewari et al., 2003). Parenting narratives could highlight patterns across generations, parenting models, paradigms of expressed emotion in the family, and explore expectations and relationships with children. The sharing of these narratives and experiences have been shown to engender closer and stronger relationships between SAAparents and children (Inman et al., 2007) and perceived as a coping strategy by South Asian adolescents (Tummala-Narra et al., 2016).

Clinicians should have an understanding of traditions within SAA culture, but also invite the family to share what the traditions uniquely mean to each of them. Pillari (2005), offered an example of the Hindu celebration, *rakhi*, a festival and tradition in which the sister(s) tie a silken thread on the wrist of their brother(s) and cousin-brothers to wish them *good health, wealth, happiness, and success*, (Pillari, 2005, p.400). The brother in return pledges his bond of protection for his sisters. The intent of the ritual is to affirm the bonds between sisters and brothers and can be effective to discuss in therapy if there is conflict between the siblings. However, if the parents have shown consistent favoritism or inequitable treatment, in favor of the male children, the ritual of rakhi may create further conflict between the siblings if the children are unable to express their experience or understanding of *rakhi*. In this case example, the exploration of Taj's name led to a deeper understanding of both the relationships with the grandparents and community expectations to have another child. With the parents not having extended family in this country, the silence of their grief affected their parenting with Taj.

Shariff (2009), identified two roles a therapist can play in family therapy involving familial conflict between first- and second-generation members with Canadian South Asians, that of a "cultural broker," (Spiegel, 1981) and "cultural systems information guide," (Bemak et al., 1996). The therapist can act as a cultural broker, by shifting the focus away from the child, and to the acculturation process, happening when the parents and youth have different experiences and expectations in the new country. This normalizes the family conflict as a transition to a new society, rather than a disobedient child. This process was exemplified in the case study, when the therapist explained to the Shahs the peer pressure to *not* report negative behavior by other students and helped the family discuss how to bring up the harassment faced by their son. Ms. Kapoor had taken the time to build the trust with the parents before sharing a perspective from a cultural lens. By building the therapeutic alliance with the parents, she avoided the pitfall some clinicians fall into of reframing a problem too quickly, which may cause the parents to feel invalidated and possibly terminate the sessions (Pandya & Herlihy, 2009).

A cultural systems information guide is when the therapist provides information to clients about the new country's dominant cultural values, behaviors, and practices that are impacting the family conflict (Bemak et. al, 1996). Before engaging in this role, the therapist must be engaged in ongoing self-reflection of their own biases, beliefs, and values, so they are not imposing cultural superiority when sharing about the new country's cultural values and practices, but rather informing how the differences could be causing a conflict in the family. Maiter and George (2003) noted that South Asian mothers in Canada identified beliefs of modesty, humility, hard work, persistence, perseverance, and having a disciplined life. While a young person might choose behaviors that seem to contradict modesty or humility, such as wearing clothing that shows their physique and using social media to share about their successes and increase their social standing among peers. This could arise in the family sessions as a conflict with the young person rejecting the mothers' values. The clinician could share the harms and benefits of social media and help the family navigate their concerns and hopes for the youth's life goals.

UNDERSTANDING HOW ACCULTURATION INFORMS PARENTAL BELIEFS AND GOALS

An assessment of how parents relate to their culture of origin relative to the host culture is important. The dissonance in acculturation between parent and child has been shown to complicate communication and mutual understanding between the two generations. Clinicians should be aware that over time these differences have created opportunities that challenge South Asian parents' ways of thinking, where they develop newer child-rearing approaches that allow them to function in two cultures with positive effects on family functioning (Farver et al., 2007). Therefore, therapists should spend time not only identifying the acculturation differences, but also guide the discussion so parents can process, reflect on these differences and decision-making in parenting, and how it relates to expectations and goals.

Clinicians should also be aware of how acculturation processes across individuals and families. Different pathways of acculturation can lead to similar outcomes. Conversely, similar trajectories can result in multiple ways to function. These complexities can occur due to a number of factors. For example, it has been noted that on one hand, the strong South Asian cultural and community network offers support and viewed as a source of resilience, but it is also possible for these networks to hinder a South Asian individual from completely assimilating or adapting to the host culture (Tewari et al., 2003). As part of acculturation discussions, clinicians should acknowledge for themselves and SAA families that there are different support and coping methods and the goal is for SAA parents to develop coping strategies that are meaningful to them. It is important for practitioners to know that the result is a much wider range of possibilities for SAA families' coping styles than simply a choice of becoming "American" or retaining only their cultural heritage (Deepak, 2005). From a strengths-based perspective, through these reflective discussions, therapists can help SAA parents identify the coping toolkit they have already developed that has been effective. SAA parents may not fully be aware of what they have accomplished navigating these processes on their own and how they can apply these approaches to other challenging parenting situations.

Lastly, acculturation processes are typically associated with those who have spent formative years in South Asia and then immigrated to the US. However, an assumption that acculturation is less of an issue for SAA parents who were raised in the US can mask information that is important to therapy effectiveness. While these parents are not "immigrants" to this country, much of their parenting dilemmas are influenced by the experience of being raised within an immigrant family, representing an intergenerational transmission of parenting values and challenges within a cultural context. In summary, consideration of acculturation processes emphasizes the need for therapists to have conversations and understanding on: the timing of immigration (for parent and child), location of extended families, activity in cultural/community organizations, value placed on South Asian values and Westernized values, goals of dual socialization and bicultural identity and inherited models of acculturative coping across generations.

Parenting Interventions

There is a dearth of research on SAA and formal parenting interventions such as parent training programs and specialized parent-child assessments and interventions. Additionally, applying interventions anchored in Westernized child rearing values to other cultural and ethnic groups is concerning. It may further reduce parent motivation to participate, and outcomes may not be as effective with a mismatch of values systems. Consideration of structured parenting interventions for use with SAA families highlights the critical question of what the right way to parent is and why (Paiva, 2008). For example, in observing SAA parent-child interactions with young children, parents appear less emotionally warm (Gibbs et al., 2017). When engaged with their preschool-aged children, British South Asian parents used instruction as the preferred parenting strategy with demonstrations of physical warmth and tangible rewards (Paiva, 2008). These parents perceive direct verbal praise as potentially leading to negative consequences (undesirable psychological attributes) and therefore used with caution. These observations through the lens of current parenting intervention models can be problematic and engender conclusions that SAA parents hold parenting deficits in expressing emotional support and affection. In the context of the case study, the clinician, Ms. Kapoor, may have formed conclusions in a similar manner leading to the development of assumptions about the Shah parents' parenting style. She recognized a bias she held, aligned with a parenting deficit, by assuming the Shahs spanked their child based on her own upbringing and a cultural assumption influenced by the "right" way to parent. Clinicians should also pay careful attention to how the information related to parenting is interpreted. By placing attention to this potential bias, Ms. Kapoor made the decision to reflect on her intake and session notes to assess for other assumptions she made with the Shahs. This practice allowed her to counter her own stereotypes, further assess parenting interpretations, and raise questions in the session that would benefit the family.

Awareness of these concerns when implementing parenting intervention programs with SAA families does not mean that therapists should refrain from using these models. Rather, therapists should consider contextual parameters for parent-child assessments and criteria on what constitutes a positive parent-child interaction. Clinicians should explore methods and meanings of expressing positive attention and guidance held by the family and community. It is suggested that therapists working with SAA families ask about parenting beliefs, expectations, and practices as they relate to children's developmental milestones and expectations (Paiva, 2008). Clinicians can also raise SAA parents' awareness that their child could be exposed to other models of supportive interactions and guidance with teachers, other parents or adults. This may impact how children interpret, receive, and reconcile parental interactions.

A review of global research on parenting interventions (Navsaria & Hong, 2016) found the following strategies for engaging and treating immigrant families and ethnic groups (not in their country of origin) to be effective: a) Translate written materials into native languages, b) Use bilingual and bicultural staff and clinicians, c) Use translators when content is presented in English, d) Give staff and clinicians cultural competency training specific to ethnicity, e) Introduce a pre-intervention motivational/supportive phase to increase potential for engagement, f) Ground key intervention components in cultural values, beliefs, and constructs by using culture-specific examples, vignettes, and visuals, g) Build trust among families, schools, and community by involving respected community agencies and trusted cultural brokers, h) Provide booster sessions, phone consultations, and home visits to provide support, reinforce information learned, and clarify misunderstandings. In summary, these guidelines can set an effective foundation for using parenting interventions with SAA families.

Community Interventions for Parents

Given the emphasis of the SAA community collective, approaching parenting support and interventions at the community level is vital. Community programs that engage parents and other family/community members should draw support from (a) multiple sources (adults and peers), (b)contexts (home and school) and (c) outreach and education (workshops, health fairs) to initiate dialogue and deepen community awareness on SAA parenting (Tummala-Narra et al., 2016). Deepak (2005) underscores the importance of finding ways to draw families into services, where community programs are created to provide concrete services (such as tutoring or activities for children) and simultaneous space for parents to discuss parenting practices or concerns. Support groups or group therapy can be perceived as useful to SAAs if the group has a specific focus on SAA parenting issues and facilitators take a more directive and facilitative role (Tewari et al., 2003). For example, a support group that explores bicultural identity, can specifically seek to help SAA families balance dual socialization struggles, address stereotypes about the model minority myth and promote successful life skills. Support groups for SAA parents that explore consequences of migration, loss of support networks and foster formation of new support networks to help strengthen parental functioning could be a much-needed community resource (Deepak, 2005; Maiter & George, 2003).

Example of a Community Outreach: The CHAI Parenting Initiative

An organization serving the South Asian community in Maryland, Counselors Helping (South) Asian, Inc. (CHAI) was awarded a grant from the Asian American Psychological Association (AAPA) and American Psychological Foundation (APF) to assess SAA parental needs to effectively plan SAA parenting resources. First, a needs assessment to understand the detailed needs of SAA parents and to inform the topics for the resource booklet created by the initiative. In general, a parenting needs assessment can help a community organization or school develop more targeted informational programming, support groups or educational resources. The needs assessment was conducted with SAA parents (n = 102) consisting of general demographic questions and an exhaustive list of parenting topics. The topic areas that generated the most interest by South Asian parents were related to healthy well-being for children, a positive parent-child relationship, and ways to maintain culture within children's identities and parenting. Focus groups may enrich and expand themes emerging from a needs assessment. Five focus groups across the US were conducted. Borrowing from the community participatory framework, the CHAI Parenting Initiative partnered with local SAA agencies to create a forum to elevate voices from the community. This partnership provided access to residents and community leaders and demonstrated the initiative's legitimacy to South Asian community members. A manual of focus group guidelines were developed specific to the parenting initiative based on a format put forth by Simon (1999) and Eliot and Associates (2007). Patterns emerged on issues important to SAA parents. Themes were categorized into the aspirations and goals of parents in order to represent the perspectives of parents. A summary of the focus group themes is listed in Table 10.1. The results of these endeavors then led to the creation of a SAA parenting resource booklet. This CHAI Parenting Initiative process of conducting a needs assessment and focus groups can be used as a template to replicate with SAA community members in a group setting.

Table 10.1 Qualitative Summary of Focus Group Themes

Parental Goals and Aspirations	Specific Themes
Who we (parents) want to be	Flexible in parenting
	Accept children's choices
	Open, build trust and understanding
	Understand children's different developmental stages
	A guide to our children rather than push ourselves on them
	A good listener in order to form the parent-child relationship
What we want for our children	Self-sufficient
	Academically strong
	Happy and well-adjusted
	Able to stand on one's own legs in the community
	Confidence, comfortable, and able to accept themselves
What we value as parents	Being a good citizen
	Respect all religions
	Well-behaved children
	Have pride & joy in culture
	Education and achievement
	Respect for elders and others
	Make religion a part of children's lives
	Connections across multiple generations
What is important in our culture	Practicing faith
	Model for children
	It is a central part of life
	Having bilingual children
	Don't forget own culture or identity
	Rituals and prayers integrated into way of life
	Navigating bicultural atmosphere successfully
	Know and respect traditions, customs and festivals
	Important to expose children to various aspects of culture (language, food etc.)
What we still struggle with	Being a good role-model
	Our own baggage and the pressures we bring
	Being patient with children and with ourselves
	Keeping children engaged in cultural traditions
	Placing too much emphasis on academic success
	Confidence to discuss difficulties in parenting with others

Critical Topics for Consideration When Working with SAA Parents

Academic Expectations

Studies have demonstrated that many SAA parents desire high education and achievement for their children. Many SAA children receive consistent parental messages that academics should have more priority over social or extracurricular activities causing significant stress on their mental health and parent-child conflict (Farver et al., 2007; Tewari et al., 2003). From the SAA parental perspective, this emphasis on academics aligns with the overall goal for migration to the US: improving their economic and social well-being and the future of their children (Walsh, 2007). There are several motivators and mechanisms by which SAA parents move toward this goal. Some South Asian parents are motivated by the principle that even if all material possessions are lost, one will always have their education (Walsh, 2007). Historically, this is particularly important as migration can lead to loss of one's belongings, finances and home. The idea that education can be a constant is salient and comforting. Another motivator relates to securing children's future social and economic standing in society. Asian-Americans (including SAAs), when facing possibilities of discrimination and lacking necessary political resources and social capital, look for strategic paths to success with the least barriers (Xie & Goyette, 2003). Therefore, education can be a feasible pathway promoted by SAA parents. Additionally, South Asian parents are driven by a sense of competition with the goal of children standing out among their peers (Dhingra, 2018). Consequently, SAA parents find that education is the best venue for their children to successfully engage in this competition.

These findings are important for a few reasons. Typically, the SAA emphasis on academics is explained as a cultural trait. However, research findings move beyond the one-dimensional stereotype of SAAs by providing a more intricate understanding of the belief systems and mechanisms that underlie this focus on academics. It is important for therapists to have a more comprehensive understanding on how cultural characteristics, family values, behavioral trends, and parental beliefs contribute to students' academic performance. Therapists and educators should anchor discussions around SAA parents' core goals related to academic expectations and better understand mechanisms guiding the parental behaviors. This discussion can lead to opportunities for SAA parents to reframe the mechanism by which children and families define and achieve goals related to future success. For example, Joshi (2005) suggests SAA parents may appreciate and benefit from information on different activities that promote children's overall development and success in life, not just academic skills.

Given SAA parents' intense emphasis on academics, schools sometimes have concerns on how to best approach and engage these parents. Many SAA parents report being highly involved in educational activities at home, but not very active in volunteering in classrooms, sports, or other events at school (Rasool & Zhang, 2020). South Asian immigrants are experiencing the US school system for the first time and are often unfamiliar with the expectations and differences in this school system versus the country of origin. Even South Asian parents who attended US schools often struggle with negotiating the demands of parenting, cultural expectations and deciding what is best for each of their children in the academic, social, and emotional realms. South Asian youth have also shared that their parents need more guidance on how to understand and navigate the US educational system (Sikh Coalition, 2016). South Asian Youth Action (2013), a social service organization based in Queens, NY, stresses the importance of parental engagement and recommends the following ways to address this issue: (a) develop a parent advocacy program to provide regular, meaningful interaction with schools and help parents successfully guide children through the system, (b) comprehensive use of interpreters for parents and development of translated resource materials, (c) South Asian community organizations can serve as a bridge between parents and schools to create workshops to engage and inform parents on the US system.

In summary, academics play an important role in the functioning of SAA families and individuals working with these families should have a clear understanding of parental beliefs, goal-directed behaviors and other factors that influence parental involvement in their children's academic achievement. In the case of the Shah family, Taj's parents may have been motivated to seek out therapy due to concerns for his academic performance. These expectations for academics were also linked to treatment goals and positive outcomes at the end of therapy. How does the motivation for Taj's grades to improve compare to their motivation for him to express himself emotionally and develop coping skills in navigating his identity? And how does the level of motivation impact progress along treatment goals? It is important for clinicians to unpack the meaning and content of parents' motivations as well as the way in which they prioritize goals in therapy.

Bullying and Discrimination

Recent economic and political shifts such as outsourcing, immigration policy, anti-immigrant sentiment, and suspicion related to 9/11 have contributed to significant numbers of racism and bias against South Asians (Tummala-Narra et al., 2016). SAA adolescents report experiences of being stereotyped by peers and adults, witnessing or hearing about family members being targets of discrimination and being victims of racism and racial violence (Tamala-Narra et al., 2016; Wang et al., 2016). SAA elementary school students have attributed the reasons for their victimization to cultural and language differences, the model minority myth and physical appearance (Wang et al., 2016). In particular, SAA Sikh and Muslim students have faced significant mistreatment (SAALT, 2011) because of their faith or religious attire. The Sikh Coalition (2016) revealed that 60% of Sikh turban wearing school students have been harassed and verbally or physically abused because of their faith or appearance and 40% of these youth were too scared to report these incidents to school officials. These patterns of constant stereotyping, bullying and harassment may convince SAA youth that they are inevitably different from mainstream Americans and negatively impact their mental health. A meta-analysis of 23 studies on Asians (including South Asians living in the US and other Westernized cultures) found that racial discrimination is significantly related to greater overall distress with stronger correlations to depression and anxiety (Lee & Ahn, 2011). Perceived discrimination has been shown to be positively associated with depression (Tummala-Narra et al., 2012) and perceived stress for SAAs (Kaduvettoor-Davidson & Inman, 2013).

When racism and discrimination is brought into the therapeutic setting, practitioners have to consider the perspective of the parents, child, and their own reactions. From the parental perspective, it is important to understand the processes by which SAA parents transmit information and perspectives relating to race and ethnicity to their children (Iqbal, 2014) and what discussions have occurred where parents make children aware of harassment, bias, and racism and how to deal with it. The review of literature suggests that South Asian parents manage these conversations in a variety of ways. Although aware of anti-Asian sentiment, a sample of Indian-American parents did not express worry for racism (Dhingra, 2018). These parents felt that Indian immigrants have been a successful and achievement-oriented group and therefore minimally impacted by racism. In addition, the cultural emphasis on academics and higher education has been shown to be part of a "strategic adaptation" used by Asian-American parents and youth to overcome their status as racial minorities and immigrants and prevent blocked mobility (Dhingra, 2018; Xie & Goyette, 2003). Some South Asian parents express fear of their children being harassed or targets of discrimination. As a result, some have suggested ways to minimize the differences (i.e., wearing a headscarf) in their appearance (Walsh, 2007). Other parents have responded to these concerns by ensuring their children understood why they wore a headscarf and instill a sense of strength and cultural pride within them to prepare for future incidents (Iqbal, 2014).

In studying British Indian and Pakistani mothers of 5- to 7-year-olds, Iqbal (2014) found that British Indian parents used less strategies to prepare their children for bias and demonstrated less reactive parenting on this topic. These mothers shared that after their children were exposed to media images related to racism, they encouraged them to ignore what they had viewed. Some mothers explained to their children that only a minority of people were racist, and that they should just ignore them. Other mothers reported feeling their child was too young to understand race and discrimination, even if the child had witnessed or been a victim of a racial incident. In contrast, British Pakistani mothers reported using more preparation strategies and parenting in a proactive manner. These mothers anticipated their children would encounter discrimination, were forthcoming in discussions on racism and used developmentally appropriate explanations of racism and discrimination. This study highlights the differences in parenting approaches within South Asian populations and the importance of considering parenting needs and vulnerabilities of specific South Asian subgroups.

As many incidents of harassment and bullying can occur at school, it is important to consider the parent and school partnerships in addressing this topic. Tummala-Narra et al. (2018), suggest considerations for school practitioners: (1) discrimination trainings for teachers, guidance counselors, and other school personnel, (2) develop an understanding that discrimination can be critical in identifying emotional distress in SA youth, and (3) creating safe spaces for dialogues focused on race, ethnicity, stereotyping, and discrimination with students and school personnel. These suggestions could complement outreach efforts to parents. The Sikh Coalition (2016) recommends that parents be informed about the process for filing bullying complaints, be given education on what bullying looks like and identify signs that their children are being bullied. Asian American parents' (including SAAs), because they view teachers as the authority, may prefer to elicit teachers' support to resolve bullying problems (Wang et al., 2016). This could result in SAA parents being less actively involved in problem-solving, which may be misinterpreted as not involved. In summary, therapists have to have therapists to have conversations with SAA parents about the extent to which they discuss bullying, harassment and racism with their children, the coping messages transmitted to children and how parental decision-making is impacted by these experiences. The school is an important arena for addressing parenting issues as they relate to this topic and SAA parents should be made aware of ways they can advocate for their child in the school setting. Lastly, the therapist themselves must be actively engaging in their own reflections and understanding about race and racism both in the states and from home countries. The prejudices and biases are woven into the societal fabric across the globe and engaging in ones' own work to surface bias, and gain further understanding about SA group and the discrimination they face both wtihin and outside of SA groups with further enhance their ability to form therapeutic alliance and trust with families.

NAVIGATING A CHILD'S INTELLECTUAL AND DEVELOPMENTAL DISABILITIES (IDD)

Parenting children with IDDs can be a stressful experience filled with a variety of emotions. To add another layer of understanding, cultural values play a significant role in how families perceive IDDs, which influences parental stress, coping strategies and from whom parents seek support. Although there is a small amount of research on how SAA parents navigate this experience, the findings converge to common themes and are summarized below. The literature presented addresses SAA parenting (one study is from Canada) in the context of IDDs which include developmental delays, Autism and Down Syndrome.

SAA parents describe the development of different coping skills in this process. They identified ways in which they engaged in ongoing adjustments in their approach to parenting a child with an IDD. These changes included adjusting academic expectations and aspirations for the child, taking a practical "1 day at a time" approach, and becoming more flexible in efforts to pass on cultural heritage (Zechella & Raval, 2016). From a religious and spiritual perspective, many viewed the IDD as a blessing from God and an opportunity to learn lessons for life with their faith as their continued source of support (Jegatheesan et al., 2010; Raghavan et al., 1999). Parents also reported a strengthening of spousal relationships because of co-parenting a child with IDDs (Raghavan et al, 1999; Zechella & Raval, 2016). Although gender role dynamics exist for many SAA families, the roles became more clearly delineated with women doing most caretaking and more easily accepting their multiple roles (i.e., parent and advocate) (Raghavan et al, 1999; Zechella & Raval, 2016). These findings highlight the strength-based perspective of the SAA parenting experience.

Across all the studies, the role of extended family and community significantly contributed to the SAA experience of having a child with an IDD. As previously mentioned, migration to another country brings about loss of extended family support, which was sorely missed in this particular context. Lack of social support, extended family arrangements and culture-sensitive childcare pose problems to family adaptation for South Asian families (Raghavan et al., 1999; Zechella & Raval, 2016). For example, it was found that the level of perceived burden of care was related to the amount of family support (Daudji et al., 2011). Some families are given information on support groups as a resource; however, they report that the culture of support groups was also alien to them (Jegatheesan et al., 2010). For example, mothers in this group feel uncomfortable voicing their concerns and feelings in front of strangers, particularly men. There were also feelings of embarrassment speaking up in what were considered to be more mainstream groups.

Families and communities could be a source of support, but could also exacerbate parents' stress. Some SAA parents did not view extended families as a resource for coping. For example, SAA families reported that they did not talk openly about their emotions and concerns because such talk could negatively impact their extended family, in particular, the elder members (Jegatheesan, et al., 2010). Traditional cultural and religious beliefs were also woven into familial and community responses and support. For example, a parent spoke about how she received messages from her family, guided in traditional beliefs, that mothers were responsible for causing children's disabilities (Daudji et al., 2011). Parents described their local community's struggles with the acceptance of the IDD being grounded in cultural and religious explanations (Daudji et al., 2011; Jegatheesan et al., 2010; Zechella & Raval, 2016). They indicated that community members' beliefs about their child's disability led to negative interactions with them and contributed to their own difficulty in diagnosis and acceptance.

Some families felt that healthcare professionals misunderstood SAA family organization and linguistic practices leading to difficulties in communication and collaboration (Jegatheesan et al., 2010). These parents report being told to speak in English only with their child and limit interactions with many relatives to simplify the child's life. Some SAA parents preferred providers who were South Asian because of the time spent conversing about families' background, immigration story and acculturation experience. They felt that these conversations provided the clinician with a comprehensive overview of the family. In comparison, SAA parents perceived European-American clinicians to be more straightforward, time conscious, and showing minimal interest in their general background.

Jegatheesan et al. (2010) highlight examples of cross-cultural communication difficulties which resulted in families ending services for their child when they disagreed with the therapists' intervention approach. South Asian mothers reported not understanding the child-centered, play-based philosophy embedded in the autism language intervention models. They characterized these interventions as too 'playful' and not directive enough. They describe that therapists did not provide more information about the intervention or respond to requests for more adult-directed teaching. Parents felt they had little or no input into the therapy goals or philosophy. As a result, parents disagreed with professionals, continued to raise children according to their beliefs and discontinued services. Children ultimately lost out on months of services during the critical early years. Some parents did report having more positive interactions with new therapists at a later time. This was attributed to a feeling that these therapists made attempts to compromise and incorporate both philosophies into the child's treatment. The issues described here speak to the importance of therapeutic alliance in establishing collaborative communication between providers and SAA parents.

To summarize, current knowledge of how SAA parents experience and perceive their child's IDDs can enable clinicians to be more cognizant of their approach in building an alliance with the family, learning family strengths, responding to SAA parents coping styles and attributions, and effectively communicating therapy goals. This can be achieved by formulating achievable expectations, minimizing parental fears, and facilitating healthy coping strategies for parents and children. Jegatheesan et al. (2010) suggests the following recommendations for health professionals who work with South Asian parents: (a) ensure immigrant community centers have resources about IDDs including information on healthy versus atypical child development and a referral process, (b) acknowledge the importance of the extended family by suggesting seminars for the entire family on basic information on IDDs to help families gain a positive interpretation of the child and their experiences, (c) acknowledge and accept the use of multiple languages within the family, (d) consider collaboration on choices of goals and teaching philosophy to sustain services. Further research is warranted to determine the best way goals may be identified and negotiated with SAA parents of children with IDDs.

Topics Requiring Further Study

Research on SAAs is in the nascent stages in the US and an exploration into parenting offers multiple topics for further study. The needs of new parents, without the support of extended family commonly provided among SA families, is worthy of further investigation. Given the crucial importance of the early years influencing a child's developmental trajectory, more research on early childhood and SAA parenting is needed. Many existing studies are from the perspective of the mother. Therefore, learning more about the specific experiences of SAA fathers can allow for a more comprehensive understanding of parents. The topic of divorce, co-parenting, and single parenting all have cultural and religious stigma within the SA community. Additionally, family and parenting are held as core values among most SA cultures and similarly SAA couples are expected to become parents. Thus, issues of infertility, miscarriage, surrogacy, and adoption are critical topics to research. Lastly, muti-racial, multi-ethnic, and multi-religious families with SAA in another area of research currently lacking.

Reflection Questions

As clinicians, we ask you to reflect on the following questions to help understand the context and case.

1   What issues can you identify that are related to SAA parenting?
2   What assumptions surfaced for you while reading the case study?
3   What strategies can clinicians use when providing support and interventions to SAA families?

Summary

A seemingly straightforward interaction between a parent and child signifies the complex interaction of numerous multigenerational factors from various ecological systems coming together. These systems include the developing child, family, schools, and communities. The goal of this chapter was to synthesize the scarce research on SAA parenting by identifying parenting goals, present a case study which explores themes in SAA parenting and family therapy, offer an example of community outreach, and emphasize the need for future research in SAA parenting.

Through exploration of various facets of SAA parenting it is clear that individuals working with families develop an understanding of cultural contexts and underlying processes that shape SAA parent goals, behaviors, and expectations of childhood. The literature presented in this chapter highlights several important points: (a) the pathways to understanding the functioning of SAA parents are complex, (b) these pathways can lead to varied outcomes and (c) there is not one "right" way to parent in the context of two cultures. Clinicians should engage in ongoing awareness of their assumptions on optimal parenting styles. Although immigrant parents might modify their parenting styles, clinicians need to respect alternative parenting styles that might have been found to be successful through years of cultural practice (Inman et al., 2007). It is also recommended that policymakers and school districts consider funding and initiatives for partnerships between parents and schools to develop more culturally informed outreach and interventions and training for educators and practitioners.

Suggested Resources

- CHAI Parenting Initiative Tree of Life Book https://probonocounseling.org/seeking-care/special-programs/

  - *A parenting resource booklet for South Asian parents created by the CHAI Parenting Initiative*

- South Asian Autism Awareness Centre (SAAAC) https://saaac.org/

  - *Provides resources and support to South Asian families (in Canada) impacted by Autism and related developmental disorders.*

- South Asian Parent https://www.southasianparent.com/

  - *An online magazine dedicated to South Asian parenting*

- Beyond the Tiger Mom: East-West parenting for the global age http://www.mayathiagarajan.info/book_beyond_the_Tiger_Mom.html
- Children's Partnership: Surrey-White Rock http://www.childrenspartnershipsurreywr.com/south-asian-ecd-task-force/resources/

  - *Resources to raise awareness about the importance of early childhood and middle childhood development within the South Asian parenting community in British Columbia, Canada.*

- *Stop Bullying: A parent's guide to keeping kids safe and happy*

  - https://www.sikhcoalition.org/wp-content/uploads/2016/12/Parent-Bullying-KYR-Postcard.pdfSikh Coalition (2016).

References

American Psychological Association, Presidential Task Force on Immigration. (2012). Crossroads: The psychology of immigration in the new century. Retrieved from http://www.apa.org/topics/immigration/report.aspx.

Bemak, F., Chung, R.C., & Bornemann, T.H. (1996). Counselling and psychotherapy with refugees. In P. B. Pedersen, J. G. Draguns, & W. J. Trimble (Eds.), *Counselling across cultures* (4th ed., pp. 243–265). Thousand Oaks, CA: Sage.

Chao, R.K. (1994). Beyond parental control and authoritarian parenting style: Understanding Chinese parenting through the cultural notion of training. *Child Development, 65*(4), 1111–1119.

Chao, R.K. (2000). The parenting of immigrant Chinese and European American mothers: Relations between parenting styles, socialization goals, and parental practices. *Journal of Applied Developmental Psychology, 21*(2), 233–248.

Dallaire, D.H., & Weinraub, M. (2005). The stability of parenting behaviors over the first six years of life. *Early Childhood Research Quarterly, 20*: 201–219.

Daudji, A., Eby, S., Foo, T., Ladak, F., Sinclair, C., Landry, M.D., ... & Gibson, B.E. (2011). Perceptions of disability among south Asian immigrant mothers of children with disabilities in Canada: Implications for rehabilitation service delivery. *Disability and Rehabilitation, 33*(6), 511–521.

Deater-Deckard, K., Ivy, L., & Smith, J. (2005). Resilience in gene-environment transactions. In Goldstein, S. & Brooks, R. (Eds.), *Handbook of resilience in children* (pp. 49–63). New York: Springer US.

Deepak, A.C. (2005). Parenting and the process of migration: Possibilities within South Asian families. *Child Welfare, 84*(5), 585–606.

Dhingra, P. (2018). What Asian Americans really care about when they care about education. *The Sociological Quarterly, 59*(2), 301–319.

Eliot & Associates (2007). Guidelines for Conducting a Focus Group [online]. available from https://datainnovationproject.org/wp-content/uploads/2017/04/4_How_to_Conduct_a_Focus_Group-2-1.pdf

Farver, J.M., & Shinn, Y.L. (1997). Social pretend play in Korean- and Anglo American preschoolers. *Child Development, 68*(3): 544–556.

Farver, J.M., Xu, Y., Bhadha, B.R., Narang, S., & Lieber, E. (2007). Ethnic identity, acculturation, parenting beliefs, and adolescent adjustment: A comparison of Asian Indian and European American families. *Merrill-Palmer Quarterly (1982-), 53*(2), 184–215.

Garg, R., Levin, E., Urajnik, D., & Kauppi, C. (2005). Parenting style and academic achievement for East Indian and Canadian adolescents. *Journal of Comparative Family Studies, 36*(4), 653–661.

Gibbs, B.G., Shah, P.G., Downey, D.B., & Jarvis, J.A. (2017). The Asian American advantage in math among young children: The complex role of parenting. *Sociological Perspectives, 60*(2), 315–337.

Inman, A.G., Devdas, L., Spektor, V., & Pendse, A. (2014). Psychological research on South Asian Americans: A three-decade content analysis. *Asian American Journal of Psychology, 5*(4), 364.

Inman, A.G., Howard, E.E., Beaumont, R.L., & Walker, J.A. (2007). Cultural transmission: Influence of contextual factors in Asian Indian immigrant parents' experiences. *Journal of counseling psychology, 54*(1), 93.

Iqbal, H. (2014). Multicultural parenting: Preparation for bias socialisation in British South Asian and White families in the UK. *International Journal of Intercultural Relations, 43*, 215–226.

Iqbal, H., & Golombok, S. (2018). The generation game: Parenting and child outcomes in second-generation South Asian immigrant families in Britain. *Journal of Cross-Cultural Psychology, 49*(1), 25–43.

Jegatheesan, B., Fowler, S., & Miller, P.J. (2010). From symptom recognition to services: How South Asian Muslim immigrant families navigate autism. *Disability & Society, 25*(7), 797–811.

Jent, J.F., Niec, L.N., & Baker, S.E. (2011). Play and interpersonal processes. In S. W. Russ & L. N. Niec (Eds.), *Play in clinical practice: Evidence-based approaches* (pp. 23–47). New York: Guilford Press.

Johnston, J.R., & Wong, M.Y.A. (2002). Cultural differences in beliefs and practices concerning talk to children. *Journal of Speech, Language, and Hearing Research, 45*(5), 916–926.

Joshi, A. (2005). Understanding Asian Indian families: Facilitating meaningful home-school relations. *YC Young Children, 60*(3), 75.

Kaduvettoor-Davidson, A., & Inman, A.G. (2013). South Asian Americans: Perceived discrimination, stress, and well-being. *Asian American Journal of Psychology, 4*(3), 155.

Lee, D.L., & Ahn, S. (2011). Racial discrimination and Asian mental health: A meta-analysis. *The Counseling Psychologist, 39*(3), 463–489.

LeVine, R. (1980). A cross-cultural perspective on parenting. In M. D. Fantini & R. Cardenes (Eds.), *Parenting in a multicultural society* (pp. 17–26). New York: Longman.

Lueck, K., & Wilson, M. (2010). Acculturative stress in Asian immigrants: The impact of social and linguistic factors. *International Journal of Intercultural Relations, 34*(1), 47–57.

Maiter, S., & George, U. (2003). Understanding Context and Culture in the Parenting Approaches of Immigrant South Asian Mothers. *Affilia*, 18(4), 411–428.

Nath, S. (2005). Pakistani families. In M. McGoldrick, J. Giordano, & N. Garcia-Preto (Eds.), (3rd Ed.), *Ethnicity and family therapy* (pp. 407–420). New York: Guilford Press.

Navsaria, N. (2011). Culture and parenting: Survey on Asian-Indian parents of young children. Unpublished raw data.

Navsaria, N., & Hong, J. (2016). Prevention in early childhood: Models of parenting interventions among immigrants. In M. Israelashvili, & J. L. Romano (Eds.), *The Cambridge handbook of international prevention science*. Cambridge, UK: Cambridge University Press.

Paiva, N.D. (2008). South Asian parents' constructions of praising their children. *Clinical Child Psychology and Psychiatry*, 13(2), 191–207.

Pandya, K., & Herlihy, J. (2009). An exploratory study into how a sample of a British South Asian population perceive the therapeutic alliances in family therapy. *Journal of Family Therapy*, 31(4), 384–404.

Parmar, P., Harkness, S., & Super, C.M. (2004). Asian and Euro-American parents' ethnotheories of play and learning: Effects on preschool children's home routines and school behaviour. *International Journal of Behavioral Development*, 28(2), 97–104.

Pillari, V. (2005). Indian Hindu families. In M. McGoldrick, J. Giordano , & N. Garcia-Preto (Eds.). *Ethnicity and Family Therapy*, Vol. 3, (pp. 395–406). New York: Guilford Press.

Raghavan, C., Weisner, T.S., & Patel, D. (1999). The adaptive project of parenting: South Asian families with children with developmental delays. *Education and Training in Mental Retardation and Developmental Disabilities*, 34(3), 281–292.

Rasool, S., & Zhang, J. (2020). Bangladeshi, Indian, and Pakistani Parents' Perceptions of Their Children's Academic Achievement in Southwest Florida. *American Journal of Qualitative Research*, 4(3), 146–160.

Shariff, A. (2009). Ethnic identity and parenting stress in South Asian families: Implications for culturally sensitive counselling. *Canadian Journal of Counselling and Psychotherapy*, 43(1), 35–46.

Sikh Coalition (2016). *How bullying affects Sikh students*. https://www.sikhcoalition.org/wp-content/uploads/2016/11/Anti-Bullying-Handout.pdf

Simon, J.S. (1999). How to conduct focus groups. *Nonprofit World*, 17, 40–43.

Sorkhabi, N., & Mandara, J. (2013). Are the effects of Baumrind's parenting styles culturally specific or culturally equivalent? In R. E. Larzelere, A. S. Morris, & A. W. Harrist (Eds.), *Authoritative parenting: Synthesizing nurturance and discipline for optimal child development* (p. 113–135). Washington DC: American Psychological Association.

South Asian American Leaders of Tomorrow (2011). *Community resilience: A South Asian American perspective on the ten-year anniversary of September 11th*. https://saalt.org/wp-content/uploads/2012/09/Community-Resilience-September-2011.pdf

South Asian Youth Action (2013). *New York City South Asian Youth: critical mass, urgent needs*. https://www.saya.org/s/Policy-Report_compressed1.pdf

Spiegel, J.P. (1981). 6. An ecological model with an emphasis on ethnic families. In Tolson E. R., & Reid W. J. (Eds.). *Models of family treatment* (pp. 121–158). New York: Columbia University Press.

Tewari, N., Inman, A.G., & Sandhu, D.S. (2003). South Asian Americans culture, concerns, and therapeutic strategies. In J. S. Mio, & G. Iwamasa (Eds.). *Culturally diverse mental health: The challenges of research and resistance*, (p. 191). New York: Taylor & Francis.

Triandis, H.C. (1994). Major cultural syndromes and emotion. In S. Kitayama, & H. R. Markus (Eds.), *Emotion and culture: Empirical studies of mutual influence* (pp. 285–308). Washington DC: American Psychological Association.

Tummala-Narra, P., Alegria, M., & Chen, C.N. (2012). Perceived discrimination, acculturative stress, and depression among South Asians: Mixed findings. *Asian American Journal of Psychology*, 3(1), 3.

Tummala-Narra, P., Deshpande, A., & Kaur, J. (2016). South Asian adolescents' experiences of acculturative stress and coping. *American Journal of Orthopsychiatry, 86*(2), 194.

Van Campen, K.S., & Russell, S.T. (2010). Cultural differences in parenting practices: What Asian American families can teach us. *Frances McClelland Institute for Children, Youth, and Families ResearchLink, 2*(1), 1–4.

Walsh, T.R. (2007). Cultural and religious contexts of parenting by immigrant South Asian Muslim mothers. In J. E. Lansford, K. D. Deater-Deckard , & M. H. Bornstein (Eds.), *Immigrant families in contemporary society*, (pp. 194–207). New York: Guilford Press.

Wang, W., Zheng, L., & Atwal, K. (2016). Justice issue: Implications with Asian American elementary school students. *School Psychology Forum, 10*(1).

Xie, Y., & Goyette, K. (2003). Social mobility and the educational choices of Asian Americans. *Social Science Research, 32*(3), 467–498.

Zechella, A.N., & Raval, V.V. (2016). Parenting children with intellectual and developmental disabilities in Asian Indian families in the United States. *Journal of Child and Family Studies, 25*(4), 1295–1309.

11 Counseling South Asian American Youth

Nina Kaur and Preet Kaur Sabharwal

Case Overview

Jaspreet Kaur is a 13-year-old Punjabi Sikh female who was born and raised in California. Jaspreet's father, Balwant Singh (aged 45), owns a trucking company and her mother, Ramanjit Kaur (aged 45) is a homemaker and seamstress. Jaspreet's parents are first generation immigrants from Punjab, India. Jaspreet has an older brother, Gurtej, aged 22, who is a software engineer, and a younger sister Manpreet, aged 10, is in the fourth grade at a public elementary school. Jaspreet also lives with her paternal grandparents, Balbir Kaur (age 70) and Parminder Singh (age 75). The family lives in a single family home that they rent in a middle -class neighborhood. Jaspreet presents with the following symptoms: depressed mood, not wanting to engage in activities she once enjoyed, having panic attacks, no appetite , fatigue, sleeping problems, and struggling to concentrate at school.

Introduction

Of the many ethnic racial minorities living in the United States, the South Asian American community is a growing minority group (South Asian Americans Leading Together [SAALT], 2019). According to 2010 U.S. Census data and the 2017 American Community Survey, there are roughly 5.4 million South Asians in the United States (SAALT, 2019). When looking at U.S. census data from 2010 and 2017, the South Asian American (SAA) community grew approximately 40% (SAALT, 2019). Given the increase in the SAA population, it is vital for clinicians to understand the clinical needs of SAA children and youth. For this chapter, South Asian American youth refers to individuals between the ages of 8–17. This chapter will focus on the psychological needs of South Asian American youth in the United States, address critical cultural factors that affect the mental health of South Asian American children and youth and its treatment implications. The chapter will provide a summary of relevant research findings and theories regarding South Asian American youth will be covered. A case study will be provided to illustrate the complexity of intergenerational conflicts between family members and the importance of providing culturally sensitive mental health services.

The South Asian American Community

The South Asian American community in the United States (U.S.) encompasses many diverse individuals from the following countries: India, Pakistan, Bangladesh, Sri Lanka, Nepal, Bhutan, and the Maldives (Kuortti, 2007). This population includes

DOI: 10.4324/9781003081548-11

different subgroups that follow various religions, speak different languages and adhere to particular cultural traditions. Along with differences, they also share some similarities. Of the many ethnic racial minorities living in the United States, the South Asian community is a growing minority group (South Asian Americans Leading Together [SAALT], 2019). According to 2010 U.S. Census data and the 2017 American Community Survey, there are roughly 5.4 million South Asians in the United States (SAALT, 2019). When looking at census data from 2010 and 2017, the South Asian community grew approximately 40% (SAALT, 2019). In regard to income, approximately 472,000 South Asians in the U.S. live in poverty and 630,000 undocumented Indian in the United States which indicate a 72% increase since 2010 (SAALT, 2019). Furthermore, the Immigration and Customs Enforcement (ICE) has detained 3,013 South Asians (dated 2017) and SAALT classified 213 incidents of hate violence towards the South Asian community. The South Asian community is seen as a model minority in the United States (Dasgupta, 2000). Model minority refers to minorities who are achieving high levels of success in the US (Cheryan & Bodenhausen, 2011). A model minority group is considered an example for other minorities regarding how they should behave in the US. Unlike the model minority image that is imposed on the South Asian community, the data from the 2010 U.S. Census data and the 2017 American Community Survey indicates the community is struggling. Given these difficulties, it is important to consider the unique challenges and needs of South Asian American children and adolescents which will be discussed later in this chapter. Each culture has its own set of beliefs, traditions, rituals and values. It is important to examine South Asian American culture in order to understand the South Asian American children's needs and experience. South Asian culture is a collectivistic culture which puts importance on the needs of others instead of focusing on the needs of the individual (Ibrahim et al., 1997). South Asian families commonly live in joint families in which two or more generations live together in one household (Abraham, 2000). The household may include parents, grandparents, parent's sons and their wives, and unmarried daughters. Furthermore, many South Asian Americans families follow a patriarchal family structure (Ahmad et al., 2004; Ayyub, 2000). Some families will continue to follow the traditional gender roles where the mother will be primarily responsible for taking care of the home and children while the father works and makes decisions in the household. While more acculturated families may have more fluid gender roles where both parents work outside of the home, grandparents become the primary care-takers. Child rearing is often a shared task amongst the various family members in the home, hence the theory that South Asian American youth are "raised by a village" (Farver et al., 2007). Early attachment patterns and styles are difficult to assess when there are multiple family members caring for the young in the home. Although there are strong emotional bonds created, children are taught to suppress their emotions and feelings (Louie, 2014). Keep in Mind: There is significant diversity in the various subgroups of South Asians and South Asian Families in terms of language, religion and traditions.

Research on South Asian American Youth

South Asian American (SAA) children and adolescents are a high risk for suicidal ideation and behavior when they are navigating family expectation, acculturative stress, discrimination stress and stigma of mental health services (Sharma & Shaligram, 2018). Acculturative stress, trauma and discrimination are found to be connected to depression, anxiety and substance abuse among SAA in the US. Furthermore, South Asian American youth's experience of dating is different than other youth in the U.S. Ragavan et al. (2021) interviewed South Asian youth to explore the connection between culture and teen dating violence. The study found that dating was stigmatized in the community which led many youth to hide their relationship from parents. Academically, South Asian children and adolescents are pressured to do well (Lee et al., 2009). While at school, South Asian youth experience racial name-calling more frequently compared to other ethnicities (Fisher et al., 2000). Atwal and Wang (2019) found 76.4% Sikh American students experienced bullying and wearing the Sikh turban was related to their perception of being stereotyped as foreigners. Furthermore, this experience led to higher victimization which was related to higher depressive and anxiety symptoms.

Although the research literature has primarily looked at South Asian women's experience of domestic violence, recent studies are now examining the experience of South Asian American children and youth in these households. Ragavan et al. (2018) interviewed staff members from South Asian Domestic Violence (DV) agencies in the United States to examine the needs of South Asian children exposed to DV. Results indicated the following components need to be taken into consideration when understanding the impact of domestic violence on South Asian children: fear about the community's thoughts, role of extended family members, difference between genders and instilling a perfect image. Mullender et al. (2002) conducted qualitative research with 14 children between the ages of 8 to 16 years of age which shows the importance of looking at culture when looking at South Asian children's experience of domestic violence. Mullender et al. (2002) examined the children's coping strategies and had them reflect on what was helpful living in their household and identified the children's extended family members to be helpful, but also the children felt they would dishonor their family if they spoke to others regarding the domestic violence in their house. It is important to keep in mind research is limited when it comes to South Asian American youth and mental health.

South Asian American Youth Identity Development

The identity of South Asian Americans is complex and impacted by many factors such as educational level, immigration status, gender identity, sexual identity, socioeconomic status, generational level, and family culture. The ecological system theory developed by Bronfenbrenner is a model which can be used to understand South Asian American youth identity development. According to Bronfenbrenner (1979), there is importance placed on viewing the interaction of various societal systems in the environment along with one's experience in their immediate family. For example the school the youth attends, cultural beliefs of the family, and historical events such as changes in immigration law that can impact the youth and their family. The Bronfenbrenner model is a lens that clinicians can use when serving South Asian American children and youth. South Asian American children and youth are impacted by the different layers of the structures throughout their development. Most importantly, by examining the interaction between the systems, a comprehensive understanding of the South Asian's American children and adolescent's experience is obtained.

Furthermore, Berry developed an acculturation model which identified four stages: assimilation, separation, integration and marginalization (Berry, 1997). Berry looked at acculturation in two dimensions: maintaining one's cultural identity and adopting identity of the dominant society. Assimilation refers to when an individual does not maintain original culture and adopts the culture of the dominant society. Separation refers to when an individual preserves one's original culture and rejects the dominant culture. Integration refers to when an individual maintains the dominant culture and original culture. Marginalization refers to when someone rejects the dominant and original culture. This model should be taken into consideration when understanding the acculturation process of South Asian American children and youth. Asian American adolescents are exposed to two different cultures and often struggle with balancing between an individualistic culture and collectivistic culture (Lee et al., 2009). The acculturation process varies for each individual and it will be discussed more in depth later in the chapter.

In South Asian American (SAA) culture, there are different expectations and roles placed on male and female identified children and youth. Sons are treated as an asset to the family due to the fact that they would be caretakers for the parents after marriage (Almeida, 2005). Furthermore, sons are considered the children who take the family's last name which allows the continuation of the family lineage. On the other hand, daughters are the holders of the family's izzat (honor) (Ayyub, 2000). There is worry that a daughter will bring shame to her family. To preserve the family reputation, many SAA families will implement stricter rules to daughters compared to sons (Netting, 2006). As SAA youth are navigating the familial gender expectations, these youth are discovering and exploring their gender identity (i.e., cisgender, transgender, gender neutral, non-binary, etc.) during this developmental stage. Depending on the biological sex, certain expectations are placed on SAA children and youth. Overall, South Asian American females have more stricter expectations and restrictions compared to South Asian American males. As clinicians it is important to keep in mind there is variability in the South Asian identity process, acculturation process, and how the South Asian culture is experienced by South Asian American children and youth.

Influences on South Asian American Youth's Help Seeking Behavior

Mental Health Stigma

The South Asian American (SAA) community like many minority communities experience stigmas and barriers around mental health which influence their help-seeking behaviors. Stigma is discussed in more depth in previous chapters. For the purpose of our work with South Asian American youth and the decisions that youth make in accessing mental health care, it is particularly important to understand the two categories of stigma: self-stigma and public or social stigma. Public or Social Stigma is when the general population discriminates against someone who has a mental health issue, and Self-stigma is when someone who has a mental health issue then internalizes messages that are endorsed by the public (Corrigan et al., 2014).

As mentioned above, SAA youth have multiple intersecting identities and may belong to multiple community groups that each carry their own Public or Social stigmas around mental health care. SAA youth not only hear messaging from the dominant American culture but also from their SAA community. Messaging around mental health within SAA families is focused around the notion that "What happens in the family stays within the family" or " Mental health issues only happen to white Americans." Table 11.1 highlights some additional messages that SAA youth have grown up hearing and internalizing which can lead to an increase in self-stigma. Table 11.1 can be used by clinicians to help SAA youth in therapy to explore the myths.

Table 11.1 Mental Health Myths

Myths	Description	Reality
Therapy is Only for Those that Are "Crazy (Pagal)"	SAA youth often think that symptoms have to be severe in order to reach out for services. Mental health services are the last resort.	Preventative Mental Health Care is possible. Just as you go in for your yearly physical to prevent physical illness you can also improve coping and strengthen supports prior to experiencing life challenges
Mental Health is a Western Disease	SAA youth are often taught that there were no mental health challenges in their parent's home countries. That these challenges are only something that white Americans face.	Although mental health theories and terminology may be based on a western lens, impacts of mental health challenges have been experienced by all communities. There are certain protective factors embedded in South Asian culture that potentially allowed the community to build resilience and cope with challenges more positively.
Family Can Solve all Problems	Coming from a collectivistic worldview, SAA youth tend to have strong family ties and rely on those ties to help work through life challenges. Youth are often told to turn to the collective in times of stress.	Although family support is a huge protective factor against mental health disease, families are not equipped to respond to all mental health challenges. Often times mental health challenges may also be perpetuated by family ties, such as in situations of domestic violence, child abuse and elder abuse.
Mental Illness is Caused by Lack of Spiritual Religious Practice	SAA families are strongly rooted in their religious practices and often will increase rituals during times of stress. They may attribute the youth's physical and emotional pain to being disconnected from god.	Spiritual and religious practices can be a part of youth's coping. However, it may become difficult to tap into spirituality and religion in the same way when they are experiencing distress. It is helpful to diversify healing practices and combine holistic and western techniques.

Model Minority Myth and South Asian American Youth

Like their Asian counterparts, South Asian Americans are often portrayed as being smart, wealthy, hard-working, self-reliant, submissive, obedient and that they voluntarily immigrated to the U.S. and have fulfilled their "American Dream." The South Asian American (SAA) community is considered a model minority in the United States (Dasgupta, 2000). Historically, the immigration of SAA professionals in 1965 contributed to images of highly successful South Asians (Das, 2002). These portrayals of the SAA community continue to enforce notions that South Asians Americans are a monolithic community and are immune to racism, discrimination, difficulties in adjusting to immigration, unemployment, poverty, and mental health issues (Tavkar et al., 2008). South Asian immigrants try to preserve this "model minority" image of themselves at all costs to avoid shame from not only the dominant community but also within their own communities (Daga & Raval, 2018). SAA youth tend to internalize these messages that have been verbally or situationally enforced in their families of what success looks like and how youth should think, feel or behave (Shankar, 2008; Thakore-Dunlap & Velsor, 2014). This leaves little room for SAA youth to develop their own sense of self. South Asian American youth also get influenced by the model minority myth coupled with parental expectations which puts undue pressures on youth to: achieve high academic success, apply and gain admission to prestigious institutions of higher learning, and to adhere to culturally determined timelines (such as college, marriage, and then have children). South Asian American parents often expect their children to be grateful for the opportunities they have given them by choosing to immigrate to the United States (Chou & Leonard, 2006). Parents may use shame, guilt and fear as a way to gain compliance from youth and also as a form of motivation to keep youth focused on goals that promote harmony within the family (Tavkar et al., 2008; Thakore-Dunlap & Velsor, 2014). SAA parents may remind youth that their actions will influence their family's image in their community. South Asian American youth will often express that their parents are always worried about, "What will others say?".

DEFINITIONS OF SUCCESS

South Asian American families define success based on academic, financial and career achievement (Chou, 2006). In South Asian American families, there is a high level of importance placed on education and academic achievement. Level of importance depends on factors such as the family's socioeconomic status, acculturation level, immigration status, gender of the adolescents, and parent's level of education and type of work. Parents that are less acculturated and have a lower level of education are not used to being proactive about their youth's academic functioning and often follow their children's lead. On the other hand, parents that are more acculturated, are financially affluent, and have a higher level of education tend to view academic success as the only determinant of overall success in life and are more work oriented. There is also an expectation that youth will surpass their parent's level of education and career.

South Asian American families define success based on academic, financial and career achievement (Chou, 2006).

South Asian American Youth and School

South Asian American (SAA) youth spend an average of 6–8 hours a day at school inter-acting with teachers, school staff and their peers. Given these numbers we can hypothesize that mental health needs will be identified at school. However, the truth is that although this is true there is a high proportion of SAA children and adolescents whose mental health needs get overlooked in academic settings because they do not display the typical red flags. When youth do struggle the first thought parents and teachers have is that the SAA youth are not trying hard enough, aren't organized, or are being lazy (Lee et al., 2009). Academic counselors, teachers and other school staff are encouraged to look beyond grades and classroom behavior when assessing SAA youths' mental health needs. It is critical school employees pay special attention to other aspects of functioning that may be determinants of a mental health need like the youth complaining of physical symptoms (headaches, stomach aches and fatigue), cross cultural communication difficulties within their family system, and difficulties in making life choices that seem to come easily to other youth. When SAA families self-refer their youth for services, they often describe having communication challenges along with concerns over academic functioning. It is also quite common for South Asian American youth to experience their first interactions with the mental health system as a result of self-harm, suicidal attempt or other behavioral health crisis.

Struggles Faced by South Asian American Youth

Acculturative Stress/Intergenerational Conflicts/ Difficulties with family

Immigrant communities experience a high level of acculturative stress which South Asian American youth internalize. As mentioned earlier, South Asian American youth are taught from an early age to suppress emotions and feelings and to show respect to their elders by not talking back or challenging any cultural values or beliefs. South Asian American youth report struggling to express themselves fully and continue to shy away from having conversations around tabooed topics such as dating or sexuality (Zaidi et al., 2016). Intergenerational conflicts are also a common struggle within SAA families, between SAA youth and caregivers. In the case study, Jaspreet watched her older brother, Gurtej going to arcades, movie theaters and parties with his friends at her age. However, Jaspreet's parents informed her she was not allowed to spend time with peers after school. When Jaspreet would question her parents, they would tell her it's different for her but not give any explanation. Jaspreet found herself getting more estranged with her brother as he would also support their parent's decision to limit her contact with peers and often take on a "parent" role with her, rather than a sibling role. This highlights the gender and power hierarchies that are present in SAA families and how these hierarchies impact South Asian American youth.

As mentioned earlier, South Asian American youth who come from immigrant parents have increased responsibilities as they are cultural brokers and interpreters for their family. These additional roles impact the youth's development and experience in the US. In the case study, Jaspreet had to interpret for her mother. As a result, she missed after school activities in order to support mother during medical appointments or house errands (i.e., going to the bank). Although she wanted to assist her mother, Jaspreet also found herself feeling resentful and frustrated for not having the opportunity to spend time with her peers.

Microaggressions, Discrimination, and Racism

South Asian American (SAA) youth experience daily microaggressions and acts of racism even if they don't always recognize it is happening. Sometimes these types of discrimination are overt, especially if youth wear articles of faith, have a audible accent and are less acculturated. Other times this discrimination can be covert and SAA youth may not be able to articulate how they are personally impacted by systemic injustices, anti-Asian hate sentiments, post 9–11 discrimination, or gender or sexuality based discrimination. Having access to the safe spaces of therapy may allow them to find the words to describe their experiences more fully. South Asian American youth may also grow up watching their parents or other family members experience discrimination or racism and hold onto anger and frustration related to those experiences. In the case study for example, Jaspreet witnessed how hard her parents had worked in order to immigrate to the US and how her father continues to be discriminated against, she would at times experience guilt and shame for feeling depressed knowing her parents experiences were far more difficult. Although she needed to seek support a lot earlier, Jaspreet had felt she needed to take care of her family instead of seeking mental health services.

DIFFICULTIES IN NAVIGATING AND BALANCING INTERSECTING IDENTITIES

Based on Erikson's developmental stages of Psychosocial Development, South Asian American youth are moving toward the stage of Identity vs Identity confusion. During this stage youth begin to question who they are and begin to formulate their sense of self in regards to values, beliefs, gender, sexuality, and career. It's also a time where they are finding their own role within the larger society. This stage of development is particularly difficult for South Asian American youth who are often not given the opportunities to explore their individual identity (Graf et al., 2008). As discussed in earlier chapters and in our introduction, South Asian communities are collectivistic in nature where there is more emphasis on the collective than on the individual. So when South Asian American youth reach this stage and begin to explore independence this is met by a lot of resistance within South Asian American families. This in turn increases the shame and guilt that South Asian American youth experience when they think, feel or behave in a way that is not congruent to the families expectations (Farver et al., 2002).

In the case study, Jaspreet grew up in a household in which her parents taught her how to speak, read, and write Punjabi. She was quite involved in the Punjabi Sikh community during her early childhood attending Sikh camps and cultural programs. However, she now did not have a desire to attend the community events which increased conflicts at home. When she would go to the cultural events she enjoyed meeting her Punjabi Sikh friends but she also wanted to do activities such as sleepovers with non-Punjabi Sikh friends. Many South Asian American youth can resonate with Jaspreet's experiences and often describe this struggle as living between two different worlds, where they act a certain way at home and act another way at school (Mittapalli, 2009; Srinivasan, 2000; Thakore-Dunlap & Velsor, 2014). Youth feel stuck and exhausted in navigating between these two worlds, "belonging nowhere and belonging everywhere" (Mittapalli, 2009).

Self-Harm (Eating Disorders, Cutting, Suicidal Ideation)

The presence of multiple protective factors and the lack of and inconsistent research around risk-taking behavior in South Asian American youth has falsely created the notion that South Asian youth do not engage in self-harm or don't experience suicidal ideation. In the author's clinical experience it is important to do a thorough risk assessment with your South Asian American youth clients on a regular basis, sometimes each session.

Anxiety and Depression

South Asian American youth often express that they are under a lot of academic stress due to the high expectations they set for themselves or are set on them by their families which has shown to lead to the development of depression and anxiety. SAA youth also exhibit shame and guilt induced anxieties around academic achievement, dual identity balance and career or life choices. Messaging within the South Asian community is that depression and anxiety are a result of character weaknesses and laziness, which perpetuates stigma around these diagnoses and keep South Asian American youth from engaging in services (Mokkarala, 2015).

Case Study Discussion

Jaspreet has been to her academic counselors 2–3 times a week the past semester and has expressed having headaches, struggles focusing in class, irritability, and feeling un-motivated to complete schoolwork. Jaspreet has recently started to share about some of her struggles at home that are impacting her ability to focus and concentrate at school. The academic counselor offers Jaspreet the option to meet with a mental health clinician to talk about her challenges at home. Jaspreet reacts indifferently to that suggestion, remarking that she isn't "crazy" or "a psycho." Jaspreet also shares that her family won't believe there is anything wrong and would just tell her that she needs to study harder to get better grades and be happy. Jaspreet also expresses feeling a lot of shame because it was already hard enough to share about her family with her academic counselor; she wasn't sure if she wanted to share this information with another adult. Jaspreet tells her academic counselor

> We don't talk about what happens at home with anyone outside of the home. I am already bringing shame onto my family by telling you these things but you promised me that no one would find out. Besides, my family doesn't believe there is anything wrong and would just blame me for feeling overwhelmed and tell me to study harder.

First Session with South Asian American Youth

When Jaspreet came into the first session with her clinician, she wasn't really sure what to expect. Jaspreet became overwhelmed when the mental health clinician shared initial paperwork which included a comprehensive clinical interview, consents, and confidentiality agreements. The clinician also mentioned to Jaspreet that they would need to gather consent from her parents as well. The mental health clinician noticed the change in Jaspreet's affect and posture so she paused and asked Jaspreet if she had any questions about what had been discussed so far. Jaspreet began to share that she didn't know why the clinician needed all this private information about her life when she wasn't even sure that she wanted to participate in services. Jaspreet also reported that she did not want her parents to find out that she was engaging in services because it would be seen as being very disrespectful and she may be sent to India. Jaspreet's mental health clinician took a pause, gathered all of the documents she had handed to Jaspreet and told her not to worry about those right now and began to talk to her about what therapy could look like for her and how it could be helpful for her. The mental health clinician gave Jaspreet a tour of the office, spoke about the logistics of the sessions and informed Jaspreet about how she could communicate with the clinician between sessions. The session ended with the mental health clinician asking Jaspreet to think about what they discussed and to come back the following week with any follow up questions or concerns.

When working with South Asian American youth, as a clinician, it is so essential to be clear about your role not only with your clients but also with their families. Mental health is a new concept for many South Asian Americans and they may not really know what the process looks like or why it is important for clinicians to gather historical information. South Asian American youth referrals tend to come from the school through teachers, counselors, or from the healthcare system through pediatricians or primary physicians. Second-generation South Asian American youth may voluntarily ask for mental health care or educated and/or acculturated South Asian American parents may self-refer their children or adolescents if they notice a mental health struggle. It is important to understand that you may have to approach the first session differently given the source of the referral and where the sessions are taking place. Based on our graduate education and our ethical and legal obligations, clinicians often are pulled into wanting to rush into going over initial paperwork and gathering consents. However, with the South Asian youth, it is essential to take your time and provide some safety and comfort first. In the Case Study, Jaspreet's clinician began with the initial paperwork but realized that Jaspreet was not familiar with the process of therapy so she made an effort to take a pause and to slow down and provide psychoeducation on what is counseling and the process including paperwork.

Explaining the Process of Therapy

When beginning therapy with South Asian American youth and their families, meet them where they are in their understanding of the process of therapy. Relying on some initial outreach and consultation can help you understand which areas of the process you need to highlight. The explanation of what therapy is and why it is important would also change based on the age of the youth. For younger children, the clinician may describe the process to the child as simply a place to come and engage in play while talking about different feelings they experience. For youth, clinicians may first have this conversation with the teen by trying to understand what they know about therapy, if they have had experience with therapy before and what their expectations of sessions may be. After initial conversations around what happens in the room, clinicians may also want to discuss the logistics of sessions. Some areas of discussion may include:

1   The duration of treatment (for example six sessions or 1 year)
2   The length and consistency of sessions (for example 50 minutes session per week)
3   Attendance Requirements (for example only three sessions can be missed)
4   Treatment Planning Process (for example collaborative vs independent, types of reports provides)
5   Types of Interventions/Orientation (such as play, art, talk therapy, story-telling, Cognitive Behavioral Therapy)
6   Expectations of family members (such as dyadic work, family sessions, home visits)
7   Clinic Information (such as hours of operation, phone number)
8   Communication Protocols (such as how and how often to communicate with clinician, phone versus email).

Beginning Treatment with South Asian American Youth

This section will explore the different aspects of therapy and how to navigate these areas when working with South Asian American youth. Depending on the age of the youth, these discussions may need to happen with the youth's parents/caregivers, with the youth directly, or with both the parents/caregivers and youth.

For the second clinical session with Jaspreet, the mental health clinician utilized the second session to go through the initial paperwork packet with Jaspreet, starting with confidentiality and it's limits. The clinician invited Jaspreet in thinking of how she could talk about the services with her family to help understand why it was important and also spoke to Jaspreet about what information she would need to share with her parents and what information she would not need to share. The clinician left room for Jaspreet to reflect on what conversations may be beneficial to have with her family. The mental health clinician clearly went over the limits to confidentiality (harm to self, harm to others, child abuse, elder abuse, and legal situations) while continuously checking in with Jaspreet to make sure she didn't have any questions. The mental health clinician also spent the session helping Jaspreet break down the messaging around mental health that she has received by providing her the knowledge to debunk some of the South Asian mental health myths. The clinician let Jaspreet know that she would contact her parents before the next sessions, inquiring if she had a preference of who she should reach out to first.

Confidentiality and Limits to Confidentiality

Going over confidentiality and limits to confidentiality is not only an ethical and legal obligation, it is also a way of building rapport with South Asian American youth and their parents/caregivers. For younger adolescents, you would most likely go over confidentiality with the youth's parents and briefly share with the youth the limitations of confidentiality in age appropriate language. For older South Asian American youth who voluntarily sought out services or who were referred to mental health clinicians at their schools, it may be more important to go over confidentiality and its limits in its entirety, leaving room for the youth to ask questions. South Asian youth will most likely be hesitant in involving their parents or their family system in the process of therapy. Thus, it is essential to describe what the parent or family system's role would be given the reason for services. The table below highlights some important areas related to confidentiality.

Table 10.2: Discussing Confidentiality Areas of Focus When Going Over Confidentiality & Limitations with South Asian American Adolescents & Parents 1) Clearly identifying your legal obligations in keeping what is shared in the session private except when certain reporting laws that pertain to mandated reporting supersede confidentiality. Other limits of Confidentiality may also apply depending on the agency or state that services are being rendered, so it's important to highlight those as well. 2) Setting clear boundaries so that the child or adolescent and parent understand what you will or will not share with the parents. Having these boundaries, especially with adolescent clients allows for a stronger therapeutic alliance and increases likelihood that the client's will be open and honest during sessions. It is important to note that with younger children, there are often fluid boundaries in treatment. 3) Preparing the child or adolescent and parent about interactions outside of the therapy room in case you are from the same community. Letting them know you will not approach them or acknowledge them in public. 4) Going over HIPPA laws and what PHI is. Providing some literacy on who has access to health records and that mental health utilization is not a part of a school transcript and does not hinder college admissions. Sabharwal & Kaur, 2021.

Keep in Mind : Don't assume that going over confidentiality in the first session is enough. You may need to go over it every session to help adolescents minimize shame and fear of what is being shared about their family will be shared with their parents or the community at large.

Gathering Information-Intake Sessions

Depending on the age of the youth , intake sessions may occur with South Asian American youth individually or with their parents or caregivers. Holding an understanding that South Asian American youth have a collectivistic upbringing is important, and to find ways of utilizing the collective and not serving the youth in a vacuum. The collective may include the South Asian American youth's parents but also may include other caregivers, grandparents, aunts, uncles, cousins, neighbors, other extended family members and friends of the family.

Concepts of parenting and supporting parents is discussed in length in a previous chapter, however we'd like to highlight briefly how to approach South Asian American parents about their youth's request to receive mental health care. It is essential to take a strength based approach when discussing the referral with a South Asian American parent. Assessing the parent's level of emotional intelligence can help a clinician identify the language to use during such discussions. For example, with a parent that has knowledge of mental health concepts, you may use more psychological, academic and research based terminology, whereas with a parent that has limited knowledge, you may focus on more preventative language, intentionally avoiding psychological jargon. The parent's linguistic needs may also help determine what language you utilize, perhaps incorporating cultural definitions and terminology in their native language. The goal of these initial contacts help parents understand the clinical process and answer questions they have, and for the youth to understand the therapeutic process.

Along with confidentiality, it is also essential for clinicians to review the ways South Asian American parents can be involved in treatment. You may have to explain why it is important for you to not share all of the content a South Asian American youth may share with you in session, emphasizing the importance of trust with the youth to help foster authenticity and transparency. To increase parent's buy-in in therapy, explaining the ways the clinician can support the parents and when it would be appropriate for them to contact the clinician (times of crisis). Although most of this information will be written in the initial intake paperwork you provide to parents, it is important to verbally explain using colloquial or informal language and have this written information translated in various South Asian languages.

INTAKE SESSION WITH JASPREET'S FAMILY

The mental health clinician contacted Jaspreet's mom and explained that Jaspreet's school had referred her to meet with the clinician for some extra support to help with stress management at school. The mental health clinician was met with initial hesitations and confusion from Jaspreet's mom. The mental health clinician held space for Jaspreet's mom to share her concerns and utilized techniques of taking pauses, providing validation, using conversational Punjabi words and phrases to explain the process of therapy, and allowed Jaspreet's mom to ask questions along the way. The mental health clinician provided psychoeducation around how psychosocial development can impact academic functioning and provided concrete examples of how developing coping strategies against stress would help strengthen Jaspreet's ability to achieve success in the future. The mental health clinician also encouraged Jaspreet's mom to use strength based language when talking to Jaspreet about services as a way of destigmatizing therapy and giving permission to Jaspreet to engage fully. Eventually Jaspreet's mom did provide consent for services and agreed to an intake session which would consist of herself, Jaspreet's father, Jaspreet's Brother and Jaspreet's grandparents.

When engaging in an intake with South Asian American youth and their families clinicians need to gather all of the typical information such as presenting symptoms and duration, prenatal history, developmental history, social history, medical history, academic history and risk factors. However you would also want to gather a thorough family history which includes an assessment of the acculturation level of the youth and also the family's acculturation level, immigration history, trauma history, and spirituality or religiosity in order to develop a cultural formulation in addition to a clinical formulation.

Once rapport was built with Jaspreet, the mental health clinician began asking her to share more during clinical sessions about her family and some of the challenges she has been experiencing which led her to services. Jaspreet described her family system consisting of her parents, older brother Gurtej, younger sister Manpreet, and paternal grandparents. She shared that her brother Gurtej recently got married to Kiran from India. Kiran will be arriving in the US in a few weeks. The marriage was arranged by extended family members. Jaspreet also spoke a lot about maternal and paternal uncles and aunts that lived nearby as well as cousins from both sides of her family, some of whom attend the same school as her. She shared that at home the family spoke mainly Punjabi but that she felt more comfortable with English so she primarily speaks English when communicating with her siblings or her father. Jaspreet shared that she has been having many arguments with her parents and feels like she is "suffocating" by the amount of responsibility and expectations from her parents. Jaspreet reported also having an additional role as an interpreter for her mom in a variety of settings. Jaspreet reported her parents are obsessed with her academics and do not allow her to choose her extracurricular activities. She felt frustrated that her parents do not want her to date or attend any of the school events/ programs (school dances, club meeting, sports, etc.). Jaspreet's symptoms started after her parents saw her in a study session at school with boys. She began to talk about feeling like she was a different person at school than she was at home which was becoming emotionally exhausting. She reported feeling comfortable sharing things with her older brother but now that he had graduated from college and gotten married, he seemed to become more authoritarian toward her. She felt pressured to maintain her grades at school while also taking on household responsibilities such as cooking dinner, cleaning the home, and making sure her younger sister was staying on top of her schoolwork. Jaspreet felt that with all these expectations she did not have enough time to be a "real teenager". Whenever she would ask to hang out with friends or to participate in school events, her parents and now her older brother would tell her to focus on academics and not to worry about socializing at this age. She felt these restrictions were unfair, as her older brother had been allowed to have friends over, participate in a multitude of afterschool activities, including being on the basketball team and he did not have as many chores at home.

Clinical Goals for Jaspreet

Jaspreet, her mental health clinician, and her family worked collaboratively to come up with a treatment plan that was clinically and culturally informed with goals that focused on Jaspreet's individual and family/collective needs.

Individual goals focused on helping Jaspreet:

a   Identify and name emotions and feelings.
b   Connect to the here and now.
c   Identify values and beliefs that are important to her as an individual to help foster a balance between intersecting identities.
d   Identify and implement coping strategies such as journaling, Sikh prayer, listening to music and spending time with her peers.
e   Increasing social engagement through participation in support groups, workshops or leadership projects with other South Asian American youth, to help normalize her experiences.

Family/Community goals focused on helping Jaspreet:

a   Reconnect with her culture and community through prayer or Seva (selfless service).
b   Establishing family routines to help foster stronger family connections and healthier family communication.
c   Identify realistic expectations in regards to household chores, academic functioning, and social engagement. Finding a balance or compromise that fits well within her family and community system.
d   Providing Psychoeducation to help increase emotional intelligence within the family system to continue to normalize mental health conversations.
e   Linkage to community resources.

Individual Clinical Interventions

Clinicians may need to spend more time in the rapport building phase, discussing confidentiality, providing psychoeducation and helping youth debunk mental health myths. Once the initial rapport is built most South Asian American youth will respond well to youth focused interventions such as play therapy and art therapy where the focus is not always on the youth talking. It can also be helpful to incorporate culturally relevant activities and discussions during session, and tapping into the youth's interests. For example, listening to

South Asian music rather than American pop, talk about cricket or football rather than baseball, and refer to bollywood rather than hollywood (Roy, 2012; Shankar, 2008). Clinicians can also intertwine a social justice focus on their work with South Asian American youth to help address the impacts of discrimination and racism on self-confidence and self-worth. Clinicians can incorporate mental health phone apps to help track emotions or thoughts, engage in mindfulness breathing and even connect with other youth experiencing mental health challenges. Youth may also ask for clinicians to share youtube videos, ted talks and information on social media influencers that speak about mental health.

Family Support and Therapy

Incorporating some level of family support is also important when working with youth. In the beginning of treatment, South Asian American youth may be hesitant to include their family, however through psychoeducation the clinician can support both the family and the youth in understanding the benefits of family sessions. In the authors' experience, psychoeducation is something that will continue to occur during the course of family work, especially around the understanding the importance of looking at the "whole child". If we think of working from a youth focused lens it is important to increase connections within the family to help promote empathy and compassion between youth and family. South Asian adolescents will often be hesitant in including their family members in their services, it may be helpful to revisit confidentiality and encourage youth to plan out the family session with you. In the author's clinical experiences, providing family members a safe space to talk about how they feel about their roles within the family, challenging un-realistic expectations and fostering active listening skills can go a long way to strengthen relationships within the family. This also helps model healthy communication for the South Asian American youth and their families which they can continue to practice outside of sessions. It helps find exceptions to the power dynamics, allowing each member to recognize external and internal pressures each member of the family may be experiencing. Introducing the importance of play can be a helpful strategy when working with youth and their families. Play is traditionally considered something that young children engage in, however research shows that play helps stimulate creativity, increases independence, promotes self-confidence and improves connection. This type of family focused work can also help the family engage in difficult conversations around tabooed topics. Clinicians are encouraged to have an understanding of some cultural norms within South Asian American communities such as differences in eye contact, importance of gift giving, tendency to under-report symptomology in the beginning of treatment and the impact of hierarchies within the family system that may prevent family members from speaking freely (Akechi, Senju, Uibo, Kikuchi, Hasegawa, & Hietanen, 2013).

Community Interventions

Goalsfocused on strengthening community engagement and leadership can help South Asian American youth find a balance between their intersecting identities, strengthen social connections and build resilience (Islam et al, 2017). Helping youth reconnect with their ethnic community can help them recognize what aspects of that identity they want to hold on to and what are the protective factors they can tap into within the community to help cope with stress and anxiety. Keep in Mind: Clinicians are encouraged to maintain participant's confidentiality during community work and help define the community's role in the treatment of the South Asian American youth.

Questions for Reflection

1 What types of psychoeducation will increase buy-in for treatment for South Asian American youth?
2 What are some ways of helping South Asian American youth break through mental health stigma, shame and resistance in telling parents that they are seeking mental health services?
3 What are 1–2 interventions that can be utilized when working with South Asian American youth?

Summary

The focus of this chapter is on counseling South Asian American youth. The chapter looked at current research, highlighted stigmas and barriers that influence help-seeking behaviors, examined presentation of symptoms and discussed clinical considerations when working with South Asian American youth in treatment. A case study that focused on a 13-year-old South Asian American female named Jaspreet Kaur was introduced to help bring to light key concepts such as how to discuss the process of therapy from a culturally informed lens. Specifically, the case illustrated how to build rapport with South Asian American youth and their families and how to help youth find a balance between their independence and interdependence. Also, the example portrayed the importance of paying attention to issues of identity development, level of acculturation and psychosomatic symptomatology. Readers are encouraged to approach work with South Asian American youth with flexibility, creativity, and meet their clients where they are in their emotional wellness journey. In the author's clinical experiences, we have found it is vital to take a slow paced, collaborative, prevention focused and culturally informed approach with South Asian American youth. It is important to provide South Asian American youth with a level of agency, making them the experts of their stories to help increase buy-in, and reduce premature treatment withdrawal. As clinicians remind yourselves to ask questions, stay curious, avoid cultural assumptions and know that the "Presenting problem is not always the problem" (Singh, 2019).

References

Abraham, M. (2000). *Speaking the unspeakable: Marital violence among South Asian immigrants in the United States*. Rutgers University Press.

Ahmad, F., Riaz, S., Barata, P., & Stewart, D.E. (2004). Patriarchal beliefs and perceptions of abuse among south asian immigrant women. *Violence Against Women*, *10*, 262–282. 10.1177/1077801203256000

Akechi, H., Senju, A., Uibo, H., Kikuchi, Y., Hasegawa, T., & Hietanen, J.K. (2013). Attention to eye contact in the West and East: Autonomic responses and evaluative ratings. *PloS One*, *8*(3), e59312. 10.1371/journal.pone.0059312

Almeida, R. (2005). Asian Indian families: An overview. In M. McGoldrick, J. Giordano, & N. Garcia Preto (Eds.), *Ethnicity and family therapy* (pp. 377–394). Guilford.

Asians and Attachment Theory by Sam Louie MA, LMHC, S-PSB (2014). Retrieved from https://www.psychologytoday.com/us/blog/minority-report/201407/asians-and-attachment-theory

Atwal, K., & Wang, C. (2019). Religious head covering, being perceived as foreigners, victimization, and adjustment among Sikh American adolescents. *School Psychology*, *34*(2), 233–243. 10.1037/spq0000301

Ayyub, R. (2000). Domestic violence in the South Asian Muslim immigrant population in the United States. *Journal of Social Distress and the Homeless*, *9*, 237–248. 10.1023/A:1009412119016

Berry, J.W. (1997). Immigration, acculturation, and adaptation. *Applied Psychology: An International Review, 46*(1), 5–68.

Bronfenbrenner, U. (1979). *The ecology of human development: Experiments by nature and design.* Harvard University Press.

Cheryan, S., & Bodenhausen, G.V. (2011). Model minority. In S. M. Caliendo & C. D. McIlwain (Eds.), *The Routledge companion to race and ethnicity* (pp. 173–176). Routledge.

Chou, W.-M., & Leonard, H.T. (2006). Fix my children: Working with strong-minded asian parents. In G. R. Walz, J. C. Bleuer, & R. K. Yep (Eds.), *Vistas: Compelling perspectives on counseling 2006* (pp. 81–84). American Counseling Association.

Corrigan, P., Druss, B., & Perlick, D. (2014). The impact of mental Illness stigma on seeking and participating in mental health care. *Psychological Science in the Public Interest, 15*(2), 37–70.

Daga, S. S., & Raval, V. V. (2018). Ethnic–racial socialization, model minority experience, and psychological functioning among south Asian American emerging adults: A preliminary mixed-methods study. *Asian American Journal of Psychology, 9*(1), 17–31. 10.1037/aap0000108

Das, S. (2002). Loss or gain? A Saga of Asian Indian immigration and experiences in America's multi-ethnic mosaic. *Race, Gender & Class, 9*(2), 131–155.

Dasgupta, S.D. (2000). Broken promises: Domestic violence murders and attempted murders in the U.S. and Canadian South Asian communities. In S. Nankani (Ed.), *Breaking the silence: Domestic violence in the South Asian-American community* (pp. 27–46). Xlibris.

Farver, J., Bhadha B., & Narang, S. (2002). Acculturation and psychological functioning in asian Indian adolescents. *Social Development, 11*, 11–29. 10.1111/1467-9507.00184.

Farver, J., Xu, Y., Bhadha, B., Narang, S., & Lieber, E. (2007). Ethnic Identity, acculturation, parenting beliefs, and adolescent adjustment: A comparison of Asian Indian and European American families. *Merrill-Palmer Quarterly, 53*(2), 184–215.

Fisher, C.B., Wallace, S.A., & Fenton, R.E. (2000). Discrimination distress during adolescence. *Journal of Youth and Adolescence, 29*(6), 679–695. 10.1023/A:1026455906512

Graf, S.C., Mullis, R.L., & Mullis, A.K. (2008). Identity formation of United States American and Asian Indian adolescents. *Adolescence, 43*(169), 57–69.

Ibrahim, F., Ohnishi, H., & Sandhu, D.S. (1997). Asian American identity development: A culture specific model for South Asian Americans. *Journal of Multicultural Counseling & Development, 25*(1), 34–51.

Kuortti, J. (2007). *Writing imagined diasporas: South Asian women reshaping North American identity.* Cambridge Scholars.

Lee, S., Juon, H.-S., Martinez, G., Hsu, C.E., Robinson, J.B., & Ma, G. (2009). Model minority at risk: Expressed needs of mental health by Asian American young adults. *J Community Health, 34*, 144–152. doi:10.1007/s10900-008-9137-1

Mittapalli, K. (2009). An Asian Indian student's identity: Living in two worlds. *The Qualitative Report, 14*, 466–477.

Mokkarala, S., O'Brien, E.K., & Siegel, J.T. (2016). The relationship between shame and perceived biological origins of mental illness among South Asian and white American young adults. *Psychology, Health & Medicine, 21*(4), 448–459. 10.1080/13548506.2015.1090615

Mullender, A., Hague, G., Imam, U., Kelly, L., Malos, E., & Regan, L. (2002). *Children's perspectives on domestic violence.* Sage.

Netting, N.S. (2006). Two-lives, one partner: Indo-Canadian youth between love and arranged marriages. *Journal of Comparative Family Studies, 37*, 129–146. https://soci.ucalgary.ca/jcfs/

Ragavan, M.I., Fikre, T., Millner, U., & Bair-Merritt, M. (2018). The impact of domestic violence exposure on South Asian children in the United States: Perspectives of domestic violence agency staff. *Child Abuse & Neglect, 76*, 250–260. 10.1016/j.chiabu.2017.11.006

Ragavan, M., Syed-Swift, Y., Elwy, A.R., Fikre, T., & Bair-Merritt, M. (2021). The influence of culture on healthy relationship formation and teen dating violence: A qualitative analysis of South Asian female youth residing in the United States. *Journal of Interpersonal Violence, 36*(7–8), NP4336–NP4362. 10.1177/0886260518787815

Roy, S. (2012). "Multiple 'faces' of Indian identity: A comparative critical analysis of identity management on facebook by Asian Indians living in India and the US." *China Media Research*, *8*(4), 6.

Shankar, S. (2008). Speaking like a model minority: "FOB" styles, gender, and racial meanings among desi teens in silicon valley. *Journal of Linguistic Anthropology*, *18*(2), 268–289.

Sharma N., & Shaligram D. (2018). Suicide among South Asian youth in America. In A. Pumariega & N. Sharma (Eds.), *Suicide Among Diverse Youth*. Springer, Cham. 10.1007/978-3-319-66203-9_6

Singh, R.K.J. (2019) *Clinical Interview and Intake Evaluation*. The Hume Center.

South Asian Americans Leading Together (SAALT). (2019). A demographic snapshot of South Asians in the United States April 2019. Retrieved from https://saalt.org/wp-content/uploads/2019/04/SAALT-Demographic-Snapshot-2019.pdf

Srinivasan, S. (2000). "Being Indian," "Being American". *Journal of Human Behavior in the Social Environment*, *3*(3–4), 135–158, DOI: 10.1300/J137v03n03_10

Tavkar, P., Iyer, S.N., & Hansen, D.J. (2008). Barriers to mental health services for Asian Indians in America. Poster presented at: The 42nd Annual Convention of the Association for Behavioral and Cognitive Therapies; Orlando, FL. [Accessed July 2021].

Thakore-Dunlap, U., & Velsor, P. (2014). Group counseling with South Asian immigrant high school girls: Reflections and commentary of a group facilitator. *The Professional Counselor*, *4*. 505–518. 10.15241/pvv.4.5.505.

Zaidi, A., Couture-Carron, A., & Maticka-Tyndale, E. (2016). 'Should I or Should I Not'?: An exploration of South Asian youth's *resistance* to cultural deviancy, *International Journal of Adolescence and Youth*, *21*(2), 232–251, 10.1080/02673843.2013.836978

12 Counseling Older South Asian Americans

Bindu Methikalam and Lavanya Devdas

Case Overview

Ammu is a 77-year-old heterosexual South Asian Cisgender female who lost her husband of 50 years, Prakash. Ammu considers herself to have been very close with Prakash and feels the grief intensely. She said that since she came to the U.S. 45 years ago he was the only consistent person in her life. Ammu lives by herself, and she has one daughter, Maya, who was also a caretaker for Prakash during his final years. Recently, Ammu tells Maya that she wanted to attend a local Indian gathering, however, nobody called her to see if she needed a ride. She says that she feels people have moved on with their lives and her life has changed. Ammu states that others are happy, and she constantly feels an emptiness after Prakash's death and the responsibility of caring for family and finances falls solely on her shoulders. Maya says she can provide Ammu with rides, her mother should feel "fine," and that maybe Ammu should move in with her. Ammu finds it frustrating when people feel that as an older widow who is completely helpless and not as intellectually capable of making decisions. She said she wants people to be considerate, but not invasive and dismissive of her capabilities and experiences.

Introduction

Data indicates that the number of people aged 65 and above in the U.S. has grown in the past century from 3 million to over 38.9 million (Sorkin et al., 2011). It is estimated that by 2030 over 72 million or one in five Americans will be over the age of 65. According to the American Psychological Association (APA) Guidelines for Psychological Practice with Older Adults (APA, 2014), the need for clinicians to understand older adults, cultural and clinical issues will continue to grow as this group shows a significant amount of hetero-geneity. However, limited information exists about this population and an even smaller amount of research exists on the South Asian older adult population. In 2007, Asian Indians over the age of 55 made up about 10% of the Asian Indian population in the U.S. (Nandan, 2007; Tummala-Narra et al., 2013). Much of the literature on South Asians focuses on identity development of adolescents, cultural conflict in the family, career concerns, and utilization of treatment; however, the aging process in South Asian American cultures is not discussed. According to Erikson et al. (1986) the goal of the stage of integrity vs. despair is quite difficult and many may struggle with fully achieving in-tegrity. More specifically, South Asians and South Asian Americans face transitions such as immigration in older age, oppression such as ageism, racism, sexism, and homophobia can exacerbate feelings of despair and disgust. Older South Asians and South Asian Americans often are navigating immigration experiences, financial and occupational concerns, as well as issues around sexuality, gender identity, and religion. The current

DOI: 10.4324/9781003081548-12

chapter will address immigration status, mental health stressors, and treatment implications for older South Asian Americans.

Immigration

Ammu's case above illustrates the nature of immigration as a long-drawn process with its beginnings embedded in the country of origin and extending onwards to the post-arrival process and experiences in the host country. Currently, about 5.4 million South Asians live in the U.S. and include individuals and families from Bangladesh, Bhutan, India, Nepal, Pakistan, Sri Lanka, and the Maldives (South Asian Americans Leading Together [SAALT], 2019) and constitute one of the largest immigrant groups in the U.S. Although the definition of immigrants encompasses voluntary migration in search of better economic and educational opportunities among other factors, the challenges of adjustment and adaptation are inevitable (Chung & Bemak, 2007) and contingent on numerous factors including the process of migration, age, and time of migration. Specifically, the immigration process can have multiple phases and each segment may bring a separate yet overlapping level of effort in preparation and adjustment. For instance, during the pre-immigration period the preparation for embarking on the journey can include anticipating the potential loss of existing family structure, family members and friends. Additionally, navigating visa issues and making related preparations including housing and finances can feel exhausting (Inman & Tummala-Narra, 2010). The second phase, which is the migration journey can be exciting and overwhelming. The third phase, which is the entry into the new country, can highlight the hardships of re-settlement such as mourning the loss of familiarity and certainty with the lifestyle in the country of origin, including social networks and relationships, alienation, feelings of uprootedness. Moreover, confusion may also arise from the host culture's influence on one's sense of well-being and collective identity (Ehrensaft & Tousignant, 2006).

In addition to the migration process, the time and age of migration also impact the cultural adjustment and adaptation for South Asians. For instance, the first and second wave of immigrants in the 1990s constituted South Asian immigrants from the northern part of rural India while those who arrived in the U.S. post 1965 were professionals from urban areas and with an educational background (Inman & Tummala-Narra, 2010). The 1980s and 1990s witnessed a shift in the trend of immigrants. South Asian immigrants from the above two decades were not as highly educated and perhaps were relatives and family members of those who immigrated in the post 1965 era (Inman & Tummala-Narra, 2010). Among family members, included were aging parents who had retired in their home countries and then traveled to the States to reunite with other family members (Nandan, 2007).

Given the diversity within and between the waves of immigration among South Asians living in the U.S., intergenerational conflicts between family members, acculturative stress, and differences in cultural values between the country of origin and the host country can be overwhelming. For instance, among the first wave of immigrants, cultural values such as filial piety, respectful for the elderly and cultural humility, children seeking their grandparents' advice and blessings frequently, and the expectation of aging parents being taken care of by their offspring were particularly prominent (Bhattacharya & Shibusawa, 2009; Nandan, 2007). As a result, the process of enculturating to the host culture that emphasizes individualism and independence can be saliently challenging for the elderly South Asian immigrants. Older Asian Americans may have limited access to resources including social support systems, social network, ability to navigate resources in the environment, income, and English language proficiency (Mui & Kang, 2006). In fact, protective factors such as access to social support and networking, support groups, mastery in relation to navigating one's immediate environment, and meaning making through collaborative spiritual or religious activities are buffers to mental health among older South Asian immigrants (Diwan et al., 2004).

Among the second wave of immigrants, the theme of bi-cultural adaptation was prominent. This meant an integration of U.S. based cultural values and the retention of values from one's indigenous culture. Various generations of family members lived under the same roof, reinforcing the values of collectivism and interdependence (Inman & Tummala-Narra, 2010; Nandan, 2007), and also making intergenerational conflicts salient, given the different levels of acculturation between family members. First-generation immigrants may look to family support to make up for the lost personal and social networks back home, endorse a preference for ethnic identification, and a collectivistic orientation (Lalonde & Cameron, 1993). In contrast, second-generation immigrants, who are born in the host country, do not experience similar losses of social connections and network, and endorse a more individualistic orientation (Merz et al., 2009), and favorable attitudes toward multiculturalism (Lalonde & Cameron, 1993). The differences in value adherence between first generation immigrants and second-generation adolescents results in increased parent-child conflict (Tsai-Chae & Nagata, 2008), differing attitudes toward family values and intergenerational solidarity (Ying, 1999) in terms of parental authority, children's rights, and obligations (Kwak & Berry, 2001). Upon arrival to the States, the Asian parent or elder may struggle with the abrupt nature of loss of power and respect as a cultural conservator/teacher in the family (Mui & Kang, 2006). This also indicates the growing dilemma of the elderly immigrants—of being independent (individualism) versus seeking interdependence from their offspring and other family members (Tummala-Narra et al., 2013). For instance, upon migrating to the U.S., the values of independence and mastery over one's environment may take precedence within the context of U.S. based Western culture. This would inform the need for independence among older South Asian immigrants as part of adapting to the United States. Simultaneously, cultural values of respect and care, and transmitting such values to the younger generation might still hold a central place based on interdependence and respect for the elders within the South Asian cultures (Tummala-Narra et al., 2013).

The aforementioned growing dilemma may especially be salient among the third wave of immigrants, where elderly immigrants retire in their home country, and join their offspring and family members living in the United States. For instance, some elderly immigrants from India who immigrated late in life to be with their children do not demonstrate proficiency in English language (Diwan et al., 2004). This creates a barrier in interfacing with their children and grandchildren and navigating resources in the host country. For example, increased caretaking responsibilities as grandparents in the United States, coupled with limited English language proficiency as "babysitters" exacerbated the nature of challenges including interactions and connection with their grandchildren (Tummala-Narra et al., 2013). Thus, among older adults who migrated to the United States, there appears to be a strong sense of dissonance when their pre-migration hopes of spending more time with their children remains unmet due to the busyness of their children's lives, coupled with their own inability to travel back to one's host country for important family occasions and festivals, among other factors (Tummala-Narra et al., 2013).

Additionally, a growing number of studies have highlighted the increased risk of isolation and psychological distress, including depression, underutilization of mental health services and limited English language proficiency among older immigrants (Diwan et al., 2004; Hernandez & Bigatti, 2010; Mui & Kang, 2006; Tummala-Narra et al., 2013). Related losses experienced by elderly South Asian immigrants include loss of hierarchy and structure in the family including family roles they imbibed in their country of origin (Bhattacharya & Shibusawa, 2009). Other losses include disconnection from children and grandchildren as a result of limited English language proficiency, loss of authority and perhaps increased dependency on family members for finances, transportation, health needs and social support, and unmet spiritual needs including peer group discourses on religion and philosophy (Balgopal, 1999; Tummala-Narra et al., 2013). The busy schedules of offspring, perceived lack of time and lack of immediate access to social support systems and networks, the loss of native language use and cultural familiarity among grand-children (Rastogi, 2007) also compounded the acculturation and adjustment process among South Asian elderly immigrants. For instance, the venerated position of elders in the family is a valued aspect of South Asian culture, where grandchildren are encouraged to seek the guidance and blessings of elders (Tummala-Narra et al., 2013). Family mem-bers continue to acknowledge the important roles that elders play in resolution of family conflicts and decision making (Rastogi, 2007). Upon migrating to the United States, the adaptation process may seem different for older South Asian adults, who prefer adhering to their Asian cultural values such as expectations of filial piety and interdependence, while second-generation family members, including adolescents, adopt a more individualistic orientation to navigate schools, colleges and other institutional settings including work-places. This implies values of autonomy, choice, and reliance on peers more than elders in the family for support and identity development (Farver et al., 2002). The widening cul-tural gap often creates an intergenerational family conflict between older South Asian immigrants and their offspring, including grandchildren.

Last but not least, the collective identity of maintaining connection between self and others in the family, the value of giving and receiving care and help from friends and family are also espoused values among the elderly Asian immigrants. In fact, ongoing engagement with peers and family members through mutual support may highlight their resonance with cultural values such as collectivism and collaboration (Inman et al., 2007). Simultaneously, the limited access to transportation, and limitations in traveling to community centers and peer group locations compound the perceived sense of helplessness and limited control ex-perienced by this immigrant group (Tummala-Narra et al., 2013). Given the multitude of factors informing the pre-immigration, migration, and post-migration cultural adjustment and adaptation process among elderly South Asian immigrants, the importance of identity and intersectionality of cultural identities warrants attention.

Intersectionality of Identities

The American Psychological Association's Multicultural Guidelines (2017) addresses the importance of examining clients from a contextual and holistic stance. Understanding intersectionality is imperative in gaining a deeper and more comprehensive awareness of others. The term intersectionality was first coined by Kimberle Crenshaw (1989) to convey how various forms of oppression, marginalization, and discrimination intersect to inform structural and systemic inequities and social positioning. Additionally, the literature emphasizes the salience of comprehending social location and how race, sexuality, religion, gender, and other cultural group memberships interface. Individuals who hold multiple minority statuses can experience various forms of discrimination, leading to decreased psychological well-being and internalized negative beliefs (Hart et al., 2021). Intersectionality is of particular importance in understanding South Asian American older adults because there are such diversity and heterogeneity of experiences. As discussed earlier, identities such as age at the time of migration, are essential vari-ables that can impact psychological well-being. Older South Asian Americans already experience a "double jeopardy" in their age and racial/ethnic identification; however, the intersectionality of religion, gender, sexual orientation, and socioeconomic status have been shown to impact the physical health of the elderly (Lai & Chau, 2007; Lai & Surood, 2013).

South Asians Americans follow a diversity of religious practices such as Hinduism, Islam, Christianity, Sikhism, Jainism, Buddhism, Judaism, and many other religious and spiritual practices. Research has shown that religious affiliation is often a protective factor correlated with better physical and mental health (Levin & Chatters, 1998). However, for many South Asians Americans who practice religion, access and availability are concerns. Older South Asian Americans might have different religious affiliation levels than their children and religious practices in the home might vary, which can cause strain. For example, older South Asian Americans may engage in more prayer practices several times a day, while their children or grandchildren might not engage in prayer rituals at all during the day. Additionally, there might not be regular access to religious places of worship, such as during the COVID-19 pandemic, which might cause distress as religious communities and physically attending services can be a source of support. Depending on where individuals are located geographically, they may not have South Asian places of worship similar to what is available in the country of origin. Social support is an essential factor in understanding an individual's well-being and a central aspect of the adjustment process, and research has suggested that gathering together as a religious community is an aspect of social support (Krause, 2006). Clement et al. (1998), found that adjustment was worse when there was no support network from the native culture. Lacking places of worship is relevant to older South Asians who are new immigrants and grieving a loss of the religious community and socialization in the country of origin. Depending on where they have migrated, older South Asians might not have others who identify with similar religions and where they can come together as a community.

Further, discrimination based on religion might become a significant concern. When compared to Hindus, Muslims South Asians reported worse physical health and engaged in less physical activities and experienced more bodily pain (Lai & Surood, 2009). The researchers stated that Muslims tend to endorse items such as "'feel pretty worthless', followed by Hindus, then Sikhs. While further research is needed in this area, it is understood that the historical and current experiences of Islamophobia and othering of the Muslim community can contribute to such differences (Lai & Surood, 2009).

South Asian American LGBTQIA+ communities are often recipients of discrimination. There is a dearth of research on older South Asians who identify as sexual minorities; however, their experiences with families and discrimination are crucial to understand. Often there are threats, physical and verbal abuse, and various forms of harassment and violence that LGBTQIA+ individuals face (Pereira & Costa, 2016). Within the South Asian community, there tend to be judgmental and negative societal views toward sexual minorities, and individuals can face homophobia from the community. Older South Asian Americans who identify as LGBTQIA+ might be ostracized by family members and the community. Further, long-term relationships and marriages might not be recognized, which can add to additional stress and strain. While many in the LGBTQIA+ community have "chosen families," which are defined as "non-biological kinship bonds, whether legally recognized or not, deliberately chosen for the purpose of mutual support and love" relational and social distress still exists (Gates, 2017). Research has also shown that South Asian LGBTQIA+ also faces a tremendous amount of racism from the LGBTQIA+ community (Sandil et al., 2015). Research has shown that Asians are racialized, ignored, and even exoticized and experience a lack of power in different spaces. For older South Asians who identify as LGBTQIA+, discrimination and multiple oppression are not a novel experience; however, managing the cumulative stressors impacts physical and mental concerns. Everett et al. (2016), noted that daily discrimination could have severe long-term physical outcomes. Further, the anticipation of discriminatory events and actual discrimination is also associated with increased levels of psychological distress (Pereira & Costa, 2016).

Regarding financial stability, there are significant differences in older South Asian Americans and finances. Older South Asians Americans who immigrated in the 1960s, 1970s, and 1980s might have had a chance to work, build pension and retirement funds; however, this is not the case for everyone. Depending on the profession's nature, individuals may not have accumulated wealth or additional income to support themselves during retirement. While many early immigrants arrived to pursue educational and employment opportunities, the third wave of immigrants arrived to join family members and were less educated (Rahman & Paik, 2017) and might have less financial stability. Additionally, many immigrants who arrived earlier might have been unable to practice the profession and trade held back in the country of origin and thus are forced to find jobs that might not provide the same financial security level. New South Asian immigrants who are older can face challenges in finding work and experience financial challenges. Older adults who also immigrated later in life lack insurance and/or quality insurance, which has shown to impact one's mental and physical health by reporting one or more health conditions or having increase in depression and anxiety symptoms (Sorkin et al., 2011). Recent immigration, low levels of acculturation, and lower proficiency in English played a significant role as a factor of depression (Casado & Leung, 2002; Lai, 2004). Diwan et al. (2004) reported that older South Asians who immigrate later in life to be with adult children typically speak limited English and have limited financial protection. Depending on their relationships with the children, financial dependency can increase strain in familial relationships and decrease autonomy. More recently, many older immigrants have children "manage" their finances, and children can withhold or steal money from parents, which ultimately has significant impacts on familial relationships and mental health. There is less freedom and flexibility with finances. Older female adults living alone with less financial security and low levels of social support were more likely to experience depressive symptoms (Lai, 2004).

Moreover, as healthcare costs soar, in particular doctor's visits, prescriptions, and receiving procedures, older individuals can fear spending a lot on medical concerns. Many older individuals' finances become a source of strain and worry because they have to consider healthcare costs and do not want to burden their children. For example, a 77-year-old South Asian first-generation male living on his own was worried about the cost of going to the ER and being admitted to the hospital or getting a live-in aide. He has been residing in the United States for 40 years, and although he was financially comfortable, as an immigrant, he was of the mindset to save and be prudent with money. He thought that a live-in aide felt too extravagant. Although his children argue with him about using his money to take care of himself, and his doctor encourages him to seek a live-in aide, he is worried about the ongoing costs and if he will struggle financially the way he did when he first came to the United States.

Psychological Concerns

South Asian American older adults have a wide-range of presenting concerns, and there are a variety of factors that can impact their psychological well-being. As a result of the immigration and aging process, many older South Asian American immigrants face various mental health problems such as acculturative stress, family and intergenerational conflict, depression, grief and loss, and elder maltreatment. As highlighted in the case of Ammu, people see her as less competent to make decisions and take care of herself because of her age and widow status.

Acculturation and Acculturative Stress

Acculturative stress is the strain one experiences as a result of trying to integrate unfamiliar cultural norms from the host culture into the norms and traditions of the culture of origin (Samuel, 2009). The greater the difference between the host culture and the culture of origin the more acculturative stress one can experience. Samuel (2009) indicated that South Asian women experienced acculturative stress as a result of intergenerational conflict at home and job stress which led to an increase in depressive symptoms. This is salient to South Asian American older adults because they are often navigating inter-generational differences. Further, acculturative stress significantly predicted depression and suicidal ideation (Hovey, 2000). Research consistently shows that depression in older adults is associated higher rates of suicide in elderly Chinese immigrants than U.S. born Chinese Americans (Yu, 1986); South Asian American elderly living in the United States with the ability to speak English, having a longer length of residency in the country, having a higher level of education, having a higher level of income, having better self-perceived health, are associated with lower levels of depression; however, this is not the case for everyone (Diwan, 2004). Olmedo and Padilla (1978) also found a relationship between acculturation and length of residence in the U.S, indicating that the longer individuals had been in the United States, the more acculturated they were. Older adults and females experience more acculturative stress than adolescents or men (Berry, 1990). Most Asian older adults have been in the United States for more than two decades (U.S. Census Bureau, 2010), increasing exposure to discrimination (Chan, 2020). Older South Asians face a "double jeopardy," which is discrimination against age and race (Dowd & Bengston, 1978; Rait and Burns, 1997). As a result, they might have to deal with the long-term and cumulative effects of dealing with multiple discrimination. Tragedies like 9–11 increased the overt and covert forms of discrimination toward the South Asian American community, and many older South Asians might have felt pressured to become naturalized citizens out of fear of deportation and being targeted (Chan, 2020).

Conversely, many recent older South Asian American immigrants have less independence and can experience more difficulty adjusting to the United States. Espin (1987) suggests that loss and mourning of the "old country" may lead to depressive symptoms. Moreover, newer immigrants can face additional challenges of language inadequacy, lack of financial resources, and a sense of anxiety about being in an unfamiliar environment (Hovey, 2000; Salgado de Snyder, 1987). There might be uncertainty and doubt regarding the decision to move from the South Asian country to the United States. There is a sense of isolation for some new older immigrants and a lack of connection with people in the same realm as in the home country. Depending on the region's weather in the host country, there might be an expectation to stay inside and not socialize like they can do back in the country of origin. In particular, if older adults stay inside while adult children are working all day and kids are at school, older adults might feel isolation, loneliness, sadness, and regret choosing or being asked to immigrate.

Family Strain

Overall within South Asian culture, strong family relationships, geographic nearness, and regular communication are emphasized and be positive contributors to overall well-being

(Kim & McKenry, 1998; Wilmoth & Chen, 2003). Therefore, when support and closeness are not received, it can also contribute to depressive symptoms in Asian older adults. While levels of intimacy and closeness vary based on factors such as immigration status and family dynamics, in many South Asian American families it is expected that all issues such as, education and job choices, financial concerns, and marriage gets discussed within the family and stays within the family (Pillari, 2005), however, many older South Asian Americans experience a significant amount of distress and stress from the family. Older South Asian Americans might have different expectations of aging and how family members will interact with them and when this perception is not a reality then it can contribute to feeling sad, hopeless, and other depressive symptoms. One should not assume that a strong bond is the case for every family. Scholars discuss how for Asians, emphasis on collectivism and familial intimacy might prevent providers from probing more about familial relationships. For example, an elderly male grandfather living with his son, daughter-in-law and children might seek treatment at the request of the family. While the son and daughter-in-law are seemingly involved, urge treatment for the father/grandfather and show care, the grandfather might feel left out in decisions and not asked about activities he is interested in doing. It is pertinent for the therapist to assess and include all voices and not assume a thorough understanding of the family from one narrative or perspective.

In some cases, older adults are seen as free babysitters, bringing joy and simultaneously placing restrictions and additional responsibilities on the older adult. In South Asian culture, there is an emphasis on indirect communication that the parents will always provide help. Therefore adult children might place expectations on the older adult without communication of expectations. Roles do not get established, and this might lead to resentment and unresolved conflict. Respect for elders, support, and a strong connection is often expected for the family; however, depending on the nature of the personalities involved, acculturation, and communication level within the family, this might not always happen.

Adult children might also make decisions without parental input and/or not share details with the parents as expected by them. Further, roles slightly reverse for older adults with adult children. Adult children might worry more about the parents, and as a result, they place more limitations and restrictions on the parents, which can frustrate parents who want independence and respect. Situations, like the pandemic and parental illness, might trigger worry in adult children which in turn impacts parent-child relationships. The parents who initially were the caretakers and capable of living independent lives are now in a place where they might need care, which might impact how the adult child(ren) views the parents. Research shows that parents can struggle with being dependent on children and losing a sense of autonomy and independence (Chappell, 1991). Therefore, feelings of bitterness and resentment might ensue. When a parent's health declines, the parent-child relationship declines as well (Kaufman & Uhlenberg, 1998). For example, in the case of Ammu while her health has not declined her daughter views her as more vulnerable and helpless which frustrates Ammu and is often a source of strain and conflict.

DEPRESSION

Research has shown (Karasz et al., 2019) that abuse, and neglect, isolation, and acculturative stress are predictors of depression in the South Asian older adult population. However, depression is often not diagnosed and expressed in the same way as with Euro-American older adults. Somaticizing is a common experience among Asians (Ladhani & Lee, 2009). Therefore it is difficult to discern whether there are actual physical ailments or emotional distress. Understanding the difference between physical and mental concerns is of particular relevance with older South Asians because there is a high likelihood physical symptoms increasing while aging while also developing psychological concerns. Depression might be described as "tension" or as headaches, "sinking heart," "hurting mind," or "hurting heart" (Krause, 1989; Rait & Burns, 1997). Chadda and Deb (2013), describe how the expectations of collectivism, such as maintaining family harmony at all costs and challenges in expressing emotions, may lead to increased stress and conflict and a higher rate of somatization. Somaticizing is the tendency to experience psychological distress in the form of physical complaints or symptoms (Al Busaidi, 2010). South Asian Americans are more likely to seek medical help from a physician or medical professional for these symptoms, However, these symptoms may in fact be a response to social, psychological, emotional, and relational strain.

Further, it should be assessed whether the depression predates immigration or if it is new onset. Diwan and colleagues found that decline in physical health and maintaining traditional South Asian ethnic identity were correlated with depressive symptoms in older South Asians Americans living in the U.S. regardless of English fluency. Further, consistent with research, women were more likely to experience depressive symptoms (Lai, 2004). There are several reasons why this has been a consistent finding. Significant discrepancies exist in gender roles for men and women in South Asian culture. Older South Asian American women might take on more responsibilities and have expectations to impart cultural values such as religious practices, language, and cultural traditions across generations. Additionally, while many earlier immigrant women and second-generation women embody a sense of empowerment and autonomy, there are subtle threads of expectations that being selfless and maintaining the family's strength and resilience are revered. Given the expectation to care and worry for various individuals, older South Asian women, compared to men over function, worry more about others, and feel guilt and more hopelessness when issues arise within the family.

GRIEF AND LOSS

Further, many South Asians experience grief and loss, which can contribute to, and impact recovery from physical ailments (Diwan et al., 2004). Bereavement is a salient concern with the older South Asians "as it can lead to psychological illness such as depression" (Hashim et al., 2013). Further, complicated grief can be expressed through somatic symptoms such as headaches and chest pain (Stroebe et al., 2007). Therefore, the physical complaints might get attention; however, the underlying emotional concerns do not get evaluated. Many South Asian American older adults are experiencing multiple losses such as the loss of an independent, autonomous life, loss of family members, and even loss of friends whom they might have immigrated with to the U.S. For many older South Asians who immigrated earlier, there is a concept of the "acquired family," a group of individuals who were part of the same immigration cohort. These individuals might have been co-workers, studied together, or part of the same religious organization. As a result of an earlier bonding experience, celebrating holidays, birthdays, and sharing babysitting responsibilities, these individuals' loss can be as painful as losing a biological relative. In particular, it should be noted that during the time of COVID-19, many South Asians Americans were not able to mourn and support one another in the same way. Many older South Asians lost family members and friends without having the opportunity to be present. Moreover, they were unable to come together to mourn and pay respect during final funeral services or ceremonies because of restrictions. Lacking the ability to come together as a collective is also a loss felt deeply by many community members. The loss also changes relationships and how people are viewed, especially for women, as seen in the case study above. Not only is Ammu grieving the loss of her husband, but because of the new role of being a widow, people including her daughter have changed their perceptions of her. They now view her as helpless and needing more support.

ELDER MALTREATMENT

Lastly, another area that often does not get openly discussed is maltreatment and abuse of the elderly. As South Asian Americans there is filial piety and respect toward the elderly, so the concept of abusing older adults seems unfathomable; however, this is a reality for many. Researchers have supported the idea that Asians are collectivistic due to the importance placed on the family and the individual's actions affect the family (Farver et al., 2002; Triandis & Gelfand, 1998). Tyyskä et al. (2013) address that many older adults do not discuss negative experiences at home because it might bring shame to the family, so they suffer in silence. Mistreatment does not always come in physical abuse; however, it can be food-related withholding, social isolation, mocking the older adult, and taking the older adult's property and assets. For example, a son manipulating a widowed mother to make him and his wife legally responsible for finances, so the mother-in-law does not have to worry. Once this legal transfer is complete, then the son and daughter-in-law can have full control over the mother's assets and in some cases, medical decisions. Therefore, medication and appropriate medical treatment can be withheld because it is seen as "too expensive." Adult children might engage in ways to Other times, older adults might want to donate funds, spoil grandchildren, or buy gifts and adult children get into arguments with their older parents about "wasting" their money in fear that there might be fewer funds in the inheritance. As a result, the older adult feels stifled and controlled by family members. Some older adults who are not naturalized citizens fear that they will be taken away by the authorities and/or deported (Alvi & Zaidi, 2017). Therefore, providers need to assess how relationships are going within the family and be able to connect with the older adult culturally and linguistically.

Treatment and Barriers

Asian immigrants are often skeptical toward the Western notion of psychotherapy as a mode of healing and support (Chung & Bemak, 2007) as a result of individual, structural/ institutional, and cultural barriers. The importance of naming each of these barriers is salient to culturally responsive treatment and access to mental health therapy among the elderly Asian immigrants in the United States.

At the cultural level, the skepticism toward mental health treatment may be informed by the limited or lack of inclusion of the cultural and religious values that are central to the daily lived experiences of Asian immigrants. For instance, treatment approaches include alternative healing remedies such as Ayurvedic or homeopathic medicine (Inman & Tummala-Narra, 2010) and the use of spiritual and religious leaders such as astrologers, and the significance of asking for "prayers or talismans" from these individuals who were viewed as pious (Inman et al., 2007). Thus, holistic, and indigenous healing strategies coupled with the incorporation of values of interdependence and collaboration and the meaning assigned to aging are important values informing the lived experiences and health related decisions among Asian immigrants. Overlooking the inclusion of such cultural values would render treatment that is not in keeping with the proposed multicultural guidelines that also stress on ecological contexts and values pertaining to the client's identity (American Psychological Association, 2014). Additionally, the lack of cultural responsiveness from therapists, verbal and non-verbal differences in communication, and culturally informed expression of presenting concerns add to barriers in accessing treatment. For example, somatic expressions of mental health concerns are common within the Asian Indian contexts (Inman & Tummala-Narra, 2010), and it is imperative that mental health service providers conduct a culturally sensitive assessment that includes somatic expression of mental health, and the meaning assigned to mental health and somatic concerns.

At the structural and institutional level, language differences between the therapist and the potential client, limited financial resources, restricted access to transportation, and playing the role of a care-taker for children and grandchildren may add to the hesitancy of elderly Asian immigrants seeking treatment (Tummala-Narra et al., 2013). As seen in the case of Ammu, the lack of transportation has prevented her from engaging in social and other obligations, so it is important for the therapist to discuss with the client how easily they can access services. Additionally, the larger values of Western based health care system (e.g., individual goals), and the preference for elderly Asian immigrants to seek support from peer groups and spiritual discourses within group also inform the underutilization of mental health services among the elderly Asian immigrants (Inman & Tummala-Narra, 2010; Mui & Kang, 2006). Furthermore, implications such as inaccurate evaluations leading to misdiagnosis due to the therapist's own blind spots and biases and being unaware of between and within group differences could further impede the trust that Asian immigrants have in the Western based mental health care system (Inman & Tummala-Narra, 2010).

Lastly, at the individual level, factors such as stigma of mental health within South Asian American cultures and families also inform the hesitancy to seek mental health services among the elderly South Asian immigrant population (Bhattacharya & Shibusawa, 2009). This stigma may be reinforced by lack of exposure to mental health counseling and limited understanding of Western views of mental health treatment (Tummala-Narra et al., 2013), and not meeting the client's preference for counselor-client ethnic matching (Uba, 1994). Additional factors contributing to the stigma of mental health and help seeking behaviors is the belief in the model minority stereotype that can lead to minimization and avoidance of one's mental health and social challenges. Moreover, the prevalence of shame and discrimination can further complicate help seeking behaviors, especially mental health treatment (Inman & Yeh, 2007; Kim et al., 2003). The different individual, structural/institutional and cultural barriers to mental health treatment warrant a more holistic, ecological, and socio-cultural lens of awareness, knowledge, and skills on the part of therapists in working with the elderly South Asian American immigrant populations in the United States (Chung & Bemak, 2007; Inman & Tummala-Narra, 2010).

Clinical Strategies

Therapists need to understand the older South Asian client from a sociocultural lens. Congruent with the APA Guidelines for Psychological Practice with Older Adults (APA, 2014) it is recommended that clinicians practice within the scope of their competence, engage in authentic and ongoing self-exploration around any biases toward this group, and engage in continuous education around the needs and sociocultural oppression and marginalization faced by this population. Integrating theories such as Feminist Psychotherapy, Family Systems, Psychodynamics, and Multicultural theories allow for a holistic understanding of the various historical experiences, oppression, and systems the person is living in. It is crucial not to assume homogeneity; however, as discussed, understanding how the person is socially located, values and beliefs, and what messages have been introjected is especially salient to older South Asian Americans. Further, it is crucial for the therapist to understand how to consider sociopolitical factors in addition to race, gender, religion, and physical health, ability status influence clients and their presenting issues. Therapists must learn to acknowledge and attend to the cultural meaning that clients attach to experiences such as loss, grief, health decline, caretaking, and being provided with care. Specifically, it is important to ask specifically about the immigration process and know when one immigrated, what choice they had in the immigration process, challenges experienced before, during, and after, positives about the immigration experience, and the sources of support the individual has in their life back in the country of origin and host country.

Further is vital to understand the differences in symptom expression. For example, as Diwan et al. (2004) suggest, South Asian Americans may not endorse positive affect and are more emotionally reserved, so it is essential to evaluate and assess based on cultural norms and emotional expression. If the clinician is evaluating depression based on Euro-American standards, the client will most likely be pathologized. Rather, assessment and treatment should prioritize what the client believes is important and what feels appropriate within the client's cultural norms. Therapy goals, expectations and informed consent should be clarified and discussed so that the older South Asian American and respective family members understand the purpose of therapy.

Community psychology is particularly impactful. For example, going into physicians' offices, senior centers, residential facilities, nursing homes, and worship places where older South Asian clients might come together allows for ease and familiarity. Rather than requiring these individuals to come to a psychology office, providing seminars, screenings, and availability in a familiar setting can make the transition and idea of psychology less threatening. For example, a group of older South Asian American men attend a community center during the day to play cards, share a meal and attend workshops on health, finances, and more recently mental health. As they attend the series of workshops, they start to discuss various issues and conflicts they have with older adult children and the loss of control around health decline. As the therapist hears these discussions, they start to consider having more workshops for families and children around aging, autonomy, and respect. This is an example of how to bring psychoeducation to the community and allow for individuals and families to gather information in a less stigmatizing manner.

It is crucial to allow older South Asians to share experiences, journeys, hopes, and dreams that might not have worked out while all validating the challenge of coming to another socioculturally different country. Further, it is essential to provide validation around experiences of discrimination. Lastly, it is essential to serve as a case manager and advocate for older South Asian clients to find resources, relationships, and books to deepen and normalize their experiences.

Case Study Discussion

Ammu is a first-generation immigrant and has been in the U.S. for 45 years. She has worked as a nurse and considers herself to be independent, however, she wants people to recognize the loss and that she is still hurting. Her frustration is that people have dichotomized her experience, that either she is a helpless widow that needs to be instructed by her daughter or she is perfectly fine and can't mourn her husband. She might not know what is appropriate given all the mixed-messages. It is often challenging for people to find a grey area, and especially an older adult who is going through a loss is trying to process grief from the cultural context of showing emotional restraint. She does not feel fine emotionally and often has stomach upsets especially around the time of dealing with any financial and estate matters. She shares that when she came to this country, she thought she would be here forever with Prakash and the country is feeling empty without him. First, it should be established Ammu has experienced a loss and what this represents to her. Clinically, it is important to provide Ammu with the opportunity to discuss her experiences with Prakash and who he was to her. For many older adults it is important to provide an opportunity to share their story. The clinician should be mindful of early migration experiences, establishing and life in the U.S., navigating two cultures, and raising children. Narratives provide the clinician the opportunity to hear about the social and familial context, roles established, while also allowing for Ammu to share her emotions regarding her loss and the life she shared with Prakash. It is important for the clinician to understand the somatic complaints and normalize and validate that we can experience strain when we are worried or upset about something, thus providing the client with the opportunity to be heard and recognized, while also sharing their concerns further.

Ammu shares that Prakash was an accountant and smart about finances better than she did. It is important for the clinician to understand why those times around financial and estate decisions bring about particular distress because of who Prakash was in her life. Ammu must miss Prakash especially during the times of handling finances because of how much she respected his expertise in finance. The clinician should help identify and normalize that those decisions seem difficult given that it reminds Ammu of Prakash's strengths and her loss. The clinician should be mindful of any internalized ageism and sexism. Does she feel as though she can make decisions? How have they made decisions in the past? What has she observed from Prakash that can empower her to feel confident knowing that these are decisions she can make as well? Secondly, the relationship with the daughter should be discussed where Maya wants Ammu to be fine and tells her what to do. Ammu finds this aggravating because now she is seen as someone who has to be told what to feel and what to do. In what ways is Maya treating her mother as someone who is incapable of being on her own? There is an intersectional oppression of age, gender and marital status which needs to be explored here. It is important to explore Ammu's acculturation, level of communication style, and how she wishes to address these concerns with Maya.

Reflection Questions

*   What might be some countertransference issues for you in this case?
*   How would things be different if Ammu was a recent immigrant?
*   What would be the pros and cons of including Maya in the treatment?

Summary

Overall, there are within and in-between group differences among older South Asian Americans contingent on the age of migration, the wave of migration, and the process of migration by itself. As clinicians and practitioners it is imperative on us to self-reflect and increase awareness of our own biases and attitudes when working with this population. In keeping with the APA Multicultural guidelines (2017) and the APA Guidelines for Psychological Practice with Older Adults (APA, 2014). This chapter also illustrates the need for an ecological approach that includes cultural values, level of acculturation between family members, a match in language proficiency between therapist and client, and taking into consideration a collectivist approach that includes holistic interventions, group support, and the potential involvement of family members based on the client's preferences. This also includes the therapist's awareness and knowledge of the use of verbal and non-verbal cues in therapy when working with older South Asian Americans in the United States this informs the holistic approach, mind and body connection, individualist and collectivist ideas, a safe space in therapy, and access to community support.

References

Al Busaidi Z.Q. (2010). The concept of Somatisation: A cross-cultural perspective. *Sultan Qaboos University Medical Journal, 10*(2), 180–186.

Alvi, S., & Zaidi, A.U. (2017). Invisible voices: An intersectional exploration of quality of life for elderly South Asian immigrant women in a canadian sample. *Journal of Cross-Cultural Gerontology, 32*(2), 147–170. 10.1007/s10823-017-9315-7

American Psychological Association. (2014). Guidelines for psychological practice with older adults. *American Psychologist, 69*(1), 34–65. 10.1037/a0035063

American Psychological Association. (2017). Multicultural guidelines: An ecological approach to context, identity, and intersectionality, 2017. *Adopted by the APA Council of Representatives in August 2017.* Retrieved from https://www.apa.org/about/policy/multicultural-guidelines

Balgopal, P.R. (1999). Getting old in the U.S.: Dilemmas of Indo-Americans. *The Journal of Sociology & Social Welfare, 26*(1), 51–68. Retrieved from https://scholarworks.wmich.edu/cgi/viewcontent.cgi?article=2544&context=jssw

Berry, J.W. (1990). Psychology of acculturation: Understanding individuals moving between cultures. In R.W. Brislin (Ed.), *Applied cross cultural psychology*, (pp. 232–253). Newbury Park, CA: Sage Publications, Inc.

Bhattacharya, G., & Shibusawa, T. (2009). Experiences of aging among immigrants from India to the United States: Social work practice in a global context. *Journal of Gerontological Social Work, 52*, 445–462. 10.1080/01634370902983112

Casado, B.L., & Leung, P. (2002). Migratory grief and depression among elderly Chinese American immigrants. *Journal of Gerontological Social Work, 36*(1–2), 5–26.

Chadda, R.K., & Deb, K.S. (2013). Indian family systems, collectivistic society and psychotherapy. *Indian Journal of Psychiatry, 55*(Suppl 2), S299.

Chan, K. (2020). The association of acculturation with overt and covert perceived discrimination for older Asian Americans. *Social Work Research, 44*(1), 59–71.

Chappell, N.L. (1991). Role of family and friends in quality of life. In J.E. Birren & J.E. Lubben (Eds.), *Concept and measurement of quality of life in the frail elderly* (pp. 171–190). San Diego: Academic Press.

Chung, R.C.-Y., & Bemak, F. (2007). Asian immigrants and refugees. In F.T.L. Leong, A.G. Inman, A. Ebreo, L.H. Yang, L. Kinoshita, & M. Fu (Eds.), *Handbook of Asian American psychology* (2nd ed., pp. 227–243). Thousand Oaks, CA: Sage Publications.

Clement, R., Michaud, C., & Noels, K.A. (1998). Acculturative effects of social support in an intergroup contact situation. *Revue Quebecoise de Psychologie, 19*, 189–210.

Crenshaw, K. (1989). Demarginalizing the intersection of race and sex: A black Feminist critique of antidiscrimination doctrine, Feminist theory and antiracist politics. *University of Chicago Legal Forum, 1989*(1), 139.

Diwan, S. Jonnalagadda, S.S., & Gupta, R. (2004). Differences in the structure of depression among older Asian Indian immigrants in the United States. *Journal of Applied Gerontology, 23*, 370–384. 10.1177/0733464804270584

Dowd, J., & Bengston, V. (1978). Aging in minority populations. An examination of the double jeopardy hypothesis. *Journal of Gerontology, 33*(3), 427–436.

Ehrensaft, E., & Tousignant, M. (2006). Immigration and resilience. In D.L. Sam & J.W. Berry (Eds.), *The Cambridge handbook of acculturation psychology* (pp. 469–483). New York: Cambridge University Press.

Erikson, E.H., Erikson, J., & Kivnick, H.Q. (1986). *Vital involvement in old age.* New York: W.W. Norton & Co.

Espin, O.M. (1987). Psychological impact of migration on Latinas: Implications for psychotherapeutic practice. *Psychology of Women Quarterly, 11*, 489–503.

Everett, B.G., Onge, J.S., & Mollborn, S. (2016). Effects of minority status and perceived discrimination on mental health. *Population Research and Policy Review, 35*, 445–469. 10.1007/s11113-016-9391-3

Farver, J.M., Narang, S.K., & Bhadha, B.R. (2002). East meets west: Ethnic identity, acculturation, and conflict in Asian Indian families. *Journal of Family Psychology, 16*, 338–350.

Gates, T. (2017). Chosen families. In J. Carlson, & S. Dermer (Eds.), *The sage encyclopedia of marriage, family, and couples counseling* (Vol. 1, pp. 240–242). Thousand Oaks, CA: SAGE Publications. 10.4135/9781483369532.n74

Hashim, S.M., Eng, T.C., Tohit, N., & Wahab, S. (2013). Bereavement in the elderly: The role of primary care. *Mental Health in Family Medicine, 10*(3), 159–162.

Hernandez, A.M., & Bigatti, S.M. (2010). Depression among older Mexican American caregivers. *Cultural Diversity & Ethnic Minority Psychology, 16*, 50–58. 10.1037/a0015867

Hovey, J.D. (2000). Acculturative stress, depression, and suicidal ideation in Mexican immigrants. *Cultural Diversity & Ethnic Minority Psychology, 6*, 134–151.

Inman, A.G., & Tummala-Narra, P. (2010). Clinical competencies in working with immigrant communities. In J.A.E. Cornish, B.A. Schreier, L.I. Nadkarni, L.H. Metzger, & E.R. Rodolfa (Eds.), *Handbook of multicultural counseling competencies* (pp. 117–152). Hoboken, NJ: John Wiley & Sons, Inc.

Inman, A.G., & Yeh, C.J. (2007). Asian American stress and coping post-9/11. In F. T. L. Leong, A. G. Inman, A. Ebreo, L. Kinoshita, & L. H. Yang (Eds.), *Handbook of Asian American psychology* (2nd ed., pp. 323–339). Thousand Oaks, CA: Sage Publications.

Inman, A.G., Yeh, C.J., Madan-Bahel, A., & Nath, S. (2007). Bereavement and coping of South Asian families post 9/11. *Journal of Multicultural Counseling and Development, 35*, 101–115. 10.1002/j.2161-1912.2007.tb00053.x

Karasz, A., Gany, F., Escobar, J., Flores, C., Prasad, L., Inman, A., Kalasapudi, V., Kosi, R., Murthy, M., Leng, J., & Diwan, S. (2019). Mental health and stress among South Asians. *Journal of Immigrant and Minority Health, 21*(1), 7–14. 10.1007/s10903-016-0501-4

Kaufman, G., & Uhlenberg, P. (1998). Effects of life course transitions on the quality of relationships between adult children and their parents. *Journal of Marriage and the Family, 60*(4), 924–938. 10.2307/353635

Kim, B.S.K., Brenner, B.R., Liang, C.T.H., & Asay, P.A. (2003). A qualitative study of adaptation experiences of 1.5-generation Asian Americans. *Cultural Diversity and Ethnic Minority Psychology, 9*, 156–170. 10.1037/1099-9809.9.2.156

Kim, H.K., & McKenry, P.C. (1998). Social networks and support: A comparison of African Americans, Asian Americans, Caucasians, and Hispanics. *Journal of Comparative Family Studies, 29*(2), 313–334.

Krause, I.B. (1989). Sinking heart: A Punjabi communication of distress. *Social Science & Medicine, 29*(4), 563–575.

Krause, N. (2006). Exploring the stress-Buffering effects of church-based and secular social support on self-Rated health in late life, *The Journals of Gerontology: Series B, 61*(1), S35–S43. 10.1093/geronb/61.1.S35

Kwak, K., & Berry, W.J. (2001). Generational differences in acculturation among Asian families in Canada: A comparison of Vietnamese, Korean, and East-Indian groups. *International Journal of Psychology, 36*, 152–162. 10.1080/00207590042000119

Ladhani, S., & Lee, S. (2009). Physical health and wellness. In N. Tewari & A. N. Alvarez (Eds.), *Asian American Psychology: Current Perspectives* (pp. 499–518). New York: Taylor and Francis Group.

Lai, D.W. (2004). Impact of culture on depressive symptoms of elderly chinese immigrants. *The Canadian Journal of Psychiatry, 49*(12), 820–827. 10.1177/070674370404901205

Lai, D.W.L., & Surood, S. (2009). Chinese health beliefs of older chinese in canada. *Journal of Aging and Health, 21*(1), 38–62. 10.1177/0898264308328636

Lai, D.W.L., & Chau, S. B. (2007). Effects of service barriers on health status of older Chinese immigrants in Canada. *Social Work, 52*, 261–269. 10.1093/sw/52.3.261

Lai, D.W.L., & Surood, S. (2013). Effect of service barriers on health status of aging South Asian immigrants in Calgary, Canada. *Health & Social Work, 38*(1), 41–50. 10.1093/hsw/hls065

Lalonde, R.N., & Cameron, J.E. (1993). An intergroup perspective on immigrant acculturation with a focus on collective strategies. *International Journal of Psychology*, *28*, 57–74. 10.1080/002075993 08246918

Levin, J.S., & Chatters, L.M. (1998). Religion, health, and psychological well-being in older adults: Findings from three national surveys. *Journal of Aging and Health*, *10*(4), 504–531.

Merz, E., Ozeke-Kocabas, E., Oort, J.F., & Schuengel, C. (2009). Intergenerational family solidarity: Value differences between immigrant groups and generations. *Journal of Family Psychology*, *23*, 291–300. 10.1037/a0015819

Mui, A.C., & Kang, S.-Y. (2006). Acculturation stress and depression among Asian immigrant elders. *Social Work*, *51*(3), 243–255. 10.1093/sw/51.3.243

Nandan, M. (2007). "Waves" of Asian Indian elderly immigrants: What can practitioners learn? *Journal of Cross-Cultural Gerontology*, *22*, 389–404. 10.1007/s10823-007-9042-6

Olmedo, E.L., & Padilla, A.M. (1978). Empirical and construct validation of a measure of acculturation for Mexican Americans. *Journal of Social Psychology*, *105*, 179–187.

Pereira, H., & Costa, P.A. (2016). Modeling the impact of social discrimination on the physical and mental health of Portuguese gay, lesbian and bisexual people. *Innovation: The European Journal of Social Science Research*, *29*(2), 205–217, 10.1080/13511610.2016.1157683

Pillari, V. (2005). Indian Hindu families. In M. McGoldrick, J. Giordano, & N. Garcia-Preto (Eds.). *Ethnicity and family therapy*, (pp. 395–406). New York, NY: The Guilford Press.

Rahman, Z., & Paik, S.J. (2017). South Asian immigration and education in the U.S.: historical and social contexts. *Social and Education History*, *6*(1), 26–52. 10.17583/hse.2017.2393

Rait, G., & Burns, A. (1997). Appreciating background and culture: The South Asian elderly and mental health. *International Journal of Geriatric Psychiatry*, *12*(10), 973–977.

Rastogi, M. (2007). Coping with transitions in Asian Indian families: Systemic clinical interventions with immigrants. *Journal of Systemic Therapies*, *26*, 55–67. 10.1521/jsyt.2007.26.2.55

Salgado de Snyder, V.N. (1987). *Mexican immigrant women: The relationship of ethnic loyalty and social support to acculturative stress and depressive symptomatology*. Spanish Speaking Mental Health Research Center. Occasional Paper No. 22.

SAALT (2019, April). *Demographic snapshot of South Asians in the United States April 2019*. Retrieved March 29, 2020, from https://saalt.org/wp-content/uploads/2019/04/SAALT-Demographic-Snapshot-2019.pdf

Samuel, T. (2009). Acculturative stress: South Asian immigrant women's experiences in canada's atlantic Provinces, *Journal of Immigrant & Refugee Studies*, *7*(1), 16–34. 10.1080/15562940802 687207

Sandil, R., Robinson, M., Brewster, M.E., Wong, S., & Geiger, E. (2015). Negotiating multiple marginalizations: Experiences of South Asian LGBQ individuals. *Cultural Diversity and Ethnic Minority Psychology*, *21*(1), 76.

Sorkin, D.H., Nguyen, H., & Ngo-Metzger, Q. (2011). Assessing the mental health needs and barriers to care among a diverse sample of Asian American older adults. *Journal of General Internal Medicine*, *26*(6), 595–602. 10.1007/s11606-010-1612-6

Stroebe, M., Schut, H., & Stroebe, W. (2007). Health outcomes of Bereavement. *The Lancet*, *370*(9603), 1960–1973.

Triandis, H.C., & Gelfand, M.J. (1998). Converging measurement of horizontal and vertical individualism and collectivism. *Journal of Personality and Social Psychology*, *74*, 118–128.

Tsai-Chae, H.A., & Nagata, K.D. (2008). Asian values and perceptions of intergenerational family conflict among Asian American students. *Cultural Diversity and Ethnic Minority Psychology*, *14*, 205–214. 10.1037/1099-9809.14.3.205

Tummala-Narra, P., Sathasivam-Rueckert, N., & Sundaram, S. (2013). Voices of older Asian Indian immigrants: Mental health implications. *Professional Psychology: Research and Practice*, *44*, 1–10. 10/1037/a0027809

Tyyskä, V., Dinshaw, F.M., Redmond, C., & Gomes, F. (2013). "Where we have come and are now Trapped": Views of victims and service providers on abuse of older adults in tamil and Punjabi families. *Canadian Ethnic Studies*, *44*(3), 59–77.

Uba, L. (1994). *Asian Americans: Personality patterns, identity, and mental health.* New York: Guilford Press.

U.S. Census Bureau. (2010). Facts for features: Asian/Pacific American heritage month: May 2011. Retrieved from https://www.census.gov/newsroom/releases/archives/facts%5ffor%5ffeatures%5fspecial%5feditions/cb11-ff06.html

Wilmoth, J.M., & Chen, P.C. (2003). Immigrant status, living arrangements, and depressive symptoms among middle-aged and older adults. *The Journals of Gerontology Series B: Psychological Sciences and Social Sciences, 58*(5), S305–S313.

Ying, Y. (1999). Strengthening intergenerational/intercultural ties in migrant families: A new intervention for parents. *Journal of Community Psychology, 27,* 89–96. 10.1002/(SICI)1520-6629(199901)27:1<89::AID-JCOP6>3.0.CO;2-O

Yu, E.S.H. (1986). Health of the Chinese elderly in America. *Research on Aging, 5*(1), 84–109.

13 Exploring the Nuanced South Asian American Therapeutic Relationship

Sheetal Shah and Munisa Haque

Case Overview

"You seem like my aunt," Sara stated as she sat down to start the intake session. The client is a 19-year-old, Muslim identified, second generation, Pakistani-American cisgendered female, who is an undergraduate student at a large university. She was referred to the college counseling center by an academic advisor because she was perilously close to being dismissed that semester for poor grades. Sara reported that she "can't focus" and doesn't want her parents to know about her academic struggles, stating, "you know how Desi parents are ..." She added that she had seen a therapist at the counseling center before for academic issues, but decided not to continue, stating "they told me I had depression, and referred me to a psychiatrist." She seemed hesitant to try therapy again but said that a friend urged her to reach out to the South Asian identified therapist on the counseling staff. During the intake session, the client commented to the therapist—"you looked so familiar, I think I've seen you at the community Iftar last year."

Introduction

Forming a good therapeutic relationship with a client is important in the process of psychotherapy (Hill & Knox, 2009), and research has shown that the therapeutic alliance is not only a strong predictor (Norcross, 2002) but a common factor that facilitates positive client outcomes (Hill & Knox, 2009). Much of the existing literature indicates that the therapeutic relationship is a key part of the change process in therapy, even more than significant techniques (Vasquez, 2007). Therapeutic relationships can be defined as "feelings and attitudes that therapists and clients have toward one another and how these are expressed" (Norcross, 2010, p. 113). A good therapeutic relationship can help a client feel understood, seen, and accepted, and hopefully to open up more as a result (Lambert & Barley, 2001). Part of having a good therapeutic relationship is having good cultural awareness and sensitivity in working with clients. This chapter will focus on the therapeutic relationship between South Asian American identified therapists working with South Asian identified clients.

South Asian Americans are a heterogeneous group, diverse in ethnic and regional identities, immigration histories, acculturation processes, languages spoken, religious practices, cultural values, socioeconomic status, and acculturation levels (Das & Kemp, 1997; Tewari, 2009). It is important in the process of therapeutic alliance building, to understand these aspects of a client who identifies as South Asian American, in addition to their demographic features, such as sexual orientation, education/job status, and more. South Asian Americans who pursue therapy prefer an active, direct, and goal-oriented approach that focuses on practical tasks (Tewari, 2009). South Asian American clients may search for and feel most

DOI: 10.4324/9781003081548-13

comfortable with a therapist who is warm, directive, and interested in establishing a therapeutic alliance similar to a relationship they may have with a respected and educated elder in the community (Das & Kemp, 1997). Depending on the client's exposure and experience with therapy, it is important for the therapist to be prepared to discuss goals and expectations from treatment with the client. Additionally, therapists will need to consider cultural adaptations to treatment. For example, adapting empirically sound techniques like Cognitive Behavior Therapy (CBT), understanding the use of emotional language, and utilizing interventions such as "positive religious coping" are ways to engage the client and foster relevancy in the therapeutic process (Mir et al., 2019). As with any therapy relationships, the therapist will want to be aware of what may be the most effective modality of treatment. Lastly, clients may have to be educated on the therapeutic process, as well as expectations of therapy, such as completing homework, dual relationships, and active participation during sessions.

This chapter will focus on specific, nuanced skills and personal factors that can influence the formation of a strong therapeutic relationship with therapists and clients that share similar identities. Salient themes that explore cultural nuances, countertransference, positive therapeutic experiences (or the joys), and shared cultural experiences that exist in the therapeutic relationship will be highlighted. The authors will share personal stories and use a clinical case example to highlight challenges, progress, and lessons learnt as well as research that can explore the impact of culture and shared cultural identities in the therapeutic dyad on the therapeutic relationship.

Cultural Competency and Humility with South Asian American Clients

Building a collaborative, trusting relationship is essential in therapy (Hovarth, 2001). As therapists consider working with South Asian American clients, therapists' cultural competency should be informed by a general understanding of South Asian American culture but also better understood by exploring clients' identities, social context, and values. The South Asian American (SAA) community, like other cultural groups, is not homogeneous: beliefs, values, and behaviors will vary based on religion, language, country of origin, social context in the host country, and individual experiences (Ibrahim et al., 1997). Kirmayer (2012) states, cultural competence must consider "how to meld recognition of, and respect for, the identity of individuals and communities with attention to the dynamic, contested, and often highly politicized nature of individuals' interactions with collectivities, both local and global" (pp. 154). Taking a cultural humility approach will make space for a collaborative, open and respectful approach to relationship building. Cultural humility is the concept that an individual engages in lifelong learning, not only about another individual, but also in examining one's self (Hook et al., 2013), which leads to more openness to diversity with clients. Cultural humility is the "ability to maintain an interpersonal stance that is other-oriented" (Tervalon & Murray-Garcia, 1998). Cultural humility is found to be attributed to "openness, self-awareness, egoless, supportive interactions, and self-reflection and critique" (Foronda et al., 2016). Additionally, these authors suggest that having cultural humility leads to "mutual empowerment, partnerships, respect, optimal care, and lifelong learning" all which enhance the therapeutic relationship. Researchers have also found that cultural humility has led to positive working alliances (Hook et al., 2013).

Thus, when working with clients who hold similar identities, the therapeutic relationship building becomes more nuanced. To practice cultural competence and cultural humility, Therapists must have a good understanding of their own identities and also be cognizant of the ways in which they present in therapy as well as identities that they may want to self-disclose or be ready to discuss. In addition, seeking the support of supervision or consultation with colleagues is a way to be self- aware and consistently check for countertransference issues, that is, therapists must have an awareness of how they may be responding to a clients' identity and be open to learning more about this process. When meeting with a client for the first time, the therapist will want to understand the client's identities stated (on paperwork) and explored (with client), taking note of similarities and differences. The more a therapist delves into the nuances of identity, we assume, the more the client will feel seen by the therapist and the more the therapist has to reflect regarding the client. For example, it may be important to not just know the country of origin, but region, languages spoken, religious orientation, and acculturation history. A therapist may be able to start to assess and understand these nuances simply by asking clients' how to correctly pronounce their names and the origin of their names. For example, a client may say "My name in Hindi means...," giving the therapist a chance to not only understand the name and how to pronounce it but also an opportunity to discuss the client's culture and ethnicity. This also sets the tone that culture will be a basis of integration for their therapy.

Cultural Considerations for Relationship Building

Paying attention to and checking in about the therapeutic relationship helps clients process their feelings, allows the client to be present with their feelings, enhances relationships, and to "transfer their learning to other relationships" (Hill & Knox, 2009). Social characteristics such as gender, age, and race/ethnicity can affect the therapeutic relationship through client attributions to themselves and others based on social expectations (Murphy et al., 2004). Furthermore, assumptions made by individuals can lead to "unexpected transference and countertransference" (Gupta, 2017). We explore some cultural considerations that should be made, with the assumption that a cultural humility stance is taken so that a therapist understands themselves as they build a relationship with their client.

For many collectivistic cultures such as South Asian American culture, "uncles and aunties" is the term denoted to anyone seen as an extension of one's community or family. It could be easy for these prescribed roles to be transferred on to the therapist, given the gender norms. For example, the terms "uncle and aunties" and the respective deviations can inadvertently be transferred to the therapist, there could be relational impacts that are important to explore. For example, is the client withholding information or are they expressing truthful reactions in therapy? Is the client afraid of being judged? Does the client worry about confidentiality? Is the client engaging in impression management? Conversely, if the therapist also starts to see the client as a part of the community, countertransference issues can also arise. A therapist will want to contemplate the potential impact on the therapeutic relationship. Is the therapist able to maintain a non-judgmental stance? Is the therapist able to separate their own values or opinions, so that they do not overlap onto the client's current struggles and needs? Essentially, the therapist should be aware of dynamics that may be created as South Asian American culture tends to be group focused (Durvasula & Mylvaganam, 1994), or *allocentric*, placing greater importance on the group or family than on the individual.

Another cultural consideration to understand is acculturative stress which is the process an individual undergoes when balancing two or multiple cultures (Cabassa, 2003). The process consists of social and psychological interactions between individuals of different cultures (Berry, 1997; Ryder et al., 2000). Our understanding of our identities and the ways we integrate or separate various aspects of culture need to be understood. A therapist working with a South Asian American client should consider the influence of culture on a person's interpersonal and intrapersonal experiences, including values orientation, acculturation status, family dynamics, relationships, and dating (Inman & Tewari, 2003).

Furthermore, there can be internal conflicts that arise between a therapist or client depending on a person's desire for belonging. This adaptive and psychological process can be further complicated if there are differences between acculturation levels, varying immigration journeys of the therapist and the client, or if the client identifies as second generation while the therapist is a first generation immigrant.

Therefore, clinicians working with South Asian Americans should have awareness and understanding of family immigration history. The experience of immigrating and settling in the United States varies for South Asian American individuals and families. Initial waves of South Asians immigrating to the United States began in 1898, largely from India, present-day Pakistan, and Bangladesh (Ibrahim et al., 1997) leading to the United States government passing the 1965 Immigration and Nationality Act that allowed South Asians to immigrant in larger numbers again (Kurien, 2005). Following the 1965 act, a large percentage of South Asians who immigrated to the United States were professionals, including doctors, engineers, scientists, academicians, and students seeking professional degrees in American universities. The 1980 Reunification Act brought a later wave of less-educated South Asian immigrants, who were less fluent in English and who were often lower wage earners (Madathil & Sandhu, 2007). The year or era of when a family or individual emigrates may likely impact their acculturation levels. Immigration experiences also impact one's identity formation. For example, a person who is a more recent immigrant entering the USA on a student or work VISA may find it harder to relate to those who identify as second or third generation South Asians. Despite having shared ethnic, religious, or cultural identity, growing up in different countries makes fitting in difficult because of the barriers in understanding mainstream culture. Life experiences in a natal country may vastly differ from those in the adoptive country, which may contribute to feelings of isolation, loneliness, and not belonging. Differences in acculturation levels need to be explored to help understand the lived experience and identify needs/concerns of the client.

Gender and sexuality are particularly important factors to consider. However, South Asian American culture also has nuanced gender expectations, usually stemming from a patriarchal value system. Traditional South Asian American families follow a patriarchal system (Durvasula & Mylvaganam, 1994) in which the head of the family is typically the eldest male of the household (Juthani, 2001). Pressures to conform to traditional gender norms can be a source of conflict but also a source of judgment. This can be particularly hard for gender-non-conforming folks, or people challenging the traditional gender norms of their heritage culture. For example, women in South Asian cultures are often reared to be more diligent and adept at housework or household chores and if they don't meet those gender expectations, there is often a judgment placed on them.

There can be countertransference or transference that occurs in the therapeutic relationship, particularly around gender roles, such as the "mother figure" or the "auntie figure" which is highlighted in the case presentation later in the text. It is common for folks with similar identities to extrapolate certain roles or expectations onto others. Many older women are considered "aunties" as a form of respect and community. So a South Asian American identified therapist who is older, can easily fit into that gendered expectation. And while a client may be swayed to show that deference, it will be important for the therapist to recognize how this nuance impacts the relational dynamic. Power differentials are also present in the room between the client and therapists. Addressing power differences as well as having awareness of the social hierarchical impact on the relationship is important. How is the client addressing the therapist? How may clients view therapists with regards to parallels in community framework, such as seeing a therapist as "auntie" as discussed previously?

Given the emphasis on heterosexuality in South Asian culture and the predominance of traditional cis-gender roles and domestic households, coming out as lesbian, gay, bisexual, transgender, or queer, can be difficult for South Asian Americans (Madathil & Sandhu, 2007). Families, especially parents, often have negative attitudes and biases toward those in the queer community (Rosario et al., 2004). Family structure and adherence to religion play large roles in coming to terms with one's sexual orientation and the coming out process for LGBTQ South Asian Americans. Social desirability and conformity are important, and someone struggling with sexual orientation issues may fear being shunned or rejected. A study by Bhugra (1997) found that siblings are more likely to be used as confidants regarding sexual orientation but that there are significant struggles in coming out to parents and extended family members. An important component when working with individuals who hold intersecting identities related to ethnicity, sexual orientation, religion, and other cultural influences is distinguishing between external stressors (i.e., familial, society, and environmental) and those that stem from maladaptive thoughts about the self. In both cases, it is important to validate a South Asian Americans' unique experience in their coming out process and assess sources of support and discord and their impact on the client's thought process. Many assumptions can be made and a therapist will want to check into the process of understanding gender and sexuality.

Culturally Relevant Assessment and Treatment

Depending on the client's exposure and experience with therapy, it is important to be prepared to discuss expectations of the therapist and treatment. Clients may have to be educated on the therapeutic process and expectations of therapy. Clients may view therapy as a form of advice seeking or may assume it is a quick process and not understand the typical therapeutic treatment trajectory, especially because there is stigma regarding accessing mental health support in the South Asian American communities.

Ethically and legally, informed consent is required prior to the commencement of therapy. With this process, a therapist's job is to assure a client of their rights and explain what they are committing to when starting therapy, as well as initiating the process of orienting a client to the therapeutic process. With the process of orienting a client to therapy, it is particularly important to emphasize the confidentiality portion and make room for questions from the client. A common question with South Asian American identified clients is about the potential of dual relationships or the worry about having people or communities in common and how that would be handled. If the client from the South Asian American community is collectivistic and community oriented, there can be increased fears and realistic chances of seeing the client at external events or having people, places, or community attachments in common. For example, a client may attend the same local temple for Diwali festivities or attend the South Asian American community Ramadan dinner. A reassurance about confidentiality and what that means needs to be emphasized. If crossed paths did occur, the therapist should assure the client that it would be explored in future therapy sessions and potential impacts to the therapeutic relationship be addressed. This is also true if the therapist works in a small setting (college counseling where they are a presence on campus) or small town. Because the South Asian American community is collectivistic there is also a fear of "gossip" therefore, assurance is needed that what is shared in therapy is the client's truth and it will not be shared elsewhere (outside of the limits of confidentiality). Therapists are encouraged to refer to their respective ethics codes and consult to assure dual or multiple relationships do not impair objectivity or cause harm to the client.

Culturally sensitive assessment and questioning is important when working with clients of similar identities, as a client may be guarded due to fear of being judged. Additionally, feelings of shame may also be a motivating factor for hesitancy in sharing sensitive information, or disclosing information usually considered taboo culturally (alcohol or drug consumption, sex or sexuality, in some instance, suicidality or self harm behaviors)—recognition of different means of expressing distress, mental health symptoms and context are critical. For example, a client may express physiological symptoms of depression such as fatigue or headaches versus sadness or disconnection. Clients need to feel comfortable answering questions so that they do not feel pathologized, but rather normalized and open. Thus, therapists need to be thoughtful in their approach to assessment, questioning, and conceptualizing a client's distress. Clients also have varied coping methods, some that may be culturally unacceptable or taboo. For example, a client may be engaging in binge drinking behaviors, which may be frowned upon by culture and family norms. Another example may be sexual behaviors such as promiscuity, whereby a client may feel the need to hide sexuality as it could be seen as demeaning to talk about. In either example, a therapist will want to take a non-judgmental stance, where they assure the client that their confidentiality is protected. If a therapist senses that a client is withholding information, they may want to clarify the role again and assure a safe space. In addition, acknowledging a lack of verbiage in native languages for taboo topics can be helpful in normalizing topics like sex and sexuality. For example, a Sikh Punjabi female client was having a hard time talking about her sexual health when it came to dating. The therapist noted that when this topic came up in therapy, the client would be less forthcoming. The therapist shared these observations with the client and reassured the client that whatever she chose to share was acceptable, and that should she want to share more, that she would be met with openness and without judgment. The therapist acknowledged that talking about these topics were considered taboo in the cultural context. The therapist used strategic self-disclosure by noting that even in her native Gujarati language, the therapist was not aware of the language for sex. The therapist did this in a humorous way, to break the tension, but also in order to acknowledge the challenge of exploring these topics within culture groups. Both assurance about therapy as a safe space and naming the taboo topics, helped normalize the client's struggle, allowing the client to explore this topic with more openness in therapy.

Additionally, the client may be worrying that their social and cultural groups are witnessing their current struggle in a certain way. A client's family/friends/community system may be a source of support but also a source of stress. Asking clarifying questions can help better assess this factor. A client's parent may be telling the client to "be strong" and "focus more," rather than empathizing with and understanding their struggles. For example, a client grew up in a devout Sri Lankan American Christian household and attended church services with their family on a regular basis but has since emigrated and is no longer as connected to the church. The client is experiencing mental health challenges in addition to loneliness, however their family sees their struggle as a disconnection from faith and religious traditions. Oftentimes, presence of mental health challenges are minimized and trivialized by family members due to cultural stigma and lack of mental health awareness. Reframing mental health challenges as due to a lack of religiosity or faith—("you should pray more") can also be shaming for the client suffering from these challenges who may then internalize these statements as a deficit within themselves. Therefore, being aware of cultural specific barriers to help seeking is important, as well as validating and normalizing mental health issues in order to break down internalized stigma and pathologizing presenting concerns.

As the therapeutic process commences, self-disclosure can be used as an important strategic intervention to facilitate rapport building, create trust, encourage engagement, validate and normalize client's experiences, as well as encourage clients to feel comfortable sharing information in sessions (Lee, 2014). Self-disclosure can be defined by the "revealing of something personal" (Hill et al., 2018). Self-disclosure by therapists happens, whether verbally (therapist verbally sharing) or non-verbally (i.e., a clothing or jewelry worn such as a Hijab or a wedding ring). There are differences in how self-disclosure is utilized by a therapist based on theoretical orientations, client considerations and therapy styles (Hill et al., 2018). When working with a South Asian American client, a therapist may choose to disclose shared or different identities, as encouraged for cultural humility and client understanding. But further, therapists may choose to self-disclose similarities or understandings of various processes that may occur for clients (Hill et al., 2018). For example, a client may inquire to see if the therapist understands them, such as "have you been to India recently?" A therapist may disclose, "yes, my family and I have often visited, and I went last December." The client in this scenario may say, "okay, you get how when we go there, my family sees me as American; and when I'm in America, I'm seen as Indian. You get that, right?" With this example, the therapist could further share and self-disclose to continue to help a client go deeper in their process of exploring their bicultural identity, if appropriate.

Case Study Discussion

As mentioned in the opening case, "Sara" grew up in a two-parent household, a couple of hours away from the university. Her parents are immigrants who grew up in Pakistan, had an "arranged marriage" (their respective families agreed on a marital alliance). She states offhandedly that she "hates the idea of this type of marriage." Sara and her younger sibling were born in America, after her parents emigrated. Her father has been employed in the tech industry for the past few years, mother has been a stay at home parent, despite completing a bachelor's degree in finance—"Mom wanted to work but my Dad's family was not happy about it, so she was not able to." Mother volunteers at the younger sibling's school. I sensed Sara's hesitancy around disclosing additional details about her family in the initial intake sessions. This is fairly common among clients who might carry shame and guilt about sharing family issues with others outside the family, fear of being judged, and stigma around seeking therapeutic support. Sara had also not completed some questions pertaining to substance use and sexual history, on the intake questionnaire. While gathering information regarding sexual history, sexual orientation, alcohol and substance use is a critical component of initial assessment, therapists should be aware that these questions can also be a source of shame, fear, hesitancy for the client, as well as seem presumptuous and judgmental for certain clients particularly when the therapist and client have a shared identity. For example, many Muslims generally abstain from alcohol and recreational drug consumption, as it is a religious taboo, therefore, when asked these questions by a Muslim identified therapist, a client who also shares that identity might feel shame at disclosing use, or conversely, may feel offended by the question if they abstain from alcohol and drugs. Establishing good rapport, trust building and approaching these questions with more sensitive and nuanced language is important. For example, normalizing the questions as part of the intake process for all clients, as well as offering the client the choice of waiting until they are ready to discuss these areas of their lives will enable them to feel less pressured.

Sara also appeared worried about confidentiality concerns, asking "where does this information go...?" She said that some of her friends had also utilized counseling services in the past, "My friend came to you last year and she recommended you." At this time, confidentiality and its limits were reviewed with Sara. Since she had already commented earlier that she had seen me at the community Iftar, this was also a good opportunity to discuss the concept of "dual relationship" that may occur in shared community spaces on campus where I am invited to conduct workshops, outreach programs which involve students, and sometimes includes current clients. Therapists should assess for client comfort in these situations, as well as offer space to process any potential concerns or issues that may occur as a result of sharing a common space outside of the therapy room. This is also a good opportunity to discuss the differences between a therapeutic relationship and a social relationship, since having shared identities can also mean shared spaces like religious or cultural centers as well as other social situations where there is a potential for client and therapist to find their paths intersecting. This enables clarity in the therapeutic relationship and sets the stage for effective boundaries during the process of therapy, as well as after termination. Sara listened intently, and appeared visibly relaxed, stating that she was "worried about sharing personal information before, but that she felt better knowing what confidentiality means in therapy."

At the conclusion of the first session, Sara was still ambivalent about therapy—"I just want some advice on how to improve my grades." However, she agreed to come back for a follow up session because she stated she was curious about how the experience might be different with a therapist from a similar cultural background "I think you get where I'm coming from..." Sara felt she did not have to explain some things to me (the therapist) because of a shared cultural identity, and acknowledged that she had been frustrated with the previous experience with a different therapist because "I felt that I had to teach them about my culture and my religion." It is important to ask for feedback continually regarding a client's experience in the ongoing therapeutic process, since it continues the trust building process, as well as offers the client agency and control. This is particularly important because there is usually a "power differential" in the therapeutic relationship.

The next couple of sessions were focused on Sara's academic struggles which she had identified as her primary concern on the intake form. She was enrolled in four classes, studying for a premedical major. In addition, Sara was involved with the school's MSA (Muslim Student's Association). When asked about specific challenges, Sara says she feels a loss of motivation and has a low frustration tolerance: "I'm irritated by everything, sometimes even my friends." Sara was expressive about her fatigue and lethargy, mental and physically; "My whole body hurts and I don't want to get out of bed." She has trouble completing her assignments for her classes, as well as fulfilling her responsibilities as a member of the MSA, "I feel so guilty for dragging my feet with this work, I feel like I'm letting people down." Her challenges were affecting multiple areas in her life, and my clinical impression was that her symptoms were consistent with mild depression. She says that her parents are "mostly supportive" of her, are very invested in her academics and career and have "high expectations." Sara feels guilty about not getting the grades they expect and has not shared her poor academic performance with them because "I don't know what will happen if they see that I have failed some classes." Sara has hinted to her parents about her academic difficulties but feels that they think she may be "distracting herself too much with extra curriculars" or is "lazy and unorganized." Sara also expressed that "they have sacrificed so much for us, but you know how Desi parents are ..."

Since Sara had commented on us (client and therapist) having a shared identity, it was a good opportunity to explore this observation with her—cultural, ethnic and religious similarities as well as differences (immigration history, age of therapist) by utilizing strategic self-disclosure. As a therapist, I chose to share that I was a first-generation immigrant, who grew up in the Indian subcontinent and emigrated to the US several years ago. I am middle aged, therefore, likely to be around her parents' age. I also shared that I identified Muslim. Sara was aware that I am involved in various community specific activities at the university since she had already seen me at an event. The conversation about our shared identities and subsequent perceptions (and even assumptions that may have been made) allowed for more comfort and trust.

In the next few sessions, while Sara continued to discuss her academic concerns, she began sharing more information about her family, although at times she appeared to stop herself, glossing over some details. While this process of building trust can be slow and painstaking, it is important for the therapist to continue to normalize general concerns, as well as utilize the unique perspective of being a "cultural insider" to discuss stigma around help seeking behavior, as well as the hesitancy and feelings of guilt around discussing challenges outside of family and in a therapeutic setting. Sara continued to open up about her family concerns, as well as her relationship with her parents. She discussed how her father is prone to sudden bursts of anger, and her mother is always worried—"I think she has some sort of anxiety." Sara's mother calls her often and will complain about her father, she feels it's her "responsibility to listen" because her mother depends on her for emotional support. She is also expected to resume her chores and responsibilities when she visits home, whereas her parents do not have these expectations from her brother. Mental health is "never talked about in her family" and her parents would "have a fit" if they knew she was seeing a counselor. "My mom always tells me I should pray more if I'm feeling sad." As part of deconstructing the stigma around mental health in South Asian American communities of all religious backgrounds, it is important to explore internalized messages around faith (or perceived lack thereof) and mental health issues and how these attitudes promote shame and guilt and hinder help seeking behaviors.

Sara recalled her parents "arguing a lot" when she was younger, she remembers most of the arguments were about family and finances. Her father was laid off from his job during the previous recession, placing a burden on the family's financial situation to the point where the parents considered moving back to Pakistan, which was "scary to think about." Sara had not visited Pakistan often, and did not have close relationships with her extended family.

Sara's experiences with having a marginalized identity were explored in depth, she felt like she "does not really belong anywhere," That is, being seen as "too American with her Pakistani family members, and "too Pakistani/Muslim/Person Of Color" within the context of American society. She stated that she was "not sure" if I understood how she felt, because as an immigrant from her parents' generation, I did not have similar life experiences as her. It is important to explore the transference occurring here. In Sara's assumptions about me, given my background and differences in life experiences as well as differences in acculturation levels (Sara is a second generation child of immigrant parents whereas I am a first generation immigrant), it was likely that she was projecting her frustrations with her parents onto me, since I served as a symbolic "stand in" for her parents- alluding to her previous observation- "you seem like an aunt." Transference concerns were addressed by validating the Sara's observation about not having this shared experience with me, discussing differences in acculturation levels between Sara and her parents, and how that informs values, expectations, and experiences, as well as adopting a stance of "humble curiosity" while inviting Sara to explore her specific experiences. While strategic self-disclosure can be used as an intervention tool as well to strengthen the therapeutic alliance, care should be taken to ensure that the attention does not shift from the client to the therapist.

Counter transference can also occur—the therapist feeling affected by client's assumptions of perceived incompetency because of not having a shared life experience or having differences in identity. There can also be a sense of protectiveness toward the client, particularly if the therapist has children/younger siblings/family members who are of a similar age or who may have experienced similar challenges in their lives. Seeking consultation with colleagues or supervisors can help the therapist work through these countertransference issues. In this instance, continual consultations with my colleague who is also South Asian identified, helped me as a therapist work through my own counter-transference during my treatment with Sara. This enabled me to process with Sara her worries regarding not being heard or understood, as well as focus the attention back on how Sara could foster more effective communication with her parents.

During one clinical session, Sara shared her thoughts about relationships within the cultural context—that she "sometimes hates the concept of marriage in the culture" especially since Sara has seen how incompatible her own parents have been in their "arranged marriage." This was a chance for the therapist to explore Sara's ideas about relationships in general, as well as the cultural norms and mores. We continued to explore differences in acculturation levels between her parents and Sara, as well as how this affects her own set of values, goals, expectations in life. In this process, Sara disclosed that she has been romantically involved with a fellow student she had met in university last year. Sara reports he was kind, funny and considerate, and she felt supported by him. She had not told her parents about him for fear of "backlash" because while he was also South Asian identified, he belonged to a different religious background than her—"my parents would freak out if they knew." She also stated that this was the first time she had "ever spoken about him to anyone, other than her one best friend." As she discussed her relationship, she asked me what I thought about it. This was another opportunity for me to explore transference issues that may be occurring for Sara. While she was appropriately using the therapeutic space to navigate her conflictual feelings including guilt and fear at this "taboo" relationship, she was also assessing for a response (approval/disapproval) from me, who was likely a "stand in" for her parents—(or an aunty from her social circle). This was another opportunity to validate Sara for forming trust in the therapeutic space to be able to share her conflict with me, as well as to bring the focus of the session back to values and expectations that Sara has about her interpersonal relationships, with her parents, as well as her partner. It was important that Sara knew she had my support in exploring her needs, but that my approval was not meant as a stand in for her parents.

Sara's case was conceptualized as stress that stemmed from financial and familial instability growing up, as well as having to take on the role of emotional caregiving for her parents which she felt was her "responsibility" being the oldest child and the only daughter in the family. In addition, her symptoms were being driven primarily by guilt and shame at breaking away from social, familial and cultural norms by dating someone who would be "unacceptable" to her family, as well as worry at potentially causing more chaos in the family as a result of her non normative relationship.

While Sara's presenting symptoms were consistent with mild depression, a referral to the psychiatrist did not seem imperative at this stage, as it would likely address the symptoms, but not the cause for the depression. Given Sara's experience with mental health, I was careful to not pathologize her challenges or concerns to avoid further exacerbating stigma around mental health. However, this did provide a good opportunity to help Sara make an informed decision about referral to a psychiatrist. By adopting a culturally curious stance, fostering trust by utilizing my unique position as the "cultural insider," using nuanced, nonjudgmental assessment and intervention techniques, I was able to facilitate Sara's comfort with processing feelings of guilt and worry which were at the root of Sara's depressive presentation. Sara was an active collaborator in her treatment plan, which also empowered her to continue her growth in therapy. The remaining sessions were utilized to work on these treatment goals.

As we discussed termination from therapy, Sara said she wanted to remain in touch with me after termination—"maybe we can have chai together sometime." Clients will often express a desire to engage in social settings with the therapist after termination, and it is important to review and reiterate the ethical boundaries of a therapeutic relationship. At the same time, the therapist can engage a client in a meaningful termination activity that celebrates the therapeutic relationship (having Chai together in the therapy room, an activity that honors shared identity of the client and the therapist such as music, art, craft).

Potential possibilities around sharing cultural space (local religious community center, university related events specific to Muslim identified students, cultural or social events outside of university setting) were also discussed in sessions during termination process.

While Sara expressed disappointment at not being able to keep a social relationship with the therapist, and sadness at the termination of therapy, she indicated understanding of confidentiality concerns and ethical taboos of maintaining a social relationship outside of the therapeutic space.

Reflection Questions

- When might a therapist choose to consult?
- What do you enjoy about your work with clients that have shared identities as you? What are some challenges?
- How would a therapist work with a client feeling "uncomfortable" talking about taboo topics such as sex?
- How might therapeutic alliance be affected if there was a possibility of a CFS referral if Sara had disclosed abuse in the family?
- How might treatment interventions be adapted if Sara was in a same-sex relationship?
- What are some cultural challenges that can arise in case of active risk issues for the client (suicidality, Homicidal ideation, active psychosis) that might result in a higher level of care?
- How might a therapist have handled the termination differently?
- How might a therapist have handled gift giving—if Sara gave the therapist a gift?
- When are times a therapist has a hard time separating their own values or opinions from that of the client?
- How might a therapist approach a client who may be engaged in impression management?
- How might a therapist approach relationship building with a client who is afraid of being judged or may be with holding reactions?

Summary

The case example highlights how paying special attention to the advantages and challenges arising from having shared identities with the client in the therapeutic dyad not only creates a safe and non-judgmental space for therapeutic change, but enhances the therapeutic work. Often clients come to therapy and struggle to feel understood. Slowing down, adjusting assessment and interventions to the client's comfort and cultural experience, acknowledging stigma with help seeking behaviors in communities, as well as taking a stance of cultural humility helps the therapist form a rich and multifaceted understanding of the client and their lived experience. It also helps provide space for the client to build trust in the therapist and the therapeutic space, allowing more room for questions, clarifications of misunderstanding and assumptions, addressing relationship dynamics and connections, thereby collaborating on culturally relevant and sensitive interventions for the client, and likely more successful therapeutic outcomes. Sara could easily have decided to not continue therapy for fear of judgment or shame. Sara could have not shared so openly with her therapist. She may have received just enough care and support around her mental health as was necessary within the confines of a brief therapy treatment model. However, we think that by building a therapeutic alliance that was safe and culturally sound, it created more meaningful and hopefully, longer lasting change. At the very least, we assume Sara would return to counseling at a future time. But at the most, we would hope that Sara's deep understanding of herself and increased insight in therapy, would contribute to her sound mental health moving forward.

As co-authors, we want to express that much of our work on this chapter stems from our consistent consultations in our work with South Asian American clients. As colleagues, who both identify as South Asian, we were in a unique situation to be working together and soon recognized the importance of consultations, given the unique nuances, challenges and joy that working with clients with shared identities affords us. This has allowed us to have deeper conversations about our work, how we are perceived as South Asian and South Asian American identified therapists and how we respond to transference and countertransference issues. These discussions and consultations have helped us form a deep trust, support, connection and respect for each other as colleagues, as well as helped us better serve a large South Asian community. We hope our observations and insights in working with clients who have a shared identity with the therapist provides opportunities for introspection, growth, and joy and inspires the reader to further explore these nuances.

Suggested Resources

- Ahmed, S., & Amer, M. M. (Eds.). (2013). *Counseling Muslims: Handbook of mental health issues and interventions.* Routledge.
- Chaudhry, T., & Chen, S. H. (2019). Mental illness stigmas in South Asian Americans: A cross-cultural investigation. *Asian American Journal of Psychology*, 10(2), 154.
- Hodge, D. R. (2004). Working with Hindu clients in a spiritually sensitive manner. *Social Work*, 49(1), 27–38.
- Inman, A. G., Devdas, L., Spektor, V., & Pendse, A. (2014). Psychological research on South Asian Americans: A three-decade content analysis. *Asian American Journal of Psychology*, 5(4), 364.
- Institute for Muslim Mental Health: muslimmentalhealth.com
- Jordan, J. V. (Ed.). (2013). The power of connection: Recent developments in relational-cultural theory.
- Kulanjiyil, T., & Thomas, T. V. (2010). Caring for the South Asian soul. Bangalore, India: Primalogue.
- Navsaria, N., & Petersen, S. (2007). Finding a voice in Shakti: A therapeutic approach for Hindu Indian women. *Women & Therapy*, 30(3–4), 161–175.
- South Asian Mental Health Initiative and Network: samhin.org

References

Berry, J.W. (1997). Immigration, acculturation, and adaptation. *Applied Psychology, 46*(1), 5–34.

Bhugra, D. (1997). Coming out by South Asian gay men in the United Kingdom. *Archives of Sexual Behavior, 26*(5), 547–557.

Cabassa, L.J. (2003). Measuring acculturation: Where we are and where we need to go. *Hispanic Journal of Behavioral Sciences, 25*(2), 127–146.

Das, A.K., & Kemp, S.F. (1997). Between two worlds: Counseling south Asian Americans. *Journal of Multicultural Counseling and Development, 25*, 23–33. 10.1002/j.2161-1912.1997.tb00313.x

Durvasula, R.S., & Mylvaganam, G.A. (1994). Mental health of Asian Indians: Relevant issues and community implications. *Journal of Community Psychology, 22*, 97–108. 10.1002/1520-6629(1994 04)22:2%3C97::AID-JCOP2290220206%3E3.0.CO;2-%23

Foronda, C., Baptiste, D.L., Reinholdt, M.M., & Ousman, K. (2016). Cultural humility: A concept analysis. *Journal of Transcultural Nursing, 27*(3), 210–217.

Gupta, R. (2017). What does being an 'American' look like in the therapy room? *Smith College Studies in Social Work*, *87*(2–3), 137–152.

Hill, C.E., Knox, S., & Pinto-Coelho, K.G. (2018). Therapist self-disclosure and immediacy: A qualitative meta-analysis. *Psychotherapy*, *55*(4), 445.

Hill, C.E., & Knox, S. (2009). Processing the therapeutic relationship. *Psychotherapy Research*, *19*(1), 13–29.

Hook, J.N., Davis, D.E., Owen, J., Worthington Jr., E.L., & Utsey, S.O. (2013). Cultural humility: Measuring openness to culturally diverse clients. *Journal of Counseling Psychology*, *60*(3), 353.

Hovarth, A.O. (2001). The alliance. *Psychotherapy: Theory, Research, Practice, Training*, *38*(4), 365.

Inman, A.G., & Tewari, N. (2003). The power of context: Counseling south asians within a family context. In G.E. Roysircar, D.S.E. Sandhu, & V.E. Bibbins Sr. (Eds.), *Multicultural competencies: A guidebook of practices* (pp. 97–107). Association for Multicultural Counseling & Development.

Ibrahim, F., Ohnishi, H., & Sandhu, D.S. (1997). Asian American identity development: A culture specific model for South Asian Americans. *Journal of Multicultural Counseling and Development*, *25*(1), 34–50.

Juthani, N.V. (2001). Psychiatric treatment of Hindus. *International Review of Psychiatry*, *13*(2), 125–130.

Kirmayer, L.J. (2012). Cultural competence and evidence-based practice in mental health: Epistemic communities and the politics of pluralism. *Social Science & Medicine*, *75*(2), 249–256.

Kurien, P.A. (2005). Being young, brown, and Hindu: The identity struggles of second-generation Indian Americans. *Journal of Contemporary Ethnography*, *34*(4), 434–469.

Lambert, M.J., & Barley, D.E. (2001). Research summary on the therapeutic relationship and psychotherapy outcome. *Psychotherapy: Theory, Research, Practice, Training*, *38*(4), 357–361. 10.1037/0033-3204.38.4.357

Lee, E. (2014). A therapist's self-disclosure and its impact on the therapy process in cross-cultural encounters: Disclosure of personal self, professional self, and/or cultural self?. *Families in Society*, *95*(1), 15–23.

Madathil, J., & Sandhu, D.S. (2007). The practice of marriage and family counseling and Hinduism. In *The role of religion in marriage and family counseling.* (pp. 134–149). Routledge.

Mir, G., Ghani, R., Meer, S., & Hussain, G. (2019). Delivering a culturally adapted therapy for Muslim clients with depression. *The Cognitive Behaviour Therapist*, 12.

Murphy, M.J., Faulkner, R.A., & Behrens, C. (2004). The effect of therapist-client racial similarity on client satisfaction and therapist evaluation of treatment. *Contemporary Family Therapy*, *26*(3), 279–292.

Norcross, J.C. (2002). *Psychotherapy relationships that work: Therapist contributions and responsiveness to patients.* Oxford University Press.

Norcross, J.C. (2010). The therapeutic relationship. In B.L. Duncan, S.D. Miller, B.E. Wampold, & M.A. Hubble (Eds.), *The heart and soul of change: Delivering what works in therapy* (pp. 113–141). American Psychological Association. 10.1037/12075-004

Rosario, M., Schrimshaw, E.W., & Hunter, J. (2004). Ethnic/racial differences in the coming-out process of lesbian, gay, and bisexual youths: A comparison of sexual identity development over time. *Cultural Diversity and Ethnic Minority Psychology*, *10*(3), 215.

Ryder, A.G., Alden, L.E., & Paulhus, D.L. (2000). Is acculturation unidimensional or bidimensional? A head-to-head comparison in the prediction of personality, self-identity, and adjustment. *Journal of Personality and Social Psychology*, *79*(1), 49.

Tervalon, M., & Murray-Garcia, J. (1998). Cultural humility versus cultural competence: A critical distinction in defining physician training outcomes in multicultural education. *Journal of Health Care for the Poor and Underserved*, *9*(2), 117–125.

Tewari, N. (2009). Seeking, receiving, and providing culturally competent mental health services: A focus on asian americans. In N. Tewari & A.N. Alvarez (Eds.), *Asian American psychology: Current perspectives* (pp. 575–606). Routledge/Taylor & Francis Group.

Vasquez, M.J. (2007). Cultural difference and the therapeutic alliance: An evidence-based analysis. *American Psychologist*, *62*(8), 878.

14 South Asian American Political Movements and Mental Health: The Importance of Advocacy, Social Justice, and Public Policy

Lakshmi Sridaran and Devika Srivastava

Case Overview

Sumana Kaluvai is a 23-year year old woman who is illustrative of the complex reality of South Asian American communities and also demonstrates how to understand barriers with a lens of solidarity. This case will address these challenges with greater clarity, success, and most importantly in transformational rather than transactional ways. Sumana Kaluvai immigrated to the United States (U.S.). from India at the age of two with her father who came on an H-1B visa and her mother who came on an H-4 visa. As a result, Sumana is categorized as a dependent visa holder, also on an H-4 visa.

It was only years later when applying to college that Sumana became aware of her status when her mother pointed out that she had answered all of the immigration questions incorrectly on her financial aid forms. Suddenly, Sumana had to list herself as an international student on her college application form and was rendered ineligible for jobs, internships, scholarships, and financial aid. She was then also competing against international students coming from abroad who often came from wealthy, upper class families and backgrounds. Despite these steep barriers, Sumana was admitted to University of California, Los Angeles (UCLA) for her undergraduate studies and found ways to earn an income to pay her tuition.

At age twenty-one, Sumana "aged out" of her dependent visa status, she was left with only one option that dependent visa children have—to switch from an H-4 to F-1 student visa or be deported. Sumana traveled to India to process her paperwork and then the application went into "administrative processing." This essentially means that an applicant cannot ask questions for 60 days. Fortunately, her application was approved after 15 days, but she missed critical time in college because of this processing delay. Since then, Sumana has been able to acquire a standard post-completion Optional Practical Training (STEM-OPT) visa as a pharmaceutical biotechnology consultant through her employer.

But, she had a pivotal moment during her sophomore year at UCLA when she found an internship posting by the UCLA Labor Center that invited students of all immigrant statuses to apply. Sumana applied and was accepted to UCLA's Development, Relief, and Education for Alien Minors Act (DREAM) Summer program in 2017. She describes this experience as a monumental summer because she realized that so many other students were going through the same thing. She also explained how she felt pressure to suppress her experience and never had this community of people facing the same issues. The internship program placed her as a fellow for the Asian Law Alliance (San Jose) where she did legal intake, developed materials for a partnership with the American Civil Liberties Union (ACLU), supported legal clinics, and ran the organization's high school internship program. It was also through UCLA's political education component that she learned about the struggle of the DREAMers, which peaked later that fall when the Trump Administration eliminated the Deferred Action for Childhood Arrivals (DACA) program.

DOI: 10.4324/9781003081548-14

It became apparent that dependent visa children and DREAMers faced nearly identical issues, particularly the threat of deportation. However, it is important to note that visa dependent children are not considered undocumented and do have the opportunity to shift to F-1 student visas, which is not afforded to those with DACA.

Introduction

Like all communities, multiple issues affect South Asian Americans, and significantly impact their mental health. Oftentimes, many South Asian American individuals in communities may hold the idea that our experiences and challenges are exceptional, unique, and an aberration rather than a necessary symptom of systemic racism and white supremacy. In turn, our community by and large, with several notable exceptions that this chapter will address, both intentionally and unknowingly uphold and perpetuate racism and white supremacy in their personal lives, which then reinforces the systems in which we operate. This is most visible in the community's anti-Black racism, which translates to support for over-policing and state violence in Black communities as one example.

Instead, if we shift our mindset to one that understands our own barriers as shared challenges with other communities of color and immigrant populations in the U.S., we can truly begin to address the mental health challenges of both suffering from, but also advancing institutionalized racism and white supremacy.

The events of 9/11 have been viewed as the watershed moment in which the mainstream South Asian American population was forced to confront the violence of racism in the U.S. on a mass scale. This is also the time that South Asian Americans Leading Together (SAALT) was catalyzed and formalized. And, in the last two decades since, has been most visible in addressing issues of hate violence and immigration at the federal level. But it is crucial to note that many South Asian American organizations existed before this time. While the majority were and continue to be focused on providing services, such as legal aid and support for survivors of domestic violence, some like Desis Rising and Up and Moving in New York City were founded specifically to organize working class South Asian American populations around domestic issues like wage theft, housing, and police brutality, not just immigration and hate violence. And, it is groups such as these which have always operated under the lens of solidarity with other communities of color who are doing the difficult work of transforming systems that would uplift all.

What we have learned from these older South Asian American organizations and movements is there is no singular South Asian American experience, but an important series of divided experiences marked by caste, class, and country of origin that define the experience of living in the U.S. As a result, it is more useful to examine the multitude of issues impacting South Asian Americans as shared challenges across communities of color and immigrant populations rather than as exceptional or unique issues. In failing to do so we exceptionalize and overrepresent the experiences of upper caste and upper class South Asian populations and erase the experiences of lower caste and working class South Asian populations in the U.S. And, we altogether fail to understand the depth and complexity of mental health challenges that our community faces.

Case Study Discussion

Sumana's internship experience and political education motivated her to join UCLA's Equity, Diversity, and Inclusion Council and fight for in-state tuition for students on DACA and dependent visas. And, upon graduation in 2019, she founded the organization, "H for Hope," to help other dependent visa children navigate the intentionally complicated immigration system.

One year later, when the Trump Administration issued its "foreign student ban," requiring international students to either transfer schools or leave the country if their colleges continued to hold classes exclusively online that Fall, Sumana founded Support Our International Students (SIOS). In particular, she created a google spreadsheet that went viral, which helped students swap classes to be able to meet the ridiculous requirements imposed by the ban. The google spreadsheet got over 26,000 hits after launching.

And, later that summer, Sumana founded the "Hidden Dream" in late June 2020 which gives young people resources, including a 30-page survival guide on navigating the immigration system. The organization also raised money for two scholarships for dependent visa children, and now has a Slack community of over 200 young people, an Instagram account with over 2,000 followers, and a board of 12 young people of mixed immigration statuses, including Sarvani Kunapareddy, who was profiled in Teen Vogue's 21 under 21. In the article, Kunapareddy says that she wants to create meaningful, widespread change. "I want to focus on fighting for comprehensive immigration reform," she explains. "Currently, there is [...] piecemeal legislation that has been pitting immigrants against one another. I hope that there can be an inclusive bill in place that helps immigrants from all communities achieve their full potential."

The piecemeal legislation that Sarvani is referencing is known as the "Fairness for High Skilled Immigrants Act" first introduced by Rep. Chaffetz of Utah and Rep. Lofgren of CA which regained momentum in 2017 by Rep. Yoder of Kansas following the murder of Srinivas Kuchibhotla by a white supremacist at a Kansas bar in his Congressional District. Srinivas' death left his widow Sunayana Dumala threatened with deportation because her H-4 dependent visa was tied to her late husband's H-1B visa.

In an attempt to clear the significant backlogs and injustices that result in the intentionally precarious circumstances for H-1B and H-4 visa holders, the Fairness for High Skilled Immigrants Act was introduced to lift the per country green card caps. However, helping clear the green card backlog that disproportionately affects Indians does not actually eliminate the backlog itself, it simply moves it around to other countries. Indians in the U.S. have among the longest wait times for green cards. The reason? Current immigration policy does not allow one particular country to account for more than 7% of visas leading to a green card in any given year. This means countries that fall below the 7% threshold have much shorter wait times than large countries like India, which has among the longest green card backlogs.

While the legislation has gained wide and even bi-partisan support, its proposal to remove green card caps does not actually increase the number of green cards available, but redistributes them by application date rather than country of origin. This inherently favors nations with much larger demand for green cards, most notably, India. But, this comes at the direct expense of countries with lower demand, who will experience higher wait times. Among South Asian countries, this puts green card applicants from Bangladesh, Pakistan, Sri Lanka, Nepal at a much greater disadvantage.

In January, 2018 a "Dear Colleague" letter circulated by Congressional co-sponsors of The Fairness for High Skilled Immigrants from both parties framed the legislation as a potential solution for the "DACA problem." In it they state,

> it can be passed along with amended language containing a fee that can be assessed upon the beneficiaries of the legislation that will raise billions of dollars. These critical

funds can be used to enhance the likelihood of passage of a DACA deal, by either enabling Congress to pay for border security or other items in a manner that does not increase deficits, burden U.S. taxpayers, or cause any opposition to the nature of the funding source.

This means the funds from additional green card processing fees would go toward further militarizing the border, possibly even funding the Trump administration's wall.

In February, 2018 hundreds of Indian-Americans rallied outside the White House supporting the Trump administration's immigration policies, drawing attention to the green card issue. In particular, they held a sign saying "Dreamers pay for the wall" and offered to pay additional fees toward their green card applications to finance a border wall by supporting The Fairness for High Skilled Immigrants Act.

These positions and actions by the Indian-American community exemplify the mindset of exceptionalism and a willingness to undermine other immigrant communities for individual benefit. This advocacy primarily led by "Immigration Voice" more recently went as far as to stage rallies in front of the home of Senator Dick Durbin (D-IL), who courageously opposed the popular legislation in the Senate. But even more notable, are the deeply flawed arguments around merit, class, and caste engrained in this fight. The founder and executive director of Equality Labs, Thenmozhi Soundararajan, writes:

> This caste-informed mindset fits neatly within the H-1B arguments that many Indian immigrants are now making. That Indian immigrants would be willing to sacrifice the immigration possibilities of all other immigrants and support the ending of family reunification and the building of the wall is the ultimate form of a casteist state of mind. It privileges their lives as Indian immigrants over the lives of other immigrants, including the other South Asian immigrant communities. Bangladeshi, Pakistani, Indo-Caribbean, and Sri Lankan immigrants all have benefited from, and would benefit from, maintaining a fair and open family reunification policy, but are not included in the vision put forth by right-wing Indian groups.
>
> It is even more heartbreaking that Indian-Americans would be willing to engage in the divisive tactic of funding the wall. These individuals are not only on the wrong side of history, but they are sowing divides between themselves and the rest of the immigration movement while feeding into the anti-immigrant racism that is part of the ecosystem of hate crimes. The violence of their choices and the willingness of Indian immigrants to throw millions of families under the bus is painful. And yet this is also part of the socialization of caste that must be fought at its core.

It was in the middle of this policy battle that Sumana first connected with other dependent visa children. Thanks in part to her experience through UCLA's Dream Summer, she knew a different, more unified advocacy strategy that collectively supported Dreamers and visa dependent children was a stronger path. And, that is what motivated her to found "Hidden Dream," which focused on resources and community building. It was challenging for Sumana to work with young people whose parents were often forcing them to portray their challenges in such a way that it prioritized visa dependent children over Dreamers.

But ultimately, the Fairness for High Skilled Immigrants Act failed to pass the Senate, and Sumana notes a huge shift even among the parents, who realized that supporting young people and students would help bring visibility to the larger structural problems with our immigration system. At the time of this interview, there was renewed hope with the new Biden administration, especially since Sumana shared that in the prior administration, everyone felt like they had to fight for themselves. However, the Biden administration has also failed to make any notable improvements in immigration and has continued with high levels of deportations.

Suman's lesson to us all is to stop using the human experience as a political pawn—leveraging pain, and pitting groups against each other, exploiting harm, etc. Although many politicians are aware of this, they wilfully ignore it.

Early Migration History and South Asian American Political Presence

Before COVID-19, before 9/11, and even before 1965, South Asians were present in the U.S. and the historical policies impacting our communities have been well documented by South Asian historians and scholars. Their work discusses these early South Asian populations and the movements they helped shape and lead in the U.S. Later, when migration flows from Asia, including South Asian countries, were intentionally shifted to meet specific demands for labor in particular industries following the 1965 Civil Rights Act, there was not only the emergence of a predominantly upper-caste population from India, but also a dominant political mindset that followed. Generally, this political mindset was characterized by a feeling that Indian-Americans were exceptional, smarter, and more hard-working than others. This changed again in the 1990s when migration flows from South Asia shifted once again to meet specific demands for labor in the service industry. And, since 2010 we have seen an increase in asylum seekers and refugees from South Asian countries, fleeing repression and state violence. Again, this was complemented by a political mindset focused on working class populations and a global struggle against authoritarian governments, primarily by those who are not from upper caste or upper-class populations.

Fewer than 5,000 South Asians lived in the United States in 1920. Today, South Asian Americans are one of the fastest growing demographic groups in the United States and approximately 5.4 million individuals identify as South Asian/South Asian American according to the 2010 United States Census and 2017 American Community Survey data. Over 31 million people of Indian birth or descent are part of the Indian diaspora spread around the world (Das, 2002). Just looking at those of Indian origin, there are 33 major languages and some 1500 minor ones, seven major religions, and six major ethnic groups in the United States and this becomes even more beautifully diverse when considering all South Asian American identities, languages, and ethnicities. South Asian Americans have a long-standing history in the United States that is often minimized or ignored completely even within our community.

The first evidence of South Asian Americans extends to the 1790 in which an Indian man came to the United States from Chennai and then chose to reside in Massachusetts (Rangaswamy, 2000). Afterward, a number of South Asians were forcibly brought into the United States by captains working for the East India Company and became enslaved or worked as servants while others chose to migrate as merchants, seaman, travelers, and missionaries. In the 1800s and early 1900s, a significant number of Punjabi Sikhs (mostly men) came to North America in response to demand for labor and to gain financial security. These early migrants were attractive to companies as cheap labor as they worked longer hours and for half the pay than white workers (Desilver, 2018). It is important to note that the demand for this Asian labor grew after the official end of enslavement of Africans in the United States in 1865 and the subsequent Jim Crow period of indentured servitude of formerly enslaved peoples. However, as seen throughout U.S. history to present day, the government has worked hard to acquire the labor of migrants without providing the rights, benefits, and protections of citizenship.

Initially, many of these Sikh men resided in the West Coast of Canada but after facing Anti-Asian racism they migrated to the West Coast of the United States. While we know that not all Indians are Hindu, these early migrants were racialized as "low-caste Hindoos," but the majority were in fact Sikh. The majority of this population were also former soldiers who had served in the British colonial army in East Asia. These men wanted to live frugally, save their wages, and return to India with greater financial means. However, history details that instead of returning home to a farming economy which was under the oppression of British rule at the time, these Sikh men settled in the West Coast of America. However, this move was not without challenges and sacrifice. These settlers faced a significant amount of Anti-Asian hate violence and state sanctioned discrimination. White communities discriminated against Chinese, Japanese, and Indians and portrayed them as threats to their employment opportunities even as the government actively re-cruited their labor. These sentiments were the strongest on the West Coast as Indian Americans soon became the newest Asian immigrant group to be targeted by the Asiatic Exclusion League, a San Francisco-based group that successfully pressured immigration officials to deny admission to Indian immigrants by describing "Hindus" as enslaved, effeminate, caste-ridden, and degraded (Maira, 2002).

Additionally, organizations such as the Asiatic Exclusion League and the American Federation of Labor stepped up their attacks in the media and lobbied for laws excluding Asians from housing, education, and labor. Sadly, many Indians were accosted with verbal taunts where they were called "ragheads" or deemed the "Hindu Menace" (Maira, 2002). Laws were also enacted to ban the wives of South Asian men from the United States, and marriage with white individuals was illegal. A unique history of marriage between Sikh men and Mexican Catholic women emerged and a community within this region arose.

Around the same time, Indian migrants were also settling on the East Coast and Bengali Muslim peddlers were arriving to New Orleans selling "exotic" products (Bald, 2013). Many of these individuals continued to live on the East Coast but others moved to cities in the Midwest and in the Deep South but later assimilated into other communities in New York, Baltimore, and Detroit. New York City, San Francisco, New Orleans, and Charleston. New Orleans and Charleston were popular destinations for many Bengali Muslim sailors who jumped British ships (Desilver, 2018). Other South Asian migrants came to work on the Western Pacific railroad and were employed in the lumber mills of Washington State (Rangaswamy, 2000) establishing the first South Asian communities in the United States.

Students seeking education in mathematics, science, engineering, medicine, and law as well as political activists from India and Sri Lanka immigrated to the United States in the early 1900s. Many of these students sought education at the University of California, Berkeley on the West Coast and several Ivy League schools on the East Coast. However, the United States and British governments started to impose restrictions on South Asian immigration further suppressing these communities.

During this time, the first organized South Asian American political presence was forming. Indian nationalist organizations calling for the Indian revolution from Britain were taking root and Indians could organize more easily in the United States than in British dominated India. In 1912, the "Hindustan Association", dedicated to supporting self-rule in India, was formed in Oregon. The Ghadar Party was also formed in San Francisco by students and expatriates in 1913 and it was in support of overthrowing the British from India. Revolutionary intellectuals, including Stanford University student Har Dayal and Taraknath Das began to organize students in Berkeley, California and supported anarchist and nationalist ideas. Its early leaders had shared leadership among Sikhs, Hindus, and Muslims. Many of its publications included the names "Ram, Allah, and Nanak." While the movement's leadership was, at first, somewhat elitist, eventually the vast majority of the members were California's rural Sikh farmers. The publicity that the group attracted in the United States was used as further justification for anti-Asian discrimination and suspicion. The racism and discrimination many South Asian Americans faced in the United States motivated their desire to end colonial rule in India and fueled a desire for change. In 1914, Canadian authorities refused the Japanese steamship Komagata Maru permission to land. The boatload of nearly 300 Punjabis was stranded for weeks in Vancouver harbor. Eventually the ship was forced to return across the Pacific. The incident sent shock waves down the West Coast to the California Sikh community.

The Ghadar party had a weekly newspaper titled *"The Ghadar,"* which did not divide Indians into categories, such as Sikhs or Punjabis but supported a unified patriotism and a fight against British rule. The first issue of *The Ghadar*, was published in 1913. The party rose to prominence in the second decade of the 20th century and expressed dissatisfaction over World War I and the lack of political reforms. International Ghadar activity in Germany and elsewhere eventually led to what the press touted as the "Hindu Conspiracy" trial in San Francisco in 1917–1918. The arrests, the trial, the shooting, and deportations all attracted sensational publicity from the American press which heightened suspicion towards Asian Indians. In the 1920s, however, the Ghadar Party was reorganized and it continued as a focal point for Punjabi and Sikh identity until the time of Indian independence in 1947.

Another Indian political organization, known as the India Home Rule League of America on Broadway which was New York based also called for India's independence from Britain. The India Home Rule League of America also had an ongoing news edition entitled "Young India" and was first published in 1918. Lala Lajpat Rai who was a social reformer founded the India Home Rule League in 1917. He also set up the "Indian Information Bureau" in New York to serve as a publicity organization for India in 1918.

Mounting anti-immigrant sentiment and violence toward Asian migrants led to the 1907 Bellingham, WA riot in which 500 white male workers attacked South Asian migrants working in local lumber mills, broke into their homes, and stole their possessions. They successfully drove out the entire South Asian population of the city within a week. But like all interpersonal attacks of hate violence, this was reinforced and reflected in the policies of the U.S. government. It began with the development of the Asiatic Exclusion League in 1905 with the goal of "driving out the cheap labor," in less than 20 years the overt racism, violence and illegal efforts of the 1907 Bellingham riot eventually found legalized and strengthened expression through the U.S. legal system and federal government. The Bellingham mob and the federal government alike both served to police and protect the boundaries of U.S. citizenship and white privilege. After being actively recruited for their labor, Asian migrants including South Asians then faced violence and exclusion through federal policies, including the Immigration Act of 1917, which defines a geographic barred zone, including what is now South Asia from which no immigrants can come to the U.S. The act also imposed a literacy test on many of the immigrants entering the country. The National Origins Act of 1924 was a component of the Immigration Act of 1924 that established a quota system for how many immigrants could enter the United States, restricted by country of origin. The quota limited immigration from any country to 3% of residents originating in that country already living in the United States. Additionally, between 1908 and 1920, U.S. immigration officials targeted Indians seeking admission to the United States and denied entry to nearly 3,500 Indians, most on the grounds that they would likely become public charges.

These anti-Asian sentiments historically were rooted in the backlash associated with the Fourteenth Amendment passed shortly after the Civil War. This Amendment extended citizenship to all African Americans and to anyone born in the United States, including children of Indians and other immigrants. However, only white immigrants could become "naturalized"—granted US citizenship after migrating to the country and fulfilling a set of eligibility criteria. For the next 50 years, very few foreign-born Indian immigrants had become United States citizens by exploiting ambiguities in the pseudoscientific race theories of the time, by claiming "north Indian Aryan" racial backgrounds inferring that they were part of the Caucasian race and as such should be considered "free whites." This loophole was closed for them in 1923 with the passage of an important US Supreme Court ruling.

In *United States vs. Bhagat Singh Thind* (1923), the Supreme Court ruled that while Indians may be Caucasian, they were not white "in the understanding of the common man," and that this prevailing view would be backed by the law. Thind argued that based on the U.S. definition of Caucasian at the time, he met the criteria that should have enabled him to acquire citizenship. This case also prevented South Asians from gaining citizenship and stripping citizenship status from those who were granted it in the years prior. Sadly, this ruling even took away citizenship from those South Asians who also served in the United States military. This law would stand for the next two decades, until President Truman signed the 1946 Luce-Celler Act which provided naturalization rights to both South Asians and Filipinos, but still limited the number of migrants allowed into the country. While small in number, the South Asians who immigrated in the following two decades started having presence in small businesses, healthcare, and engineering. After two decades, the South Asian population in the United States had reached an all-time low after steady growth prior to 1924. Not only were the numbers low in relation to the general population but so was their educational attainment, as they ranked the lowest among all racial and ethnic groups.

In a 2018 Scroll Magazine article, SAALT's Founding Executive Director, Deepa Iyer, writes about Thind's case:

Perhaps because of this political context, Thind chose to frame his arguments for naturalization through a particular racial lens. In his brief to the U.S. Supreme Court, he identified himself as "… a high caste Hindu of full Indian blood, born at Amritsar, Punjab, India". He argued that since he came from "… the original home of the Aryan conquerors …, it must be held that [he] belongs to the Caucasian or white race".

In relying on arguments based in caste, bloodline and color, Thind did not challenge the racial prerequisite of whiteness for naturalization as the unconstitutional, discriminatory and morally abhorrent qualification we now know it to be. Nor did he choose to align himself with persons of African descent who were eligible for naturalization.

Iyer notes in her piece that Thind

> did not choose to align himself with persons of African descent who were eligible for naturalization. A nuanced historic understanding of the desperate political circumstances that Thind and other Asian immigrants faced in the 1920s may provide some balance to the legitimate critiques we can make today about his reliance on caste and color arguments, his choice to identify as white rather than black or African, and his decision not to question the racial premise behind naturalization laws.

The fight for citizenship for South Asian immigrants did not end here, but unfortunately the decision not to challenge the premise of racist immigration and naturalization laws continued among South Asian leaders visible in this fight. In the Introduction to Bengali Harlem, where author and historian Vivek Bald documents the lost histories of South Asians in the East Coast and South, he begins with the contrasting 1945 Congressional testimonies of two men from India before the House Committee on Immigration and Naturalization, Mubarek Ali Khan, a farmer in Arizona and J.J. Singh, an entrepreneur in New York City. Bald writes:

> The two men had been lobbying Congress over several sessions, each advocating a different approach to redressing India's exclusion. Khan's proposed legislation was focused and practical; it sought naturalization rights for the roughly three thousand Indians who were estimated to have settled in the United States prior to the Supreme Court decision of 1923 in the Thind case. Most of these immigrants were farm and factory laborers – exactly the population of 'undesirable aliens' that the 1917 Immigration Act had sought to keep out of the country. Singh's bill was more extensive and more ambitious. It would repeal the very logic of exclusion, making Indians racially eligible to become U.S. citizens, and it would create a quota allowing one hundred Indians per year to naturalize. His legislation, however, was focused primarily on the future; it would favor new, and presumably more highly qualified, immigrants over pre-1923 settlers, and reserve seventy-five of each year's naturalization for such applicants. (p. 2–3)

Much like today, both men employed arguments that touted the contributions of Indian immigrants, highlighting the accomplishments of scientists, engineers, and scholars to justify their right to citizenship. They both also downplayed and essentially erased the experiences of the majority of Indians who were actually living in the U.S. at that time, which were farm laborers and industrial and service workers. However, in Bald's extensive research, he unearthed written testimony from a third man, a Bengali immigrant from New York City named Ibrahim Choudry, who served as secretary of the India Association for American Citizenship. His letter lifted the shroud over the South Asian working-class population that Khan and Singh had overlooked and excluded in their testimonies. Choudry's testimony in part read

> I speak for the many. I am not speaking for the transient element – the student, the business man, the lecturer, the interpreter of India's past and present, whose interests and ties in this country are temporary, the man or the woman whose roots are in India and who eventually returns home. I talk for those of us who, by our work and by our sweat and by our blood, have helped build fighting industrial America today. I talk for those of our men who, in factory and field, in all sections of American industry, work side by side with their fellow American workers to strengthen the industrial framework of this country ... .

This ruling and subsequent application greatly impacted the daily lives of many naturalized Indian American citizens. They were shut out of white-only schools, swimming pools, and barbershops. White American women who had married Indian men lost their citizenship, becoming stateless in their own country. In turn, this led to many couples not being allowed to marry due to statutes banning marriage between white people and non-white people. Congress went one step further by passing the Immigration Act of 1924, which instituted race-based quotas for immigrants and entirely banned the immigration of Indians as well. In the face of this discrimination and limited opportunities in the United States, many Indians returned to India. President Truman's 1946 legislation, the Hart-Cellar Act did make all Indians already residing in the U.S. eligible for citizenship, but solidified future immigration policy to continuously bend in the favor of scientists, engineers, and businesspeople.

As political calls for change grew and the Civil Rights movement proceeded, the 1965 Immigration and Nationality Act, which did eliminate the racial/nationality based discrimination in immigration quotas, triggering the second wave of South Asian migration which overwhelmingly favored this population, largely excluded working class immigrants. These crucial policy decisions over time shaped the political mindset of the majority of South Asians in the U.S. and provide important context for why Indian immigrants would support the construction of a border wall in exchange for green cards in 2018. Even since 1965, the demographics of South Asian America have become increasingly diverse: documented and undocumented immigrants, refugees and asylum seekers, second, third, and even fourth-generation South Asian Americans now comprise this community (Arora, 2017).

Post-9/11 Policies, Immigration and Hate Violence

This history sheds important light on how September 11, 2001 drastically changed the South Asian American community, but very simply uncovered the truth: the same working-class immigrants who bore the brunt of violence from white supremacy in the early 1900s, and were overlooked in federal immigration legislation, were the same populations who were overwhelmingly impacted by the interpersonal violence and government surveillance of South Asian American communities following 9/11. Desis Rising Up and Moving (DRUM), founded in 2000, was the first and one of the only organizations in the U.S. to mobilize these low-wage members and workers of the South Asian community in New York City to question, challenge, and transform the very root of racist education, economic, and immigration policies. In a 2012 report titled "In Our Own Words," by DRUM and other members of the National Coalition of South Asian Organizations coordinated by SAALT, the 10-year timeline below of "Selected Policies Resulting in Profiling of the South Asian Community in New York City Since September 11th" details the precision with which the federal government targeted South Asian, Muslim, and Arab communities with surveillance and deportation.

Timeline of Selected Policies Resulting in Profiling of the South Asian Community in New York City since September 11th

- September 2001: The Federal Bureau of Investigation (FBI) created a national tip line where ordinary citizens call in to report evidence of terrorist activity. Within a week of its launch, the FBI received tens of thousands of tips from New York, many based on irrational fears of Muslims, Arabs, and South Asians.
- September 2001: The then-Immigration and Naturalization Service (INS) is-sued a rule allowing immigrants to be detained 48 hours without charge, which could be extended in the event of an "emergency."
- September 2001: Chief Immigration Judge Michael Creppy issued a memorandum allowing Immigration Courts to close deportation proceedings for "special interest" detainees.

- September 2001 through February 2002: Attorney General John Ashcroft ordered the FBI to inform the INS to arrest any men found in violation of immigration law. In all, according to government figures, at least 762 South Asian, Muslim, and Arab men—including 491 in New York (the "New York Detainees")—were arrested by the FBI and referred to INS for detention, based on their national origin and immigration status. Community organizations reported that actually over 1,200 men were rounded up in these raids. No one arrested as a part of these sweeps was ever charged with terrorist activity or linked to the September 11th attacks.
- September 2001: The FBI arrested individuals deemed "of interest;" even if suspicion was based solely on alleged immigration status, religious beliefs, ethnicity, national origin, and skin color. New York Detainees deemed of "high interest" by the FBI were held for further questioning at the Metropolitan Detention Center (MDC) in Brooklyn. Detainees were often held for lengthy periods of time without charge, denied access to attorneys or family members, and had daily prayers interrupted. Some also endured threats, racist slurs, strip searches, and physical abuse by MDC staff. Ultimately, almost all of the men arrested in New York were deported to their home countries.
- October 2001: President George W. Bush signed the USA PATRIOT Act into law, which increased the government's ability to conduct searches and surveillance and enhanced detention powers.
- November 2001: Attorney General Ashcroft ordered "volunteer questioning" of over 5,000 men who came from countries where al-Qaeda had a "terrorist presence." A second round of questioning began in March 2002. Of the 2,261 men who were actually interviewed nationwide, the Department of Justice (DOJ) reported that none were charged with crimes related to the September 11th attacks.
- 2002: New York City Police Department (NYPD) Commissioner Raymond Kelly established the Department's Counter-terrorism Bureau, the first of its kind in the country. It also began engaging in a Joint Terrorism Task Force (JTTF) partnership with the FBI.
- March 2002: NYPD Commissioner Kelly promulgated Operations Order 11, prohibiting racial profiling by NYPD officers. The order does not explicitly include religion within its definition of "racial profiling." It does prohibit police officers from relying on race, ethnicity, religion, or national origin as a "determinative factor" in initiating law enforce-ment action.
- April 2002: DOJ's Office of Legal Counsel issued its "inherent authority" opinion used as a basis for allowing state and local law enforcement to carry out federal immigration laws, a practice that results in profiling.
- May 2002: Attorney General Ashcroft issued revised FBI investigative guidelines relating to domestic terrorism that allow agents to attend public events without evidence of suspicious activity; and diminish oversight from FBI head-quarters over the activities of field offices in terrorism-related cases.
- June 2002: DOJ rolled out the Special Registration program as part of the National Security Entry-Exit Registration System (NSEERS). Aspects of the program required males over the age of 16 on non-immigrant visas and from 24 Muslim-majority countries, including Pakistan and Bangladesh, (plus North Korea) to report to local immigration offices for fingerprinting and interrogation. Nationwide, over 83,000 individuals registered of which 13,000 individuals were placed in deportation proceedings. The NSEERS program failed to identify any terrorism suspects or uncover any terrorism-related evidence.

- November 2002: The Department of Homeland Security (DHS) is formed with authority over both immigration and national security policy in the country.
- December 2002: The U.S. and Canada signed the Safe Third Country Agreement which requires most refugee claimants to request protection in the first safe country they arrive in. As a result, many South Asians, Arabs, and Muslims were forced to turn back to the U.S. after at-tempting to seek asylum in Canada from post-September 11th blanket round-ups in the U.S.
- 2003: Courts loosened rules under the Handschu Guidelines which, in 1985, established a three-member panel to oversee NYPD surveillance operations and allowed detectives to start an investigation only when they had "specific information" about a future crime. Under the Modified Handschu Guidelines, NYPD intelligence authorities can act alone to authorize investigations for certain periods of time; it also lowered the threshold standard to merely showing that the facts "reasonably indicate" the commission of crime.
- June 2003: DOJ issued its Guidance on the Use of Race by Federal Law Enforcement Agencies. Its anti-profiling measures include broad exceptions for national security and border integrity; fails to prohibit profiling on the basis of religion or national origin; does not apply to state or local law enforcement agencies; and lacks meaningful enforcement mechanisms.
- September 2003: President Bush signed the homeland Security Presidential Directive-6 creating the Terrorist Screening Center responsible for the Terrorist Screening Database. The database included various watchlists, including the "no-fly list" (including names of passengers not allowed to board planes) and the "selectee list" (including names of passengers required to undergo additional screening prior to boarding).
- Fall 2004: DHS instituted Operation Frontline designed to "detect, deter and disrupt terrorist operations" immediately prior to the 2004 presidential elections. Relying upon NSEERS databases, the government investigated individuals from primarily Muslim-majority countries.
- July 2004: New York City Mayor Michael Bloomberg signed legislation codifying Operations Order 11, prohibiting racial profiling. Advocates have called for this law to be strengthened, specifically in terms of its enforcement mechanisms.
- July 2005: The NYPD announced it would commence random searches of bags and packages carried by individuals entering the city's subways. This announcement was condemned by advocates as it would result in profiling.
- February 2006: Reports released that about 90% of all individuals subjected to NYPD's stop-and-frisk activities were engaged in no unlawful activity what-soever, and nearly 86% of all persons stopped were African-American or Latino.
- May 2006: An internal NYPD intelligence strategy report was issued to Commissioner Kelly calling for targeted surveillance of Shia Muslims and their mosques in New York, New Jersey, and Connecticut based solely on their religion. These secret documents became public through the Associated Press (AP) in January 2012.
- February 2007: DHS instituted the Traveler Redress Inquiry Program (TRIP) intended to allow travelers to submit complaints with watchlists and heightened screening. Yet many individuals reported that the program failed to provide any meaningful recourse.
- August 2007: The NYPD released the report "Radicalization in the West: The Homegrown Threat," asserting that radicalization is widespread among Muslims in New York and that law enforcement must mobilize to combat it. The report was heavily criticized for its failure to provide any evidence of increasing radicalization

while it listed benign behaviors, such as engaging in group outdoor activities and giving up smoking, as evidence of the phenomenon.

- August 2007: The Transportation Security Administration (TSA) issued guidelines stating that Sikh turbans and Muslim headscarves should be subjected to additional screening. In October 2007, such searches were no longer mandatory under TSA's "bulky clothing" policy, but instead left it to the discretion of screeners; passengers were also offered additional screening options providing increased privacy. Sikh and Muslim community members still continued to frequently be pulled out for security screening because of their attire.

- July 2008: U.S. Customs and Border Protection (CBP) was given greater authority to search and seize the belongings of passengers entering the United States, even absent evidence that an individual poses a threat.

- December 2008: DOJ issued the FBI's Domestic Investigative Operative Guide (DIOG) that relaxed restrictions on federal law enforcement to conduct threat assessments using factors based on religion and ethnicity. It also lowered the threshold to commence threat assessments without requiring an adequate factual basis or supervisory approval for national security cases.

- January 2010: TSA began requiring U.S.-bound passengers who were nationals of or travelling from/through 14 Muslim-majority countries, including Pakistan, (plus Cuba) to receive full body pat-downs and searches of all carry-on items. This policy was rescinded in April 2010 and replaced with a "real-time threat-based" screening system.

- July–September 2010: Debate across the country focused on the proposed construction of the Park51 Muslim community center in Lower Manhattan. Numerous elected officials and political candidates made statements opposing the establishment of Park51 because of a Muslim center's perceived proximity to Ground Zero. Within this climate, several hate crimes occurred, including the vicious assault of a Bangladeshi taxi driver in New York, Ahmed Sharif, whose attacker was a passenger who asked if Sharif was Muslim.

- October 2010: Following the initial roll-out of new Advanced Imaging Technology (AIT) machines in airports across the country, DHS and TSA informed Sikh advocacy groups that turbaned Sikh travelers at U.S. airports should always expect to undergo secondary screening in the form of a turban pat-down and/or a metallic detector wand over the turban.

- October–December 2010: The NYPD screened the film The Third Jihad to its Chemical, Ordinance, Biological, and Radiological (COBRA) Unit, which provides terrorism awareness training for patrol forces. Screened before 1,500 officers, the film included numerous Islamophobic messages, including that Muslims aim to "infiltrate and dominate" the United States. NYPD Com-missioner Kelly also played a role in its production, including being interviewed for the film. News about the film's use came to light in 2011, after which Kelly initially denied involvement with the film and minimized its widespread use during police training.

- January 2011: New York Governor Andrew Cuomo issued a letter to DHS indicating that the state would be sus-pending its participation in Secure Communities, a program where participating jails submit arrestees' fingerprints to the FBI and immigration databases, allowing Immigration and Customs Enforcement (ICE) access to information on individuals held in jails. Concerns remain as DHS has since asserted that states and municipalities will be unable to elect out of the initiative.

- March 2011: Peter King, a Congressional representative from Long Island and chair of the house Committee on homeland Security, commenced a series of Congressional hearings focused on radicalization within the Muslim community. In New York City, as well as elsewhere in the country, community members mobilized to raise concerns regarding the hearings' exclusive focus on the Muslim community.

- April 2011: DhS announced modifications to NSEERS, specifically "delisting" the list of countries whose nationals were subject to registration requirements. Despite the announcement, individuals remain affected by adverse immigration consequences as a result of the program and the program's underlying regulatory framework also remains intact.

- April 2011: The New York State Senate's Committee on Veterans, homeland Security, and Military Affairs convened a hearing on national security issues, which included topics such as "the culture of jihad" and "Sharia law."

- August 2011: An AP investigation revealed that the NYPD developed programs, with the assistance of the Central Intelligence Agency (CIA), using informants, known as "mosque crawlers," to spy on communities often absent any evidence of wrongdoing; and engaged in surveillance of neighborhoods, often solely on the basis of religion or ethnicity.

- November 2011: The U.S. Citizen-ship and Immigration Services (USCIS) issued a policy memorandum with directions to "refer all cases in which an application is denied based on an NSEERS violation to ICE for possible Notice to Appear (NTA) issuance." NTAs are charging documents that initiate deportation proceedings.

- November 2011: The New York City Department of Education released its first public data in compliance with the Student Safety Act reporting 73,441 suspensions in schools, an increase from 21,396 in 2002. Community groups site the parallel 65% increase in New York City's budget for police (including 200 armed NYPD officers and 5,200 School Safety Agents) and security equipment in schools (metal detectors and scanners) since 2002.

- February 2012: The AP published its investigative report on NYPD officers infiltrating Muslim Student Associations at universities throughout the north-eastern U.S. Another AP investigation revealed that the NYPD has been building secret files on mosques outside of its jurisdiction in New York City, including in New Jersey and New York's Suffolk and Nassau Counties. Police also photographed and mapped mosques, listing them as "Islamic Religious Institutions."

- December 2014: DOJ issued revised Guidance on the Use of Race by Federal Law Enforcement Agencies after years of advocacy by communities of color. The revised guidance expands the definition of profiling to prohibit the improper consideration of gender, national origin, religious, sexual orientation, or gender identity—in addition to race and ethnicity. However, it failed to prohibit profiling at ports of entry, including airports and the border and continued to allow mapping based on protected characteristics, as well as recruitment of informants.

- 2016: The Department of Homeland Security institutes the Countering Violent Extremism Program framed as a congressional mandate to help states and local communities prepare for, prevent, and respond to emergent threats from violent extremism. The Brennan Center breaks down the reality of this program: CVE is a counterterrorism strategy that recruits community leaders, social workers, teachers, and public health providers ostensibly to assist the government in identifying individuals that may be "at risk" of becoming violent extremists. But the idea that there are predictive risk indicators has been discredited by decades of scholarly research. They have been targeted almost exclusively at Muslims and employ spurious criteria, such as religiosity and political activism and vague feelings of alienation, as proxies for violent tendencies.

- January 2017: President Donald Trump signed an Executive Order that banned foreign nationals from seven predominantly Muslim countries from visiting the country for 90 days, suspended entry to the country of all Syrian refugees indefinitely, and prohibited any other refugees from coming into the country for 120 days.

Case Study and Mental Health Challenges

While we know that the COVID-19 pandemic, white supremacy, institutionalized racism, and constant discrimination have an immense toll on individual mental health, we are not always aware of the full impact in the South Asian American community. However, psychological research has time and time again found an association between depression, anxiety, and PTSD when an individual is faced with chronic stress linked to discrimination and acculturative stress.

Sumana detailed her mental health challenges not only with fighting for changes in the immigration system and consistently producing resources for others, but also fighting her family's personal battles, which included her own visa. When her father was finally allowed to return to the U.S. 8 months later in November 2020, she finally let herself feel everything. Thankfully her parents were very supportive of her pursuing therapy, which she began in the Fall of 2020, but it took time for her to feel an improvement in her mental health. When Sumana's group "Hidden Dream" released the 30-page survival guide, they asked for feedback and the number one request was for mental health resources. Many young people shared that their parents tell them to keep fighting as they wait for decades for a resolution on their immigration status and that it will work out if they just do their best. Not only does that continue to reinforce a merit-based argument as the solution to overcome systemic racism and discrimination, it fails to explain why they keep hearing "no" if they are supposedly doing everything right.

Sumana also importantly identifies that there is a lot of rightful attention placed on the interpersonal domestic violence that many women on H-4 visas face from their spouses. However, this tends to overlook the abuses faced by young H-4 dependent visa holders because they are often seen as privileged. She states there is emotional and mental abuse resulting from having their immigration status constantly dangled in front of them. Even citizen children like Sumana's younger brother feel this toll as their parents face wage theft and uncertainty around job security as a result of their immigration status. The same drive for cheap labor in the service industry is the same drive for cheap labor in industries that are considered "high skill" such as information technology. It is more beneficial to see these struggles as linked rather than drive a wedge that is centered around a flawed perception of merit.

In September, 2020, South Asian Americans Leading Together (SAALT) released the report *Unequal Consequences: The Disparate Impact of COVID-19 Across South Asian Americans*, highlighting the urgent need for funders and policy makers to gather accurate disaggregated data on South Asian communities in the U.S. to be able to understand and respond to the needs that have emerged since the onset of the pandemic. The report examines areas of the U.S. with among the largest South Asians populations including New York, Chicago, Houston, Atlanta, and the Bay Area and Central Valley in California and draws primarily on interviews with community leaders who are members of the National Coalition of South Asian Organizations (NCSO), a national community survey, and media reports. SAALT also launched an interactive map and video testimonials to further highlight the impact of the pandemic on South Asians.

The vast majority of the 50+ member organizations of the National Coalition of South Asian Organizations are domestic violence survivor support service organizations. During interviews with their staff for this report, the most common theme was the lack of mental health support for survivors during the Covid-19 pandemic, specifically as a result of isolation and often being trapped at home with abusers. Two other major themes that emerged from the community surveys were the mental health challenges of isolation faced by South Asian elders as well as the fear of applying for public benefits, specifically the Covid-19 stimulus payments, because of the possibility of losing immigration status.

These significant challenges require not just individual support from mental health practitioners, but also a political understanding that ties them back to unjust systems.

There were also significant findings and changes related to mental health policies and services impacting different racial and ethnic groups in the United States, also involving South Asian Americans.

Timeline of Mental Health Policy Impacting South Asian Americans

- 1960–1970s: The civil rights movement helped highlight mental health needs of people of color, including South Asian Americans.
- 1963: Community Mental Health Centers Act: It helped make mental health services accessible to a broader range of people including Asian Americans and other people of color and targeted those most in need of clinical services, regardless of their ability to pay. This led to the creation of community mental health centers. Increased numbers of people began to utilize mental health services including Asian Americans and other people of color (Kiesler, 1992; Stockdill, 2005). Asian Americans and other people of color fared worse in the community mental health system than White Americans, in terms of underutilization and premature termination (Sue, 1977). Thus, there was more work to be accomplished to ensure that Asian Americans received much-needed mental health services.
- 1981: The Omnibus Budget Reconciliation Act of 1981 repealed the 1963 CMCH Act. Many community mental health centers were subsequently closed, resulting in persons needing mental health services no longer receiving them. There was an independent mindset emerging during this time which was in contrast to community support and responsibility and this furthered inequality for people of color. This notion also dismissed systemic inequalities facing people of color which were viewed as violations of fairness.
- 1980s: A shift in mental health to private mental health care services, which excluded those who were unable to afford them including many Asian Americans (Kiesler, 1992). A managed care model for those with private health insurance coverage became where most mental health services were provided.
- 1989: Congress passed a resolution by President George H. W. Bush that proclaimed the 1990s to be the "Decade of the Brain". This initiative focused on the biological basis of mental disorders came from special interest groups whose goal was to de-stigmatize mental disorders and to conceptualize them as diseases that were not the fault of the person experiencing them. Biological science also became more valued compared to psychological science and an emphasis on psychological or behavioral approaches became apparent when looking at funding towards different programs and policies. The emphasis on the brain and the biological bases of behavior continued at the NIMH during the 2000s and into the current decade. As part of President George W. Bush's New Freedom Commission on Mental Health, NIMH Director Thomas Insel (2003) indicated that mental illnesses are "brain illnesses". Although former

Surgeon General David Satcher (2003) acknowledged on the Commission the role of culture in the diagnosis and treatment of mental disorders, he also referred to the connection between mental disorders and changes in the brain. When viewing mental illness in this light, cultural stigma may decrease for Asian Americans who report greater stigma associated with psychological disorders as they were viewed similar to other medical conditions and had a biological basis. However, emotions and the complexity of psychological states could not be totally accounted for by biological mechanisms or brain activity and did not capture cultural and sociocultural influences very much impacting Asian Americans. This view did not consider cultural components commonly affecting Asian Americans such as acculturation or family separation and community support.

2001: In the U.S. Surgeon General released a report, *Mental Health: Culture, Race, and Ethnicity,* substantial differences in mental health service utilization between non-Hispanic white adults and other racial/ethnic groups. This valuable report noted racial/ethnic differences in the types of services that are used. However, what was important about this report was that the majority of the differences in mental health service utilization were not from personal preference. Significantly, many of the racial/ethnic differences in mental health service utilization resulted from structural barriers, such as lack of transportation, low availability of care providers, cost, and insurance barriers.

- Past year mental health service use findings from 2008–2012 included:

  1 Estimates of any mental health service utilization among adults were similar for adults reporting two or more races, whites, and American Indian or Alaska Natives compared to for Black, Hispanic and Asian adults.
  2 The estimate of service utilization among black adults was higher than the estimate for Hispanic and Asian adults.
  3 Racial/ethnic differences among adults also were observed for the utilization of different types of mental health services. Estimates of prescription medication use were highest among white adults, adults who reported two or more races, and American Indian or Alaska Native adults.
  4 Asian adults had the lowest percentage of prescription medication use.
  5 Asian adults had the lowest percentage of outpatient service use.
  6 Estimates of inpatient mental health service use among Asian adults.
  7 Asian females had the lowest percentage of mental health service use compared to females in other racial/ethnic groups.
  8 Among those aged 18 to 25, estimates of mental health service utilization were similar among black, Asian, and Hispanic adults.
  9 Among adults aged 50 or older, the estimate of past year service use was higher among black and Hispanic adults than among their Asian counterparts.
  10 Within each insurance group, Asian adults had the lowest estimate of mental health service use, with one exception—Asian and black adults with private insurance had similar estimates of mental health service use.
  11 The belief that mental health services would not help was the least frequently cited reason for not using mental health services among members of each racial/ethnic group. This reason for not using services was more likely to be reported by white adults with an unmet need than among their black or Hispanic counterparts.
  12 Asian adults with an unmet need for mental health services were more likely than their black counterparts to believe that mental health services would not help.

13 Asian adults with any mental illness were the least likely to use any mental health services, prescription medication, or outpatient services.

14 Service cost or lack of insurance coverage was the most frequently cited reason for not using mental health services across all racial/ethnic groups. The belief that use of mental health services would not help was the least frequently cited reason for not using mental health services across all racial/ ethnic groups. Among all adults and adults with AMI or SMI, white adults were generally the most likely to cite cost or insurance and believing that services would not help as reasons for not using mental health services compared with other racial/ethnic groups.

- 2008: Mental Health Parity and Addiction Equity Act of 2008: Increased insurance coverage for mental health care and access to care for different racial/ethnic groups.
- 2010: This act provided health insurance to many who were previously uninsured and allowed a greater number of people the ability to pay for existing health care services including mental health care services. The health care reform law also resulted in the establishment of the National Institute on Minority Health and Health Disparities at the NIH. The mission of the NIMHD is to promote minority health and to eliminate health disparities for ethnic minority groups and they push for research associated with societal, cultural, and environmental dimensions of health.

The New York Police Department's Muslim Surveillance and Mapping program, launched in 2001 by Mayor Michael Bloomberg was a massive and organized effort to infiltrate and profile New York City's Muslim communities. "In Our Own Words" details how this program resulted in South Asians being stopped by law enforcement without cause, questioned about their faith, national origin and immigration status, and being approached by law enforcement to spy on their own communities (often threatened with immigration consequences for not complying), as well as interactions with law enforcement harming their relationships with government, friends, and family members.

In parallel, the federal government launched the notorious National Security Entry Exit Registration System (NSEERS) in 2002. This program required all non-citizen, non-immigrant, men and boys above the age of 16 from 25 Muslim-majority countries and North Korea to report to their local immigration offices. After hours of waiting, hours more interrogation about their immigration status, employment, faith, political beliefs, etc. many would be asked to surrender all of their belongings and placed into deportation proceedings. Most of the men had no opportunity to notify their families and the entire process was intentionally unclear and terrifying. Ultimately, over 80,000 men went through this unnecessarily torturous program, and over 13,000 were deported all under the false premise of identifying "homegrown terrorists," and resulted in zero terrorism related convictions. What actually resulted was the devastation of New York City's Muslim communities who lost thousands of men to deportation. The mental health toll of this erasure and destruction of families has yet to be quantified and addressed, but we continue to see the cumulative cost it claims. During Covid, it is these same communities who were racked with death due to a lack of access to proper healthcare and PPE for essential workers; it is these same communities who have gone without any stimulus checks in every iteration of federal recovery legislation because of their immigration status; and it is these same communities who continue to suffer the mental health consequence of isolation and unemployment.

Often 9/11 is seen as the horrifying and yet unifying event that brought the South Asian American community together, awakened a political consciousness that did not exist before, and catalyzed the creation of multiple community organizations. However, this is only a small part of the story that highlights the perspectives of the doctors, engineers, and scholars who have always been the focus of U.S. immigration policy, and not the focus of its dark surveillance and profiling underbelly. In 2014, 2017, and 2018, SAALT published a series of reports detailing its documentation of incidents of hate violence and xenophobic political rhetoric alongside an analysis of federal policies that continued to target South Asian, Muslim, and Arab American communities long after 9/11. A salient theme across all the reports is that these federal policies span Democratic and Republican presidential administrations alike, and thus our work cannot be limited to legislative advocacy alone.

SAALT's 2014 report, "Under Suspicion, Under Attack," firmly rooted in data collected during the Obama administration showed that over 80% of the incidents of hate violence documented were motivated by anti-Muslim sentiment and that over 90% of the political rhetoric, mostly heard on a national platform, was also motivated by anti-Muslim sentiment. The 2017 report, "Power, Pain, Potential," which highlights data collected starting from the Paris and San Bernardino attacks at the end of 2015, through the 2016 election cycle, up to the election of President Trump show that the number of hate violence incidents and instances of racist political rhetoric sharply increased by 34% in less than a third of the time covered in the 2014 report. In particular, this report found that one in five of the documented instances of xenophobic political rhetoric could be directly attributed to candidate and ultimately President Donald Trump. However, the real violence our communities experienced as a result of the 2016 election stage crosses party lines. Debates, public discourse, and candidate talking points were full of threats of mass deportations, loyalty checks, and false equivalencies between combating Islamophobia and combating terrorism. In addition, the divisions in our community became exposed as candidates on both sides of the aisle also capitalized on largely anti-Muslim rhetoric and policy proposals in an effort to win over non-Muslim South Asians. SAALT's 2018 report "Communities on Fire" further documents incidents of hate violence and xenophobic political rhetoric in the first year after Trump's election, which saw a 45% increase from the previous analysis in just 1 year alone. And, this report shows how one in five perpetrators of hate violence incidents explicitly referenced President Trump, a Trump policy, or Trump campaign slogan while committing the act of violence, underlining a strong link between President Trump's anti-Muslim agenda and hate violence post-election.

It is important to note that SAALT's data includes hate violence and rhetoric, which meets a lower threshold than the legal definition of a hate crime, but nonetheless paints a fuller picture of the xenophobia our communities face, which is steeped in anti-Muslim sentiment. We caveat this with the importance of acknowledging that not all South Asians are Muslim, and not all Muslims are South Asian. Yet it is enough simply to be perceived as Muslim to be a target of hate violence and xenophobic political rhetoric. SAALT's reports illustrate how the federal government has repeatedly failed to accurately document the level of hate violence against our communities and communities of color at large, which is glaringly obvious with the annual release of the FBI's hate crime statistics. This is due to poor directives and data collection from the FBI itself, a complete lack of incentive for local law enforcement to report the data to federal agencies, and deep lack of trust among our communities to report incidents of violence to local law enforcement. This is also coupled with the dissonance of law enforcement itself being the arbiters of deadly violence as non-Black communities across the nation finally awakened to this reality with the brutal murder of George Floyd in June 2020.

This level of suspicion and violence from the government and law enforcement certainly has deep, lasting, and recurrent consequences on the mental health of our communities. This in addition to the process of acculturation, intergenerational family differences and conflict, and legal status has great impact on psychological well-being.

The National Latino and Asian American Study (NLAAS) found that Asian Americans have a 17.30% overall lifetime rate of any psychiatric disorder and a 9.19% 12-month rate, yet Asian Americans are three times less likely to seek mental health services than Whites. Abe-Kim and colleagues also found that in general, only 8.6% of Asian-Americans sought any type of mental health services or resource compared to nearly 18% of the general population nationwide (Spencer et al., 2010).

Research also indicates a significant relationship between experiences of discrimination and poor mental health among Muslims populations. Nadal (2012) identified that individuals, including Muslim Americans, could experience intersectional microaggressions in which overlapping identities (gender, religion, race, gender identity) can produce complex overt and covert forms of discrimination. Unfortunately, some of the racist stereotypes involving Muslim men may be that they may be viewed as terrorists, a threat, or aggressive and found a common stereotype for Muslim women may be that they lack control over their own lives Nadal (2012). However, Muslim Americans who are South Asian may have stigma in accessing treatment for fear of what the community may say knowing if they have psychological issues. Additionally, depending on worldview, they may not view Western therapy as effective for their problems. Additionally, they may also find mental health providers that also may be Islamophobic or not culturally responsive further causing a barrier to help them resolve symptoms.

Hodge and colleagues (2015) conducted a studies based in two different cities in the United States and found that discrimination due to Muslim identity was associated with increased depressive symptoms. In California and Chicago, South Asian Americans who were perceived to have experiences of discrimination were found to have greater symptoms of depression, anxiety, and anger (Nadimpalli et al., 2016). South Asian American teens who also had experiences of perceived racism were also found to have poor mental health but religious support and religious coping were associated with positive mental health (Ahmed et al., 2011).

Research also indicates that chronic and continued exposure to discrimination can lead to psychopathology and mental distress. Discrimination has consistently been associated with psychopathology for Asian Americans and other groups of color in the U.S. (Hall & Yee, 2012). Depressive symptoms were also linked to discrimination for Asian American students (Romero et al., 2007), Asian American international students (Wei et al., 2010), Asian American college students (Wei et al., 2010; Yoo et al., 2009), Asian American adults generally (Srivastava, 2012), and Asian American older adults (Jang et al., 2010). Discrimination has also been found to be associated with internalizing and externalizing disorders and with psychological distress among Asian American college students (Hwang & Goto, 2009).

Acculturation impacting immigrants and subsequent generations of immigrant populations has also been linked to mental distress. Low levels of acculturation for Asian Americans has been found to be associated with depression (David et al., 2009; Srivastava, 2012). However, another study suggests that high levels of acculturation is negatively associated with depression among Asian American college students (Hwang & Ting, 2008) however, this may be moderated by ethnic identity, social support, and family cohesion. Asian Americans culture-bound syndromes also may arise in which mental health symptoms may appear differently or due to different causes and based on cultural beliefs and this may also impact the accuracy of incidences of mental illness as they may not be accurately diagnosed and considered. Additionally, Asian Americans may experience mental disress, including depression, which manifest as physical symptoms like GI issues, pain, or neurasthenia syndrome (Zheng et al., 1997).

Additionally, the evidence observing the underutilization of mental health services by Asian Americans, including South Asian Americans, is that mental health services may also not be culturally competent (Sue et al., 2009). Culturally responsive mental health services have been found to result in better outcomes for Asian Americans and other persons of color than services that are not culturally responsive (Sue et al., 2009). Another aspect to consider is that Asian Americans may use alternative medicine or other forms of support, perhaps the use of prayer or guidance from a religious or spiritual advisor, a healer, a chiropractor, or a spiritualist and this may also be something to consider when trying to understand and integrate the Asian American client's views into mental health treatment (Meyer et al., 2009).

There are many factors that are critical to consider, such as the impacts of discrimination and acculturation when trying to understand mental distress of South Asian Americans. There is even more research to be conducted to observe how mental health issues develop within intergenerational populations of South Asian Americans further elucidating barriers and access to care issues. This is very important as we move forward in identifying the needs of South Asian American communities and as we call for efforts against discrimination and policies ensuring programing that can provide support and culturally responsive mental health services to these important yet often neglected populations of our American society.

Advocacy/Next Steps

It is critical to examine how a systems approach to understanding the racism, discrimination, and mental health needs we face as South Asian Americans merits not only policy solutions, but shared community organizing strategies and regular practices of solidarity. This also informs how we understand and approach our own mental health.

One example is the successful, collaborative, and shared campaign strategy in the fight to repeal Trump's Muslim Ban: the "No Ban, No Wall, No Raids" campaign combined efforts to reverse the Muslim Ban, resist the border wall, and draw attention to the mass immigration raids by the same administration. Ultimately, while this did not prevail during the Trump Administration, it set an important stage for the Biden Administration to make this a priority within their first 100 days in office. And, while the total repeal of the Muslim Ban is a major victory, it only scratches the surface of the deeply embedded anti-Muslim infrastructure in our government. For example, the notorious NSEERS program mentioned earlier, formally ended in 2002, but the regulations permitting the program to exist were not dismantled until DRUM, SAALT, and other civil rights and advocacy organizations appealed directly to DHS Secretary Jeh Johnson in the very final days of the Obama Administration in 2016.

Engaging in policy change is one critically important way to support our South Asian American communities. Research finds that there is significant disparity when observing the utilization of care for South Asian American populations further complicated by unique mental health needs. To efficiently serve and help these populations, comprehensive systemic efforts to mold programming, policy, and training for cultural competency is needed. Additionally, we must address social justice issues, access to care, language justice, and cultural responsiveness in mental services. We must identify ways to collect accurate data, which includes disaggregating data so we can gain a clearer picture of mental health disorders, psychological issues, hospitalizations, and psychological services needed. To better gauge the needs for services, we need to understand physical and mental health disorders and further support, fund, and mandate training for culturally responsive mental health services. We must also work with cultural community centers, enabling a supportive and open network, where South Asian Americans can feel comfortable receiving continued mental health care. Additionally, expanded and flexible coverage for telehealth services should be considered for South Asian American populations as there are many barriers to care and finding a culturally responsive provider who may also speak their language, and who can also understand unique and intersecting cultural issues. This is further heightened by the negative stigma associated with seeking mental health support, and the telehealth medium may make many South Asian American individuals more comfortable and safe in receiving care. There must be a greater effort to mandate language justice policies in providing mental health information and increasing access to resources. Many South Asian American individuals may not be fluent in English and knowledge about mental health should be translated and made accessible for those who have fluency in different South Asian American languages. This is critical for public health guidance. According to the American Psychological Association (APA) Commission of Ethnic Minority Recruitment, Retention, and Training, "1 in 2 Asian Americans suffering from mental illness will not seek help due to a language barrier." Additionally, many cognitive screening tests have cultural and linguistic bias, making it difficult to diagnose Asian American patients. (Sue et al., 2009).

Further, mental health concepts and issues should be tailored for different populations in how they express symptoms or presented in a culturally appropriate manner. To have further connection for South Asian Americans to access care we must also link with different centers of religion and faith, such as mosques, temples, gurdwaras. Places of worship and community can help dispel stigma and support individuals needing help to find providers who are versed in culturally responsive and effective care. We must also have policies and funding directed towards helping populations of South Asian Americans of varying immigration statuses find support, as well as programming for intergenerational South Asian American families so conflict can be reduced and a sense of community and support is further enhanced.

Reflection Questions

1   Upon reading the case study, what came to your mind in terms of symptomology that would emerge for Sumana and H-4 visa holders? How would older South Asian Americans be expressing mental health symptoms given their challenges?
2   How would these immigration policies impact the family system and mental health?
3   What would culturally responsive treatment look like? What factors should be considered?
4   As a mental health provider, what could you do to impact systemic change to help this population gain more access to mental health care and advocate for policy changes?

Summary

This important chapter is unlike the others, and provides historical context of South Asian American populations and traces the history of South Asian Americans from early migration in the early 1800s to the 1960s to the present. This chapter focuses on how racism and discrimination have evolved and impacted intergenerational populations. It covers historical U.S. discrimination against early Sikh, Hindu, Muslim, and other South Asian populations dating back to the early 1800s and leading into the 1960s civil rights movement to the present. This chapter also highlights the importance of advocacy, social justice, and public policy relevant to addressing South Asian American mental health issues and needs. Past and current policies are explored, in addition to community organizing efforts to improve mental health care for South Asian Americans, making it an important priority. Finally, this section provides future policy recommendations to support South Asian American mental health needs.*

Note

* mental health, mh policy-federal; themes of south asian on communities, indiv, future direction: mh policies for saa; immigration, hate crimes, solidarity; training-systemic; access to care; language equity; cultural responsiveness; systemic.

References

Ahmed, S.R., Kia-Keating M., & Tsai, K.H. (2011). A structural model of racial discrimination, acculturative stress, and cultural resources among arab American adolescents. *American Journal of Community Psychology*, 48(3–4), 181–192.

American Civil Liberties Union. (2017). Washington. *Timeline of the Muslim Ban.* https://www.aclu-wa.org/pages/timeline-muslim-ban

APA Commission on Ethnic Minority Recruitment, Retention, and Training in Psychology Task Force (CEMRRAT2). (2017). Asian Americans need culturally competent mental health care. Retrieved from https://www.apa.org/advocacy/civil-rights/diversity/asian-american-health

Arora, N. (2017). *Political reviews and essays. Coming to America: The making of the South Asian diaspora in the United States.* Caravan Magazine.

Bald, V. (2013). *Bengali Harlem and the lost histories of South Asian America.* Harvard University Press.

Brennan Center. (2019, September). *Why Countering Violent Extremism Programs are Bad Policy.* https://www.brennancenter.org/our-work/research-reports/why-countering-violent-extremism-programs-are-bad-policy

Cahn, D. (2008). The Seattle civil rights & labor history Project, university of Washington. *The 1907 Bellingham Riots in Historical Context.* https://depts.washington.edu/civilr/bham_history.htm

Das, S. (2002). Loss or gain? A saga of Asian Indian immigration and experiences in America's Multi-ethnic mosaic. *Race, Gender & Class*, 9(2), 131–155.

Daum, C.W., & Ishiwata, E. (2010). From the myth of formal equality to the politics of social justice: Race and the legal attack on native entitlements. *Law & Society Review*, 44, 843–876.

David, E.J.R., Okazaki, S., & Saw, S. (2009). Bicultural self-efficacy among college students: Initial scale development and mental health correlates. *Journal of Counseling Psychology*, 56, 211–226.

Department of Homeland Security. (2019, May). *Countering Violent Extremism Grant Program.* https://www.dhs.gov/publication/countering-violent-extremism-grant-program

Desilver, D. (2018). *5 Facts about Indian Americans.* Pew Research Center.

Hall, G. C. N., & Yee, A. (2012). U.S. mental health policy: Addressing the neglect of Asian Americans. *Asian American Journal of Psychology*, 3(3), 181–193. 10.1037/a0029950. PMID: 24490000; PMCID: PMC3905325.

Hodge, D.R., Zidan T., & Husain A. (2015). Modeling the relationships between discrimination, depression, substance use, and spirituality with muslims in the United States. *Social Work Research*, 39(4), 223–233.

Hwang, W., & Goto, S. (2009). The impact of perceived racial discrimination on the mental health of Asian American and Latino college students. Asian. *American Journal of Psychology*, 1, 15–28.

Hwang, W., & Ting, J.Y. (2008). Disaggregating the effects of acculturation and acculturative stress on the mental health of Asian Americans. *Cultural Diversity and Ethnic Minority Psychology*, 14, 147–154.

Iyer, D. (2018, February 22). Scroll. In. *An Indian Immigrant's Fight for US Citizenship in 1923 Holds Lessons in Trump's America.* https://scroll.in/article/869304/bhagat-singh-thinds-fight-for-citizenship-in-1923-holds-lessons-for-immigrants-in-trumps-america

Jang, Y., Chiriboga, D.A., Kim, G., & Rhew, S. (2010). Perceived discrimination, sense of control, and depressive symptoms among Korean American older adults. Asian. *American Journal of Psychology*, 1, 129–135.

Kiesler, C.A. (1992). U.S. mental health policy: Doomed to fail. *American Psychologist*, 9, 1077–1082.

Kiesler, C.A. (2000). The next wave of change for psychology and mental health in the health care revolution. *American Psychologist*, *55*, 481–487.

Maira, S.M. (2002). *Desis in the house: Indian American youth culture in New York city*. Philadelphia: Temple University Press.

Meyer, O.L., Zane, N.W., Cho, Y.I., & Takeuchi, D.T. (2009). Use of specialty mental health services by Asian Americans with psychiatric disorders.*Journal of Consulting and Clinical Psychology*, *77*, 1000–1005.

Miles, E., & Crisp R.J. (2014). A meta-analytic test of the imagined contact hypothesis. *Group Processes & Intergroup Relation*, *17*(1), 3–26.

Nadal, K.L., Griffin, K.E., Hamit, S., Jayleen Leon, J., Tobio, M., & Rivera, D.P. (2012). Subtle and overt forms of Islamophobia: Microaggressions toward Muslim Americans. *Journal of Muslim Mental Health*, *6*(2), 15–37. http://hdl.handle.net/2027/spo.10381607.0006.203

Nadimpalli, S.B., Kanaya, A.M., McDade T.W., & Kandula, N.R. (2016). Self-reported discrimination and mental health among Asian Indians: Cultural beliefs and coping style as moderators. *Asian American Journal of Psychology*, *7*(3), 185–194.

New York City Profiling Collaborative, Desis Rising Up and Moving, The Sikh Coalition, South Asian Youth Action, Coney Island Avenue Project, Council of Peoples Organization, South Asian Americans Leading Together. (2012). *In Our Own Words: Narratives of South Asian New Yorkers Affected by Racial and Religious Profiling*. https://saalt.org/wp-content/uploads/2012/09/In-Our-Own-Words-Narratives-of-South-Asian-New-Yorkers-Affected-by-Racial-and-Religious-Profiling.pdf

Rangaswamy, P. (2000). *Namaste America: Indian immigrants in an American Metropolis*. University Park: The Pennsylvania State University Press.

Romero, A.J., Carvajal, S.C., Volle, F., & Orduña, M. (2007). Adolescent bicultural stress and its impact on mental well-being among Latinos, Asian Americans, and European Americans. *Journal of Community Psychology*, *35*, 519–534.

Soundararajan, T. (2018, February 14). Rewire news group. *Why Are Some South Asian Immigrants Offering to Pay for Trump's Wall?* https://rewirenewsgroup.com/article/2018/02/14/south-asian-immigrants-offering-pay-trumps-wall/

South Asian Americans Leading Together. (2014). *Under Suspicion, Under Attack: Xenophobic Political Rhetoric and Hate Violence against South Asian, Muslim, Sikh, Hindu, Middle Eastern, and Arab Communities in the United States*. https://saalt.org/wp-content/uploads/2014/09/SAALT_report_full_links.pdf

South Asian Americans Leading Together. (2015). *Issue Brief: Department of Justice Guidance on Law Enforcement Profiling—History and Current State of Play*. https://saalt.org/wp-content/uploads/2015/07/SAALT-DOJ-Guidance-Issue-Brief.pdf

South Asian Americans Leading Together. (2017). Power, pain, potential: South Asian Americans at the forefront of growth and hate in the 2016 election cycle. https://saalt.org/wp-content/uploads/2017/01/SAALT_Power_rpt_final3_lorez.pdf

South Asian Americans Leading Together. (2018). *A Guide to Advocacy for Legal Immigration Reform: H-1B and H-4 visas and the South Asian American Community*. https://saalt.org/advocacy-for-legal-immigration-reform-h1b-and-h4-visas/

South Asian Americans Leading Together. (2018). *Communities on Fire: Confronting Hate Violence and Xenophobic Political Rhetoric*. https://saalt.org/wp-content/uploads/2018/01/Communities-on-Fire.pdf

South Asian Americans Leading Together. (2019, April). *Demographic Snapshot of South Asians in the United States*. https://saalt.org/wp-content/uploads/2019/04/SAALT-Demographic-Snapshot-2019.pdf

South Asian Americans Leading Together. (2020). *Unequal Consequences: The Disparate Impact of Covid-19 Across South Asian American Communities*. https://saalt.org/wp-content/uploads/2020/09/Unequal-Consequences_SAALT-2020.pdf

Spencer, M., Chen, J., Gee, G., Fabian, C., & Takeuchi, D. (2010). Discrimination and mental health–related service use in a national study of Asian Americans. *American Journal of Public Health, 100*(12), 2410–2417.

Srivastava, D. (2012). *The effects of ethnic identity, family conflict, and acculturation on racial discrimination and mental distress of second generation Asian Americans.* Fordham University ProQuest Dissertations Publishing.

Stockdill, J.W. (2005). National mental health policy and the community mental health centers, 1963–1981. In W. E. Pickren & S. F. Schneider, (Eds.), *Psychology and the National Institute of Mental Health: A historical analysis of science, practice, and policy* (pp. 261–293). Washington, DC: American Psychological Association.

Sue, S., Zane, N., Hall, G.C.N., & Berger, L.K. (2009). The case for cultural competency in psychotherapeutic interventions. *Annual Review of Psychology, 60*(60), 525–548.

Sue, D.W. (1977). Counseling the culturally different: A conceptual analysis, *The Personnel and Guidance Journal, 55*(7), 422–425.

Teen Vogue. (2020, November 24). *Teen Vogue's 21 Under 21, 2020: The Girls and Femmes Building a Better Future.* https://www.teenvogue.com/story/21-under-21-2020

Vasquez, M.J.T., & Jones, J.M. (2007). Diversity is a compelling interest, and affirmative action is an important strategy for achieving it. *American Psychologist, 62*, 146–147.

Wei, M., Liao, K.Y., Chao, R.C., Mallinckrodt, B., Tsai, R., & Botello-Zamarron, R. (2010). Minority stress, perceived bicultural competence, and depressive symptoms among ethnic minority college students. *Journal of Counseling Psychology, 57*, 411–422.

Yoo, H.C., Gee, G.C., & Takeuchi, D. (2009). Discrimination and health among Asian American immigrants: Disentangling racial from language discrimination. *Social Science & Medicine, 68*, 726–732.

Zheng, Y.P., Lin, K., Takeuchi, D., Kurasaki, K.S., Wang, Y., & Cheung, F. (1997). An epidemiological study of neurasthenia in Chinese-Americans in Los Angeles. *Comprehensive Psychiatry, 38*(5), 249–259.

Index